Stroke Imaging

Guest Editor

PAMELA W. SCHAEFER, MD

NEUROIMAGING CLINICS OF NORTH AMERICA

www.neuroimaging.theclinics.com

Consulting Editor
SURESH K. MUKHERJI, MD

May 2011 • Volume 21 • Number 2

SAUNDERS an imprint of ELSEVIER, Inc.

W.B. SAUNDERS COMPANY
A Division of Elsevier Inc.

1600 John F. Kennedy Boulevard • Suite 1800 • Philadelphia, Pennsylvania 19103-2899

http://www.theclinics.com

NEUROIMAGING CLINICS OF NORTH AMERICA Volume 21, Number 2
May 2011 ISSN 1052-5149, ISBN 13: 978-1-4377-2693-0

Editor: Joanne Husovski
Developmental Editor: Donald Mumford

Neuroimaging Clinics of North America (ISSN 1052-5149) is published quarterly by Elsevier Inc., 360 Park Avenue South, New York, NY 10010-1710. Months of issue are February, May, August, and November. Business and editorial offices: 1600 John F. Kennedy Blvd., Suite 1800, Philadelphia, PA 19103-2899. Business and editorial offices: 6277 Sea Harbor Drive, Orlando, FL 32887-4800. Periodicals postage paid at New York, NY, and additional mailing offices. Subscription prices are USD 314 per year for US individuals, USD 436 per year for US institutions, USD 158 per year for US students and residents, USD 363 per year for Canadian individuals, USD 546 per year for Canadian institutions, USD 461 per year for international individuals, USD 546 per year for international institutions and USD 226 per year for Canadian and foreign students and residents. To receive student/resident rate, orders must be accompanied by name of affiliated institution, date of term, and the *signature* of program/residency coordinator on institution letterhead. Orders will be billed at individual rate until proof of status is received. Foreign air speed delivery is included in all *Clinics* subscription prices. All prices are subject to change without notice. POSTMASTER: Send address changes to *Neuroimaging Clinics of North America*, Elsevier Health Sciences Division, Subscription Customer Service, 3251 Riverport Lane, Maryland Heights, MO 63043. Telephone: 1-800-654-2452 (U.S. and Canada); 314-447-8871 (outside U.S. and Canada). Fax: 314-447-8029. E-mail: journalscustomerservice-usa@elsevier.com (for print support); journalsonlinesupport-usa@elsevier.com (for online support).

Reprints. For copies of 100 or more of articles in this publication, please contact the Commercial Reprints Department, Elsevier Inc., 360 Park Avenue South, New York, NY 10010-1710. Tel.: 212-633-3812; Fax: 212-462-1935; E-mail: reprints@elsevier.com.

Neuroimaging Clinics of North America is covered by *Excerpta Medical/EMBASE,* the RSNA Index of Imaging Literature, *MEDLINE/PubMed (Index Medicus),* MEDLINE/MEDLARS, SciSearch, Research Alert, and Neuroscience Citation Index.

Printed and bound by CPI Group (UK) Ltd, Croydon, CR0 4YY

Transferred to Digital Print 2011

GOAL STATEMENT

The goal of *Neuroimaging Clinics of North America* is to keep practicing radiologists and radiology residents up to date with current clinical practice in radiology by providing timely articles reviewing the state of the art in patient care.

ACCREDITATION

The *Neuroimaging Clinics of North America* is planned and implemented in accordance with the Essential Areas and Policies of the Accreditation Council for Continuing Medical Education (ACCME) through the joint sponsorship of the University of Virginia School of Medicine and Elsevier. The University of Virginia School of Medicine is accredited by the ACCME to provide continuing medical education for physicians.

The University of Virginia School of Medicine designates this educational activity for a maximum of 15 *AMA PRA Category 1 Credits*™ for each issue, 60 credits per year. Physicians should only claim credit commensurate with the extent of their participation in the activity.

The American Medical Association has determined that physicians not licensed in the US who participate in this CME activity are eligible for a maximum of 15 *AMA PRA Category 1 Credits*™ for each issue, 60 credits per year.

Credit can be earned by reading the text material, taking the CME examination online at http://www.theclinics.com/home/cme, and completing the evaluation. After taking the test, you will be required to review any and all incorrect answers. Following completion of the test and evaluation, your credit will be awarded and you may print your certificate.

FACULTY DISCLOSURE/CONFLICT OF INTEREST

The University of Virginia School of Medicine, as an ACCME accredited provider, endorses and strives to comply with the Accreditation Council for Continuing Medical Education (ACCME) Standards of Commercial Support, Commonwealth of Virginia statutes, University of Virginia policies and procedures, and associated federal and private regulations and guidelines on the need for disclosure and monitoring of proprietary and financial interests that may affect the scientific integrity and balance of content delivered in continuing medical education activities under our auspices.

The University of Virginia School of Medicine requires that all CME activities accredited through this institution be developed independently and be scientifically rigorous, balanced and objective in the presentation/discussion of its content, theories and practices.

All authors/editors participating in an accredited CME activity are expected to disclose to the readers relevant financial relationships with commercial entities occurring within the past 12 months (such as grants or research support, employee, consultant, stock holder, member of speakers bureau, etc.). The University of Virginia School of Medicine will employ appropriate mechanisms to resolve potential conflicts of interest to maintain the standards of fair and balanced education to the reader. Questions about specific strategies can be directed to the Office of Continuing Medical Education, University of Virginia School of Medicine, Charlottesville, Virginia.

The faculty and staff of the University of Virginia Office of Continuing Medical Education have no financial affiliations to disclose.

The authors/editors listed below have identified no professional/financial affiliations for themselves or their spouse/partner:
Hakan Ay, MD; William A. Copen, MD; Josser E. Delgado Almandoz, MD; Steve H. Fung, MD; Mikayel Grigoryan, MD; Jason Hom, MD; Daniel P. Hsu, MD; Joanne Husovski, (Acquisitions Editor); Andrea Kassner, PhD; Puneet Kochar, MD; Angelos A. Konstas, MD, PhD; Carlos Leiva-Salinas, MD; Daniel M. Mandell, MD, FRCPC; Bijoy K. Menon, MD; David J. Mikulis, MD, FRCPC; Volker Puetz, MD; Luca Roccatagliata, MD; U. Sadat, MRCS, MPhil; Pamela W. Schaefer, MD (Guest Editor); Lubdha M. Shah, MD (Test Author); Christie E. Tung, MD; Steven Warach, MD, PhD; Ona Wu, PhD; Hooman Yarmohammadi, MD; and Victoria Young, MRCS, MPhil.

The authors listed below have identified the following professional/financial affiliations for themselves or their spouse/partner:
Gregory W. Albers, MD is on the Advisory Board/Committee for Lundbeck and Genetech.
Andrew M. Demchuk, MD, FRCPC is on the speakers bureau and advisory committee/board for Sanofi-Aventis and Boehringer Ingelheim, and owns stock in Calgary Scientific Inc.
J. H. Gillard, MD, FRCR, MBA is an industry funded researcher/investigator and consultant for GlaxoSmithKline; is on the speakers bureau and advisory committee/board for Bayer Schering; and is an industry funded researcher/investigator and on speakers bureau for Guerbet.
R. Gilberto Gonzalez, MD, PhD is an industry funded research/investigator for NIH and Penumbra.
Michael H. Lev, MD receives research support from GE Healthcare, SPOTRIAS - NIH/NINDS, and NBIB/NIH through U. Cincinnatti.
Suresh K. Mukherji, MD (Consulting Editor) is a consultant for Philips.
Javier M. Romero, MD is a consultant for Lundbeck.
Gurpreet Sandhu, MD is an industry funded research/investigator for Siemens Medical Solutions.
Lee H. Schwamm, MD is a consultant for the Mass Department of Public Health and is on the Advisory Board for Lunbeck, Inc.
A Gregory Sorensen, MD is a consultant for ACRIN Image Metrix, Siemens Medical Solutions, Genzyme, Bayer, Mitsubishi Pharma, and Biogen Idec, Inc.; receives research support from NIH, Genzyme, Exelixis Inc., Schering Plough, and Millennium.
Jeffrey L. Sunshine, MD, PhD is an industry funded research/investigator for Siemens Medical.
Max Wintermark, MD is an industry funded research/investigator for GE Healthcare and Philips Healthcare.
Greg Zaharchuk, PhD, MD is an industry funded research/investigator and is on the Advisory Board for GE Healthcare.

Disclosure of Discussion of Non-FDA Approved Uses for Pharmaceutical Products and/or Medical Devices.
The University of Virginia School of Medicine, as an ACCME provider, requires that all faculty presenters identify and disclose any off-label uses for pharmaceutical and medical device products. The University of Virginia School of Medicine recommends that each physician fully review all the available data on new products or procedures prior to clinical use.

TO ENROLL

To enroll in the Neuroimaging Clinics of North America Continuing Medical Education program, call customer service at 1-800-654-2452 or sign up online at http://www.theclinics.com/home/cme. The CME program is available to subscribers for an additional annual fee of USD 196.

Neuroimaging Clinics of North America

RELATED INTEREST

Neurologic Clinics, November 2008
Stroke
Sean D. Ruland, DO and Philip B. Gorelick, MD, MPH, FACP, *Guest Editors*
www.neurologic.theclinics.com

THE CLINICS ARE NOW AVAILABLE ONLINE!

Access your subscription at:
www.theclinics.com

Contributors

CONSULTING EDITOR

SURESH K. MUKHERJI, MD, FACR
Professor and Chief of Neuroradiology and
Head, and Neck Radiology; Professor of
Radiology, Otolaryngology Head and Neck
Surgery, Radiation Oncology, Periodontics and
Oral Medicine, University of Michigan Health,
System, Ann Arbor, Michigan

GUEST EDITOR

PAMELA W. SCHAEFER, MD
Associate Director of Neuroradiology; and
Neuroradiology Fellowship Director,
Massachusetts General Hospital, Department
of Radiology, Division of Neuroradiology;
Associate Professor of Radiology, Harvard
Medical School, Massachusetts General
Hospital, Boston, Massachusetts

AUTHORS

GREGORY W. ALBERS, MD
Professor of Neurology and Neurological
Sciences; Director of the Stanford Stroke
Center, Department of Neurology and
Neurological Sciences, Stanford University
Medical Center, Palo Alto, California

HAKAN AY, MD
Stroke Service, A.A. Martinos Center for
Biomedical Imaging, Massachusetts
General Hospital, Harvard Medical School,
Boston, Massachusetts

WILLIAM A. COPEN, MD
Director of Advanced MR Neuroimaging,
Massachusetts General Hospital,
Department of Radiology, Division of
Neuroradiology; Instructor in Radiology,
Harvard Medical School, Massachusetts
General Hospital, Boston, Massachusetts

JOSSER E. DELGADO ALMANDOZ, MD
Division of Neuroradiology, Massachusetts
General Hospital, Boston, Massachusetts;
Clinical Fellow in Diagnostic and Endovascular
Surgical Neuroradiology, Division of
Neuroradiology, Mallinckrodt Institute of
Radiology, Washington University School of
Medicine, Saint Louis, Missouri

ANDREW M. DEMCHUK, MD, FRCPC
Director, Calgary Stroke Program; Associate
Professor, Department of Clinical
Neurosciences, Foothills Medical Centre,
University of Calgary, Calgary, Canada

STEVE H. FUNG, MD
Assistant Professor of Radiology; Chief of
Clinical MRI Research, Neuroradiology
Section, Department of Radiology, The
Methodist Hospital, Weill Cornell Medical
College, Houston, Texas

J.H. GILLARD, MD, FRCR, MBA
Professor of Neuroradiology, University
Department of Radiology, Addenbrookes
Hospital, Cambridge, United Kingdom

R. GILBERTO GONZALEZ, MD, PhD
Professor of Radiology; Director of
Neuroradiology, Neuroradiology Division,
Department of Radiology, Massachusetts
General Hospital, Harvard Medical School,
Boston, Massachusetts

MIKAYEL GRIGORYAN, MD
Cerebrovascular Fellow, Stanford
Stroke Center; Department of Neurology
and Neurological Sciences, Stanford
University Medical Center,
Palo Alto, California

JASON HOM, MD
Research Fellow, Neuroradiology Section,
Department of Radiology, University of
California, San Francisco, California

DANIEL P. HSU, MD
Department of Radiology, University
Hospitals—Case Medical Center,
Cleveland, Ohio

ANDREA KASSNER, PhD
Assistant Professor & Co-Director of
Research; Canada Research Chair in
Neuroimaging, Department of Medical
Imaging, University of Toronto, Toronto,
Ontario, Canada

PUNEET KOCHAR, MD
Department of Radiology, Foothills
Medical Centre, University of Calgary,
Calgary, Canada

ANGELOS A. KONSTAS, MD, PhD
Department of Radiology, Massachusetts
General Hospital, Boston, Massachusetts

MICHAEL H. LEV, MD
Department of Radiology, Massachusetts
General Hospital, Boston, Massachusetts

CARLOS LEIVA-SALINAS, MD
Research Fellow, Neuroradiology Division,
Department of Radiology, University of
Virginia, Charlottesville, Virginia; Departamento
de Medicina, Universidad Autónoma de
Barcelona, Barcelona, Spain

DANIEL M. MANDELL, MD, FRCPC
Chief Fellow, Diagnostic Neuroradiology,
Department of Medical Imaging,
Toronto Western Hospital, Toronto,
Ontario, Canada

BIJOY K. MENON, MD
Calgary Stroke Program, Department of
Clinical Neurosciences, University of
Calgary, Calgary, Canada

DAVID J. MIKULIS, MD, FRCPC
Professor, Department of Medical Imaging,
Toronto Western Hospital, University of
Toronto, Toronto, Ontario, Canada

VOLKER PUETZ, MD
Department of Neurology, Dresden
University Stroke Centre, University of
Technology Dresden, Dresden, Germany

LUCA ROCCATAGLIATA, MD
Assistant Professor of Neuroradiology,
Department of Neuroscience, Ophthalmology
and Genetics, University of Genoa,
Genoa, Italy

JAVIER M. ROMERO, MD
Instructor of Radiology, Harvard Medical
School; Director, Ultrasound Imaging
Services; Associate Director, Neurovascular
Laboratory, Division of Neuroradiology,
Massachusetts General Hospital,
Boston, Massachusetts

U. SADAT, MRCS, MPhil
Clinical Research Associate, University
Department of Radiology, Addenbrookes
Hospital, Cambridge, United Kingdom

GURPREET SANDHU, MD
Department of Radiology, University
Hospitals—Case Medical Center,
Cleveland, Ohio

PAMELA W. SCHAEFER, MD
Associate Director of Neuroradiology; and
Neuroradiology Fellowship Director,
Massachusetts General Hospital,
Department of Radiology, Division of
Neuroradiology; Associate Professor of
Radiology, Harvard Medical School,
Massachusetts General Hospital, Boston,
Massachusetts

LEE H. SCHWAMM, MD
Vice Chairman, Neurology Service,
Department of Neurology; Professor of
Neurology; Director, TeleStroke & Acute
Stroke Services, MGH, Boston,
Massachusetts

A. GREGORY SORENSEN, MD
Professor of Radiology, Department of
Radiology, MGH/MIT/HMS; Co-director,
Athinoula A. Martinos Center for Biomedical
Imaging, MGH, Charlestown, Massachusetts

JEFFREY L. SUNSHINE, MD, PhD
Department of Radiology, University
Hospitals—Case Medical Center,
Cleveland, Ohio

CHRISTIE E. TUNG, MD
Resident Physician, Department of Neurology
and Neurological Sciences, Stanford University
Medical Center, Palo Alto, California

STEVEN WARACH, MD, PhD
Chief of the Section on Stroke Diagnostics
and Therapeutics, National Institute of
Neurological Disorders and Stroke,
National Institutes of Health,
Bethesda, Maryland

MAX WINTERMARK, MD
Associate Professor of Radiology,
Neurology, Neurosurgery and Biomedical
Engineering; Chief of Neuroradiology,
Neuroradiology Division, Department of
Radiology, University of Virginia,
Charlottesville, Virginia

ONA WU, PhD
Assistant in Neuroimaging, MGH/MIT/HMS
Athinoula A. Martinos Center for Biomedical
Imaging, Charlestown; Assistant Professor of
Radiology, Harvard Medical School, Boston,
Massachusetts

HOOMAN YARMOHAMMADI, MD
Department of Radiology, University
Hospitals—Case Medical Center,
Cleveland, Ohio

V.E.L. YOUNG, MRCS, MPhil
Clinical Research Associate, University
Department of Radiology, Addenbrookes
Hospital, Cambridge, United Kingdom

GREG ZAHARCHUK, PhD, MD
Assistant Professor of Radiology,
Stanford University, Stanford University
Medical Center, Stanford, California

Contents

> Multidetector computed tomographic (CT) angiography is rapidly becoming a pivotal examination in the initial evaluation of patients with hemorrhagic stroke. This article provides an update of the literature on this dynamic topic, focusing on (1) the utility of CT angiography in the identification of hemorrhagic stroke patients who harbor an underlying vascular etiology and the role of the secondary intracerebral hemorrhage score, as well as (2) the clinical value of the CT angiography spot sign and spot sign score in patients with primary intracerebral hemorrhage.

> Computed tomographic perfusion (CTP) imaging is an advanced modality that provides important information about capillary-level hemodynamics of the brain parenchyma. CTP can aid in diagnosis, management, and prognosis of acute stroke patients by clarifying acute cerebral physiology and hemodynamic status, including distinguishing severely hypoperfused but potentially salvageable tissue from both tissue likely to be irreversibly infarcted ("core") and hypoperfused but metabolically stable tissue ("benign oligemia"). A qualitative estimate of the presence and degree of ischemia is typically required for guiding clinical management. Radiation dose issues with CTP imaging, a topic of much current concern, are also addressed in this review.

> Although acute stroke imaging has made significant progress in the last few years, several improvements and validation steps are needed to make stroke-imaging techniques fully operational and appropriate in daily clinical practice. This review outlines the needs in the stroke-imaging field and describes a consortium that was founded to provide them.

> After onset of ischemic stroke, potentially viable tissue at risk (ischemic penumbra) may be salvageable. Currently, intravenous alteplase is approved for up to 4.5 hours

after symptom onset of acute ischemic stroke. Increasing this time window may allow many more patients to be treated. The ability to use MRI to help define the irreversibly damaged brain (infarct core) and the reversible ischemic penumbra shows great promise for stroke treatment. Recent advances in penumbral imaging technology may enable a phase III trial of an intravenous thrombolytic to be performed beyond 4.5 hours using techniques to select patients with penumbral tissue.

Magnetic resonance (MR) perfusion imaging offers the potential for measuring brain perfusion in acute stroke patients, at a time when treatment decisions based on these measurements may affect outcomes dramatically. Rapid advancements in both acute stroke therapy and perfusion imaging techniques have resulted in continuing redefinition of the role that perfusion imaging should play in patient management. This review discusses the basic pathophysiology of acute stroke, the utility of different kinds of perfusion images, and research on the continually evolving role of MR perfusion imaging in acute stroke care.

Since acute stroke and transient ischemic attack (TIA) are disruptions of brain hemodynamics, perfusion neuroimaging might be of clinical utility. Recently, arterial spin labeling (ASL), a noncontrast perfusion method, has become clinically feasible. It has advantages compared to contrast bolus perfusion-weighted imaging (PWI) including lack of exposure to gadolinium, improved quantitation, and decreased sensitivity to susceptibility and motion. Drawbacks include reduced signal-to-noise and high sensitivity to arterial transit delays. However, this sensitivity can enable visualization of collateral flow. This article discusses ASL findings in patients with acute stroke and TIA, focusing on typical appearances, common artifacts, and comparisons with PWI.

Transient ischemic attack (TIA) can convey a high imminent risk for the development of a major stroke and is therefore considered to be a medical emergency. Recent evidence indicates that TIA with imaging proof of brain infarction represents an extremely unstable condition with early risk of stroke that is as much as 20 times higher than the risk after TIA without tissue damage. The use of neuroimaging in TIA is therefore critical not only for diagnosis but also for accurate risk stratification. In this article, recent advances in diagnostic imaging, categorizations, and risk stratification in TIA are discussed.

The blood-brain barrier (BBB) is a functional concept to describe unique features of intracranial blood vessels that prevent many substances in the systemic circulation from entering the brain. In the setting of acute ischemic stroke, loss of blood-brain barrier (BBB) integrity is believed to be a precursor to hemorrhagic transformation.

CT and MR imaging may evaluate BBB integrity by detecting leakage of intravenously administered contrast media into the extravascular space. In its simplest form, BBB integrity is assessed qualitatively, by determining the presence or absence of contrast enhancement on structural images of the brain. When dynamic contrast-enhanced (DCE) MRI or CT is combined with a suitable pharmacokinetic model, one can quantify and spatially map BBB integrity throughout the brain.

Stroke is a leading cause of death and adult morbidity worldwide. By defining stroke symptom onset by the time the patient was last known to be well, many patients whose onsets are unwitnessed are automatically ineligible for thrombolytic therapy. Advanced brain imaging may serve as a substitute witness to estimate stroke onset and duration in those patients who do not have a human witness. This article reviews and compares some of these imaging-based approaches to thrombolysis eligibility, which can potentially expand the use of thrombolytic therapy to a broader population of acute stroke patients.

Diffusion-weighted MRI provides image contrast that is dependent on the molecular motion of water. Diffusion-weighted imaging is the most reliable method for early detection of cerebral ischemia, for the definition of infarct core, and for the differentiation of acute ischemia from other disease processes that mimic stroke. Diffusion tensor imaging and diffusion kurtosis imaging may offer additional diagnostic information on the microstructural status of tissue. This review discusses the development and applications of diffusion-weighted imaging, diffusion tensor imaging, and diffusion kurtosis imaging in acute and chronic ischemia.

With more than 700,000 strokes per year resulting in greater than 160,000 deaths per year, stroke remains the leading cause of disability and third leading cause of death in the United States. Despite an overall decline in stroke mortality over the past 40 years, the total number of stroke deaths continues to increase, suggesting an increase in stroke incidence. The last 20 years of neuroscience advances have moved stroke from a condition that is monitored clinically and imaged serially as it evolves to an entity that can be treated acutely, with remarkable alterations in its natural history.

Currently carotid imaging has 2 main focuses: assessment of luminal stenosis and classification of atherosclerotic plaque characteristics. Measurement of the degree of stenosis is the main assessment used for current treatment decision making, but an evolving idea that is now driving imaging is the concept of vulnerable plaque, which is where plaque components are identified and used to define which plaques are at high risk of causing symptoms compared with those at low risk. This review

Foreword

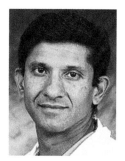

Suresh K. Mukherji, MD
Consulting Editor

It is both and honor and a privilege to have Dr Pam Schaefer edit this edition of *Neuroimaging Clinics of North America*. Dr Schafer is a recognized expert on stroke imaging and is a member of the world-renowned stroke team at the Massachusetts General Hospital. She has invited a fantastic group of authors who are all recognized experts in their respective areas of stroke imaging. I think the timing of this issue is excellent and I am very confident that this volume will be a state-of-the-art reference on stroke imaging for many years to come.

On a personal note, I was delighted when Pam agreed to guest edit this edition. I have been a great admirer of her scientific work and her leadership abilities for many years. She will soon be President of the American Society of Neuroradiology and I know our society will continue to prosper and flourish under her guidance and exceptional leadership.

Suresh K. Mukherji, MD
Department of Radiology
University of Michigan Health System
1500 East Medical Center
Ann Arbor, MI 48109-0030, USA

E-mail address:
mukherji@med.umich.edu

Neuroimag Clin N Am 21 (2011) xiii
doi:10.1016/j.nic.2011.05.013
1052-5149/11/$ – see front matter © 2011 Elsevier Inc. All rights reserved.

Imaging Acute Stroke is Rapidly Evolving

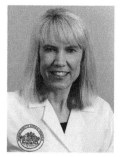

Pamela W. Schaefer, MD
Guest Editor

With the advent of advanced MR and CT techniques and new endovascular procedures, diagnosis and management of acute stroke are a rapidly evolving field. It would be impossible to cover all the important aspects of acute stroke in a single edition of *Neuroimaging Clinics of North America*, and I have focused on selected topics.

Since atheromatous disease is a major cause of acute ischemic stroke, one article includes a review of noninvasive imaging of the carotid artery with a focus on vulnerable plaque imaging.

Five articles address advanced CT and MR techniques such as CTA, CT perfusion, diffusion-weighted imaging, diffusion tensor imaging, dynamic susceptibility perfusion-weighted imaging, arterial spin labeling perfusion-weighted imaging, and permeability imaging for evaluating acute ischemic stroke.

Three articles address intravenous and intra-arterial therapies and the use of advanced imaging to guide patient selection. One reviews intra-arterial recanalization strategies. One addresses the role of diffusion and perfusion MRI in selecting patients for IV therapy and reviews major trials to date. An additional article reviews ASPECTS and other neuroimaging scores that are used in the acute setting to guide patient selection for intravenous and intra-arterial therapies and to help predict outcome.

Two articles address specific clinical syndromes to which our imaging approach and treatment are rapidly changing: wake-up strokes and transient ischemic attacks.

Another article on acute ischemic stroke addresses the need for a stroke imaging research roadmap; that is, the need to share data and standardize and validate imaging techniques.

While I have focused mostly on acute ischemic stroke, I did include one article on advanced CT imaging of hemorrhagic stroke since, in the emergency room setting, CTA has markedly improved our ability to rapidly diagnose underlying vascular lesions and predict who is at risk for subsequent rebleeding.

I am indebted to all of the authors for their invaluable contributions and I thank all of them for spending so much time and effort on their individual topics. I hope that readers find the articles in this issue interesting, informative, and thought-provoking.

Pamela W. Schaefer, MD
Department of Radiology
Massachusetts General Hospital
55 Fruit Street
Boston, MA, 02114

E-mail address:
pschaefer@partners.org

Neuroimag Clin N Am 21 (2011) xv
doi:10.1016/j.nic.2011.05.012

Advanced CT Imaging in the Evaluation of Hemorrhagic Stroke

Josser E. Delgado Almandoz, MD[a,b,*],
Javier M. Romero, MD[a]

KEYWORDS

- Multidetector CT angiography • Hemorrhagic stroke
- Secondary intracerebral hemorrhage score
- CT angiography spot sign

According to the National Stroke Association 2009 Fact Sheet, hemorrhagic stroke accounts for 13% of cases of acute stroke in the United States, with approximately 100,000 hospital admissions per year. Hemorrhagic stroke has a worse prognosis than ischemic stroke, with up to 50% 30-day mortality and very high rates of severe neurological disability among survivors.[1] There are 2 major types of hemorrhagic stroke: (1) those that are due to an underlying vascular lesion such as an arteriovenous malformation (AVM), aneurysm with intraparenchymal rupture, dural venous sinus (or cerebral vein) thrombosis (DVST), vasculitis, and Moya-Moya disease, which represent a minority of cases and are potentially treatable (secondary intracerebral hemorrhage [ICH]); and (2) those that are not due to an underlying vascular lesion (primary ICH).

Timely and accurate identification of patients with secondary ICH is important because these patients may benefit from prompt surgical or endovascular intervention once an underlying vascular abnormality has been identified, since rates of rehemorrhage, with increased morbidity and mortality, can be as high as 18% per year.[1–5] Although conventional catheter angiography remains the gold standard for the detection of underlying vascular etiologies in patients with hemorrhagic stroke, thanks to its widespread availability, rapidity of acquisition, lower cost, and favorable risk profile, multidetector CT angiography (MDCTA) is rapidly becoming the favored diagnostic tool in the initial evaluation of this patient population.

For patients with primary ICH, the total volume of extravasated intracranial blood is the most potent predictor of mortality and poor outcome among survivors, and those patients who develop hematoma expansion after admission have a worse prognosis than those who do not.[6] Although current treatment options for primary ICH consist primarily of supportive measures, emerging hemostatic therapies aiming to reduce the extent of hematoma expansion such as recombinant activated factor VII or intensive blood pressure reduction may be able to decrease the dreadful morbidity and mortality of this disease.[7,8] Nevertheless, given that most patients with primary ICH do not experience hematoma expansion after admission, accurate patient selection to target hemostatic therapy only to those patients who are actively bleeding at the time of presentation—and hence are most likely to benefit from hemostatic therapy—is imperative.

[a] Division of Neuroradiology, Massachusetts General Hospital, Gray 2, Room 273A, 55 Fruit Street, Boston, MA 02114, USA
[b] Division of Neuroradiology, Mallinckrodt Institute of Radiology, Washington University School of Medicine, Campus Box 8131, 510 South Kingshighway Boulevard, Saint Louis, MO 63110, USA
* Corresponding author. Division of Neuroradiology, Massachusetts General Hospital, Gray 2, Room 273A, 55 Fruit Street, Boston, MA 02114.
E-mail address: josser.delgado@gmail.com

Neuroimag Clin N Am 21 (2011) 197–213
doi:10.1016/j.nic.2011.01.001

Table 1
Accuracy of MDCTA compared with catheter angiography for the detection of vascular etiologies in patients with hemorrhagic stroke

Study	N	Sensitivity	Specificity	Accuracy
Yeung et al[14]	55	89	92	91
Romero et al[15,a]	43	96	100	98
Yoon et al[16]	78	96	100	99
Delgado Almandoz et al[17,a]	210	96	98	98

Abbreviations: MDCTA, multidetector CT angiography; N, number of patients in study.
 [a] These studies also included findings of surgical evacuation and autopsy in addition to catheter angiography as gold standards.

Importantly, several recent studies with large cohorts of acute hemorrhagic and ischemic stroke patients evaluated with MDCTA on admission, have found that the incidence of acute contrast-induced nephropathy in this patient population is low, ranging from 2% to 7%, and that this risk is not higher in patients whose baseline creatinine value is unknown at the time of scanning.[9–13]

ACCURACY OF MULTIDETECTOR CT ANGIOGRAPHY FOR THE DETECTION OF UNDERLYING VASCULAR LESIONS IN HEMORRHAGIC STROKE

Several recent studies comparing the accuracy of MDCTA to the gold standards of conventional catheter angiography as well as findings of surgical hematoma evacuation and autopsy have demonstrated that MDCTA can accurately identify those patients with hemorrhagic stroke who have an underlying vascular etiology (secondary ICH),

with sensitivities ranging from 89% to 96% and overall accuracy rates of 91% to 99% (Table 1).[14–17] Thus, MDCTA is an accurate diagnostic tool that allows for the rapid identification of the important minority of patients with hemorrhagic stroke who have secondary ICH, which, in turn, allows for the prompt institution of endovascular or surgical treatment in suitable patients in order to prevent rebleeding from the causative vascular lesion.

Frequency of Secondary ICH in Patients with Hemorrhagic Stroke Evaluated with MDCTA

The incidence of underlying vascular etiologies for an ICH varies significantly according to the patient's clinical characteristics and noncontrast CT (NCCT) findings, with patient age being one of the most important variables. Indeed, in recent MDCTA studies the frequency of secondary ICH has ranged from 13% to 28% in patients older than 18 years[16–19] to 65% in patients 40 years

Table 2
Frequency of secondary ICH in patients with hemorrhagic stroke evaluated with MDCTA

Study	N	Age Range (Years)	ICH Location	Secondary ICH (%)
Gazzola et al[18,a]	96	16–86	All	25.0
Romero et al[15,b]	43	4–40	All	65.1
Yoon et al[16,a]	78	21–86	Lobar	28.2
Delgado Almandoz et al[17,b]	623	18–94	All	14.6
Delgado Almandoz et al[19,b]	222	18–94	All	13.1

Abbreviation: ICH, Intracerebral hemorrhage.
 [a] These studies excluded patients with primarily/predominantly subarachnoid hemorrhage.
 [b] These studies excluded patients with any subarachnoid hemorrhage in the basal cisterns.

Table 3
Relative frequency of different vascular etiologies in a cohort of 845 hemorrhagic stroke patients evaluated with MDCTA

Vascular Etiology	N	%
Arteriovenous malformation	55	45.8
Aneurysm with purely intraparenchymal rupture	26[a]	21.7
Dural venous sinus/cortical vein thrombosis	20[b]	16.7
Arteriovenous fistula	11	9.2
Vasculopathy	4[c]	3.3
Moya-Moya	4	3.3

[a] Includes 3 pseudoaneurysms.
[b] Includes 2 cases of isolated cortical vein thrombosis.
[c] Includes a patient in whom vasculitis led to pseudoaneurysm formation and rupture.

or younger (**Table 2**).[15] **Table 3** provides a summary of the different types and relative frequencies of causative vascular lesions in a cohort of 845 ICH patients evaluated with MDCTA at the authors' institution over a 10-year period.[19]

Practical Risk Stratification for the Presence of Underlying Vascular Lesions in Patients with Hemorrhagic Stroke: The Secondary ICH Score

In a recent series of 623 consecutive patients who presented with hemorrhagic stroke at the authors' institution over a 9-year period, several independent clinical and NCCT predictors of a higher incidence of a causative vascular lesion were identified in ICH patients evaluated with MDCTA: (1) age younger than 46 years (47%), lobar (20%) or infratentorial (16%) ICH location, female sex (18%), and absence of known hypertension or impaired coagulation at presentation (33%).[17]

In addition, the authors devised a system to categorize the NCCT according to the probability that an underlying vascular etiology would be found on the subsequent MDCTA examination. In this system, a high-probability NCCT was defined as an examination in which there were either (1) enlarged vessels or calcifications along the margins of the ICH, or (2) hyperdensity within

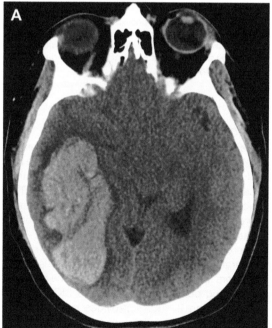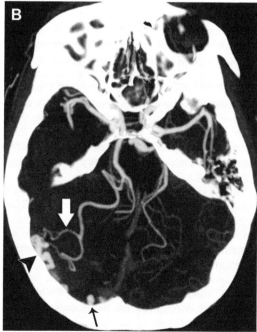

Fig. 1. A 59-year-old woman with a history of hypertension and daily aspirin use presents with headache and worsening left-sided weakness. (*A*) Indeterminate NCCT demonstrates a right temporo-parieto-occipital ICH (SICH score 3). (*B*) Axial maximum intensity projection (MIP) image of a CTA demonstrates a right temporo-parieto-occipital AVM (*arrowhead*) with arterial supply from the right posterior cerebral artery (*white arrow*) and venous drainage to the right transverse sinus (*black arrow*).

a dural venous sinus or cortical vein along the presumed venous drainage path of the ICH. A low-probability NCCT was defined as an examination in which (1) none of the findings of a high-probability NCCT were present, and (2) the ICH was located within the basal ganglia, thalamus, or brainstem. An indeterminate NCCT was defined as an examination that did not meet criteria for a high- or low-probability NCCT (most commonly, lobar or cerebellar ICH).[17,19] Of note, in multivariate analysis the authors found that the NCCT categorization according to this system superseded ICH location (defined as lobar, cerebellar, or deep gray matter) as a predictor of an underlying vascular etiology for the ICH.[19]

Although a hemorrhagic stroke patient presenting with any of the aforementioned clinical or NCCT characteristics would be at a significantly increased risk of having secondary ICH, the clinical scenario encountered is often complex. For example, one may be presented with a male patient younger than 46 years who has a history of hypertension and presents with a basal ganglia hemorrhage; or, alternatively, a female patient in her 50s or 60s who has a history of hypertension and impaired coagulation but presents with a lobar ICH (Fig. 1). Hence, a scoring system that integrates a given hemorrhagic stroke patient's risk of harboring an underlying vascular etiology for the ICH would be desirable and clinically valuable. The authors have recently devised such a scoring system based on the aforementioned independent predictors of a higher incidence of secondary ICH, utilizing the NCCT categorization rather than ICH location, and have designated it the Secondary ICH (SICH) Score (Table 4).[19] Table 5 provides the predictive value of the SICH score in the retrospective derivation cohort of 623 patients as well as in a prospective validation cohort of 222 patients. Figs. 2, 3, and 4[19] depict patients with high SICH scores and secondary ICH demonstrated by MDCTA.

The SICH score is advantageous because it can be rapidly calculated immediately after the NCCT examination has been performed, while the patient is still on the CT scanner table, and thus serves as a valuable tool in the clinical decision as to whether to perform MDCTA. Indeed, this scoring system would be most useful at institutions where neurovascular imaging is not performed in all ICH patients but is reserved for those patients who are deemed most likely to harbor an underlying vascular abnormality. However, given the relatively high positive rate of MDCTA for the presence of an underlying vascular etiology in patients with hemorrhagic stroke (14.2% in the authors' cohort), some institutions (including the authors') perform

MDCTA in all patients with this condition. Hence, the usefulness of the SICH score at the latter institutions lies in selecting ICH patients for more invasive diagnostic tests such as conventional catheter angiography when the initial MDCTA is either negative or inconclusive but the patient's pretest probability of harboring an underlying vascular lesion—as determined by the SICH score—is high. Of importance, results of receiver operating characteristic (ROC) analysis in the authors' patient cohort showed that the maximum operating point was reached at a SICH score of greater than 2. Fig. 5 provides proposed algorithms for the diagnostic workup of patients with hemorrhagic stroke based on the admission SICH score at institutions that perform neurovascular imaging selectively (see Fig. 5A) as well as at institutions that perform MDCTA in all patients (see Fig. 5B).

Table 4
Calculation of the SICH score

Parameter	Points
NCCT categorization[a]	
High probability	2
Indeterminate	1
Low probability	0
Age group (years)	
18–45	2
46–70	1
≥71	0
Sex	
Female	1
Male	0
Neither known HTN nor impaired coagulation[b]	
Yes	1
No	0

The SICH score is calculated by adding the total number of points for a given patient.

Abbreviations: aPTT, activated plasma thromboplastin time; HTN, hypertension; INR, international normalized ratio; NCCT, noncontrast CT; SICH, secondary intracerebral hemorrhage.

[a] High-probability NCCT: an examination with either (1) enlarged vessels or calcifications along the margins of the ICH, or (2) hyperdensity within a dural venous sinus or cortical vein along the presumed venous drainage path of the ICH. Low-probability NCCT: an examination in which neither (1) nor (2) are present and the ICH is located in the basal ganglia, thalamus, or brainstem. Indeterminate NCCT: an examination that does not meet criteria for a high- or low-probability NCCT.

[b] Impaired coagulation defined as admission INR >3, aPTT >80 seconds, platelet count <50,000, or daily antiplatelet therapy.

Table 5
Predictive value of the SICH score

Score	Retrospective Cohort (N = 623)		Prospective Cohort (N = 222)		All Patients (N = 845)	
	N (%)	% Positive CTAs	N (%)	% Positive CTAs	N (%)	% Positive CTAs
0	37 (5.9)	0	15 (6.8)	0	52 (6.1)	0
1	145 (23.3)	1.4	67 (30.2)	1.5	212 (25.1)	1.4
2	209 (33.5)	5.3	68 (30.6)	4.4	277 (32.8)	5.1
3	138 (22.2)	18.1	40 (18.0)	20	178 (21.1)	18.5
4	61 (9.8)	39.3	21 (9.5)	38.1	82 (9.7)	39
5	28 (4.5)	85.7	10 (4.5)	80	38 (4.5)	84.2
6	5 (0.8)	100	1 (0.4)	100	6 (0.7)	100
AUC (95% CI)	0.86 (0.83–0.89)		0.87 (0.82–0.91)		0.87 (0.84–0.89)	
MOP	>2		>2		>2	
Sensitivity	85.7		86.2		85.8	
Specificity	71.1		75.6		72.3	
P value	<.0001		<.0001		<.0001	

Abbreviations: AUC, area under the curve after receiver operating characteristic analysis; CI, confidence interval; CTA, CT angiogram; MOP, maximum operating point after receiver operating characteristic analysis.

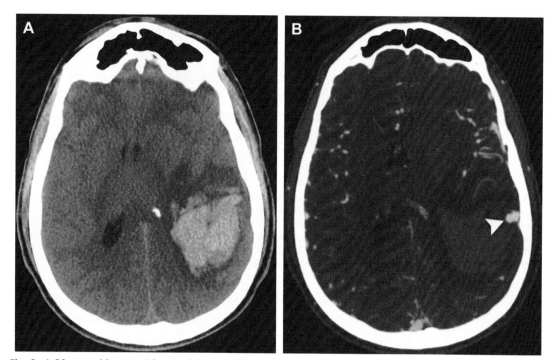

Fig. 2. A 28-year-old man without a history of hypertension or impaired coagulation presents with right-sided hemiparesis. (*A*) Indeterminate NCCT demonstrates a left parietal ICH (SICH score 4). (*B*) Axial CTA source image demonstrates a 9-mm outpouching arising from a distal branch of the left middle cerebral artery (*arrowhead*), consistent with a pseudoaneurysm. The patient was later found to have a history of intravenous drug use.

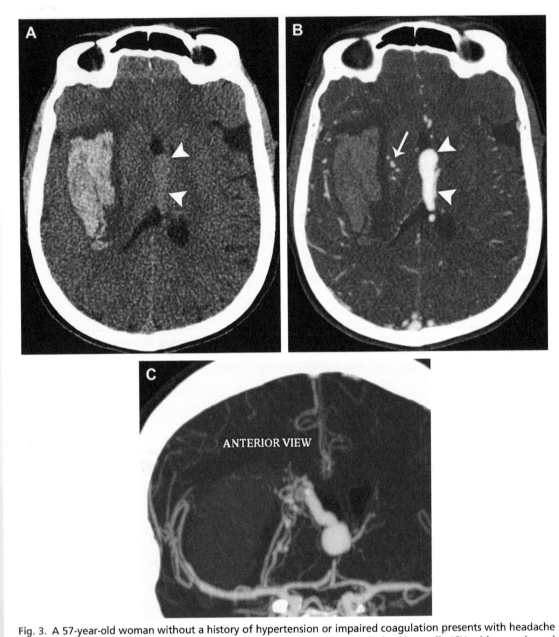

Fig. 3. A 57-year-old woman without a history of hypertension or impaired coagulation presents with headache followed by obtundation. (A) High-probability NCCT demonstrates a right basal ganglia ICH with an enlarged vessel medial to the ICH in the region of the third ventricle (arrowheads, SICH score 5). (B) Axial CTA source image demonstrates abnormal vessels in the right basal ganglia (arrow) as well as a markedly enlarged right internal cerebral vein (arrowheads), consistent with an AVM. (C) Coronal CTA MIP image redemonstrates the right basal ganglia AVM with venous drainage to the right internal cerebral vein and straight sinus.

Potential Pitfall in the Diagnosis of Dural Venous Sinus Thrombosis

There is an important potential pitfall to be aware of when making the diagnosis of DVST as the ICH etiology, which is of utmost clinical importance because its treatment may entail the institution of anticoagulation (despite the presence of ICH) and mechanical thrombectomy. Since the introduction of 64-slice CT scanners, the time

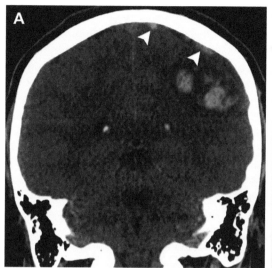
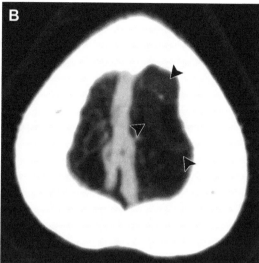

Fig. 4. A 21-year-old woman without a history of hypertension or impaired coagulation presents with worsening headaches for the past week. (*A*) High-probability coronal NCCT demonstrates a left parietal ICH with hyperdensity within a cerebral vein in the expected venous drainage path of the ICH (*arrowheads*, SICH score 6). (*B*) Axial CTA source image demonstrates nonopacification of several cerebral veins in the left cerebral hemisphere near the vertex (*arrowheads*), consistent with cerebral vein thrombosis as the ICH etiology. The patient was later found to have stopped oral contraceptives 1 week prior to admission.

delay from contrast injection to scanning has decreased and, as a result, the normal dural venous sinuses may or may not be adequately (ie, homogeneously) opacified at the time of CT scanning. Indeed, at institutions where MDCTA is performed from the skull base to the vertex, this phenomenon may occur as frequently as 40% to 60% of the time for the transverse and sigmoid sinuses (**Fig. 6**).[20] Thus, if in the first-pass CT angiogram (CTA) a dural venous sinus is homogeneously opacified, then DVST can be effectively ruled out. However, if a dural venous sinus is either inhomogeneously opacified or nonopacified in the first-pass CTA, then it could be due to scan timing or partial/complete DVST. Hence, identification of inadequate contrast opacification of a dural venous sinus during review of the first-pass CTA in a distribution that may explain the ICH should prompt acquisition of an immediate delayed scan to confidently make (or exclude) the diagnosis of DVST as the ICH etiology. In the authors' experience, the delayed scan can be obtained up to 7 minutes after the first-pass CTA.

THE CT ANGIOGRAPHY SPOT SIGN IN PRIMARY ICH

In the past decade, several studies have shown that the presence of active contrast extravasation at MDCTA, known as the spot sign, is an indicator of ongoing hemorrhage and, as such, is an accurate and powerful predictor of hematoma expansion, mortality, and poor outcome among survivors in patients with primary ICH (**Table 6**).[21–29] Of importance, these studies have also shown that the frequency of spot signs varies considerably according to the time from ictus to MDCTA evaluation, ranging from 66.2% in patients imaged within 3 hours of ictus to 13.5% in those patients imaged after 6 hours from ictus.[28]

Criteria for the Identification of a Spot Sign and the Spot Sign Score

In a recent series of 573 consecutive patients with primary ICH from the authors' institution (367 of whom had a follow-up NCCT examination), strict radiological criteria for the identification of a spot sign in the CTA source images were developed (**Box 1**).[27,28] The first 2 criteria in **Box 1** allow the reader to make the important differentiation between "true" spot signs and spot sign "mimics" such as choroidal calcifications, aneurysms, and AVMs,[18] while the third criterion minimizes the likelihood that hematoma heterogeneity and inherent CTA source image noise is misdiagnosed as a spot sign.

In addition, the authors systematically characterized this MDCTA finding and demonstrated

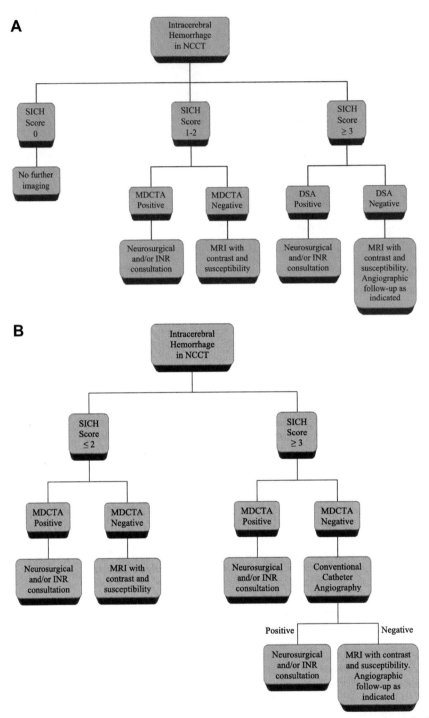

Fig. 5. Proposed diagnostic algorithms for the workup of patients with hemorrhagic stroke. (*A*) Algorithm for institutions that perform neurovascular imaging selectively. (*B*) Algorithm for institutions that perform MDCTA in all patients. NCCT, noncontrast CT; SICH, secondary intracerebral hemorrhage; MDCTA, multidetector CT angiography; DSA, digital subtraction angiography; INR, interventional neuroradiology; MRI, magnetic resonance imaging.

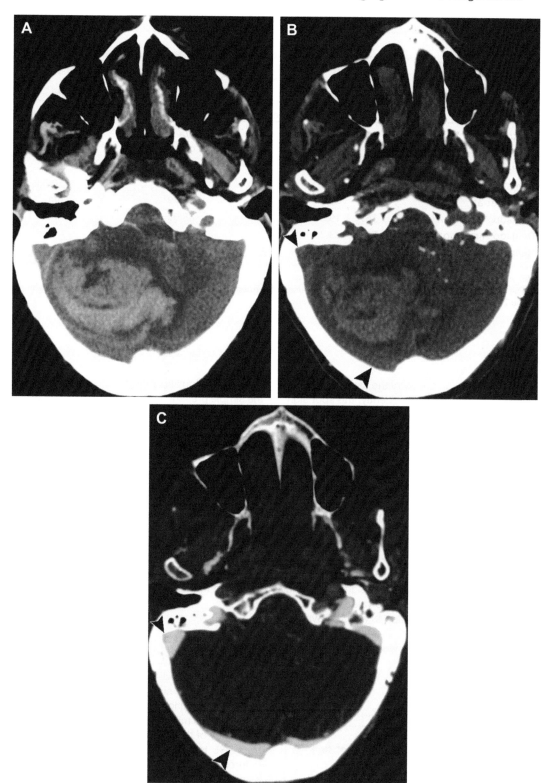

Fig. 6. A 67-year-old woman presents with unresponsiveness. (*A*) NCCT demonstrates a right cerebellar intracerebral hemorrhage with intraventricular extension. (*B*) Axial source image of a first-pass CTA performed in a 64-slice CT scanner demonstrates nonopacification of the right transverse and sigmoid sinuses (*arrowheads*), which may be related to scan timing or DVST. (*C*) Delayed CTA performed 27 seconds after the first-pass CTA demonstrates homogeneous opacification of the right transverse and sigmoid sinuses (*arrowheads*), which excludes DVST as the ICH etiology.

Table 6
Frequency and accuracy of the spot sign for the prediction of hematoma expansion and mortality in primary ICH

| | | | Sensitivity/Specificity | |
| | | | Hematoma Expansion | Mortality |
Study	N	Spot Sign Frequency (%)		
Becker et al[21]	113	46.0	n/a	77/73
Wada et al[22]	39	33.3	91/89	43/69
Goldstein et al[23]	104	55.8	92/50	73/50
Kim et al[24,a]	56	26.8	n/a	50/83
Ederies et al[25,a]	61	42.6	94/79	n/a
Delgado Almandoz et al[27,a]	367	19.3	88/93	n/a
Delgado Almandoz et al[28,a]	573	23.2	n/a	41/85
Hallevi et al[29,a]	27	48.1	100/100	n/a

Abbreviation: n/a, not applicable (not a study end point).
[a] The results in these studies include delayed spot signs identified in a delayed acquisition of the head typically performed 2 to 3 minutes after the first-pass CT angiogram.

that all spot signs do not carry the same predictive value (**Figs. 7** and **8**). Subsequently, the spot sign characteristics that independently predicted the likelihood of hematoma expansion (ie, the number of spot signs, maximum axial dimension, and maximum absolute attenuation) were utilized, and a spot sign scoring system developed (**Table 7**), which further refined the spot sign's predictive value for the aforementioned outcome measures (**Table 8**).[27,28] Furthermore, the spot sign score also explained why a spot sign's predictive value for hematoma expansion decreases as time from ictus increases: in patients with spot signs and an exact known time from ictus, the mean and median spot sign score (and hence, the spot sign's predictive value) decreases significantly as time from ictus to MDCTA evaluation increases. Indeed, in the authors' study, when the spot sign score was entered into the multivariate logistic regression model instead of the simple presence of a spot sign as a binary variable, time from ictus to MDCTA evaluation was no longer an independent predictor of hematoma expansion.[27]

Thus, as accurate indicators of ongoing hemorrhage, the presence of a spot sign and spot sign score could serve as triage tools to target early hemostatic therapy for those patients with primary ICH who are most likely to benefit from treatment, regardless of time from ictus to MDCTA evaluation. Future research may also help elucidate whether patients with different spot sign scores will derive the same clinical benefit from these emerging therapies.

Value of Delayed MDCTA Acquisitions in Patients with Primary ICH

Several recent studies have found that a significant minority of spot signs are found on the delayed MDCTA acquisitions only, which are typically performed 2 to 3 minutes after the first-pass CTA. The frequency of these delayed spot signs has ranged from 8% to 23% of all spot signs identified in different series.[21,24,25,27–29] Nevertheless, these delayed spot signs carry the same predictive value as the spot signs identified in the first-pass CTAs and, when coupled with the spot signs identified in the first-pass CTAs, increase this finding's sensitivity and negative predictive value for hematoma expansion.

Box 1
Criteria for the identification of a spot sign

≥1 focus of contrast pooling within the ICH

Discontinuous from normal or abnormal vasculature adjacent to the ICH

Attenuation ≥120 Hounsfield Units

Any size and morphology

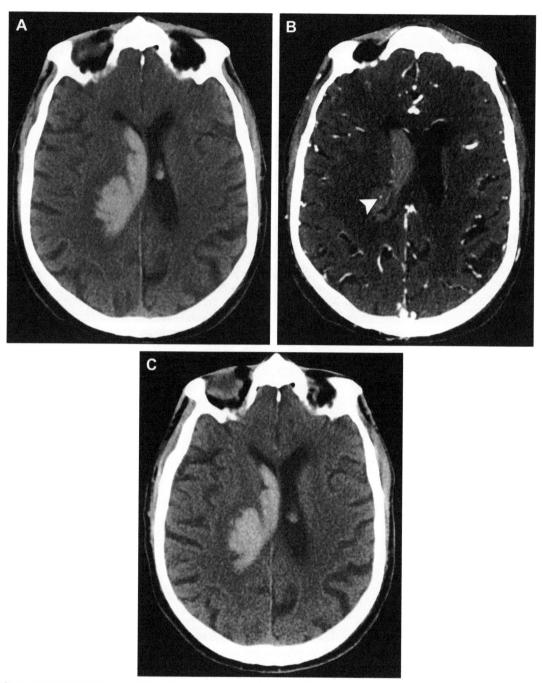

Fig. 7. An 87-year-old man with a history of hypertension and daily aspirin intake presents with left-sided numbness and confusion for the last 5 hours. (*A*) NCCT demonstrates a right thalamic ICH with intraventricular extension. (*B*) Axial CTA source image demonstrates a single focus of contrast pooling within the ICH with a maximum axial dimension of 2 mm and attenuation of 128 Hounsfield Units (*arrowhead*), consistent with a spot sign (spot sign score 1). (*C*) Follow-up NCCT performed 18 hours after the baseline CTA demonstrates no interval change in the ICH or intraventricular hemorrhage. The patient was discharged to a rehabilitation facility after a hospital stay of 7 days.

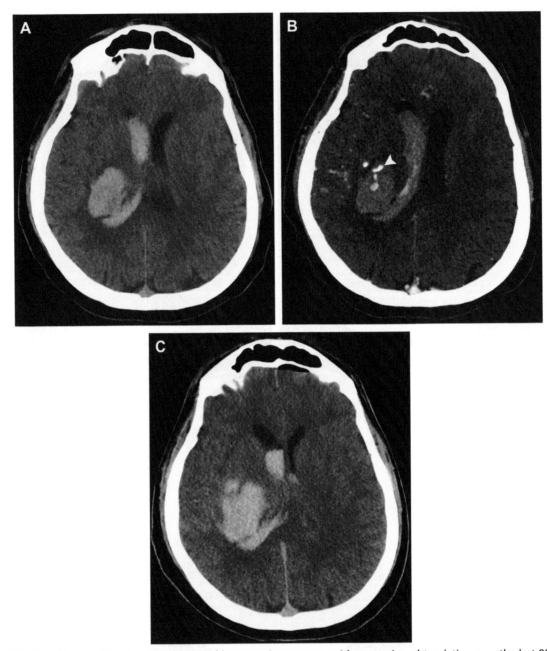

Fig. 8. A 44-year-old man with a history of hypertension presents with worsening obtundation over the last 80 minutes. (A) NCCT demonstrates a right thalamic ICH (15.4 mL) with intraventricular extension (24.3 mL). (B) Axial CTA source image demonstrates at least 4 foci of contrast pooling within the ICH, consistent with spot signs. The largest spot sign had a maximum axial dimension of 7-mm and an attenuation of 218 Hounsfield Units (arrow-head, spot sign score 4). (C) Follow-up NCCT performed 4.5 hours after the baseline CTA demonstrates interval expansion of the right thalamic ICH (26.9 mL) and intraventricular hemorrhage (27.8 mL). The patient was discharged to a rehabilitation facility after a hospital stay of 23 days.

Table 7
Calculation of the spot sign score

Spot Sign Characteristic[a]	Points
Number of spot signs	
1–2	1
≥3	2
Maximum axial dimension	
1–4 mm	0
≥5 mm	1
Maximum attenuation	
120–179 HU	0
≥180 HU	1

Abbreviation: HU, Hounsfield Unit.
[a] The spot sign characterization is performed in the first CTA acquisition in which a spot sign is identified. For CTAs with more than 1 spot sign, the maximum dimension in a single axial CTA source image and maximum attenuation of the largest spot sign is determined. The spot sign score is obtained by adding the total number of points for the CTA.

Delayed MDCTA acquisitions are also extremely useful in cases where differentiating a spot sign from an aneurysm or small AVM is challenging. By definition, spot signs are extravascular collections of contrast and aneurysms or AVMs are intravascular structures. It follows that on a delayed MDCTA acquisition, a spot sign should change in configuration and attenuation relative to the vasculature adjacent to the hematoma because the extravasated contrast mixes with the blood within the hematoma; indeed, the contrast often layers in the dependent portions of the hematoma. However, an intravascular structure, such as an aneurysm or small AVM, should maintain its morphology and have the same attenuation as the vasculature adjacent to the hematoma on the delayed MDCTA acquisition (Fig. 9). Distinguishing spot signs from aneurysms or small AVMs is important because the treatment implications are vastly different.

Nevertheless, the clinical benefits derived from improving (1) the spot sign's sensitivity and negative predictive value for the prediction of hematoma expansion as well as (2) the ability to accurately make the distinction between spot signs and aneurysms or small AVMs must be carefully weighed against the additional radiation exposure incurred from performing a delayed CT examination of the head—approximately 2.5 mSv at the authors' institution, which is slightly less than the estimated average annual radiation dose for a person living in the United States (3 mSv).

THE CT ANGIOGRAPHY SPOT SIGN IN SECONDARY INTRACEREBRAL HEMORRHAGE

Although an initial report suggested that spot signs were uncommon in patients with secondary ICH and the spot sign may be a finding specific to patients with primary ICH,[18] a recent study of 173 patients with secondary ICH from the authors' institution demonstrated that, utilizing the strict radiological criteria delineated in Box 1, spot signs can be identified in this patient population.[30] Indeed, spot signs were less common in secondary ICH than in primary ICH, occurring in approximately 14.5% of secondary ICH patients

Table 8
Predictive value of the spot sign score for hematoma expansion, in-hospital mortality, and poor outcome among survivors in primary ICH

Spot Sign Score[a]	Hematoma Expansion (%)	In-Hospital Mortality (%)	Poor Outcome[b] (%)
0	2	24	29
1	33	41	42
2	50	59	47
3	94	61	54
4	100	64	75
AUC (95% CI)	0.93 (0.89–0.95)	0.64 (0.60–0.68)	0.56 (0.51–0.61)
P value	<.0001	<.0001	0.04

[a] A score of zero indicates that no spot sign is identified in the CT angiogram.
[b] Defined as a modified Rankin Scale ≥4 at 3-month follow-up.

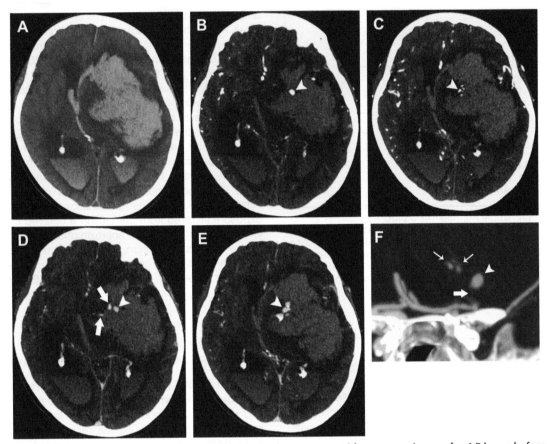

Fig. 9. A 92-year-old woman with a history of hypertension presents with unresponsiveness for 4.5 hours before presentation. (*A*) NCCT demonstrates a large left thalamic ICH with intraventricular extension. (*B*) Axial first-pass CTA source image demonstrates a rounded 6-mm collection of contrast within the ICH (*arrowhead*), which demonstrated a connection to a small lenticulostriate branch of the left middle cerebral artery, consistent with an aneurysm. (*C*) Axial first-pass CTA source image at a slightly higher level demonstrates 5 discrete foci of contrast pooling within the ICH, which were not connected to any vessels outside the ICH, consistent with spot signs. The largest spot sign measured 5 mm and had an attenuation of 192 Hounsfield Units (*arrowhead*, spot sign score 4). (*D*) Delayed axial CTA image obtained 34 seconds after the first-pass CTA demonstrates that the lenticulostriate aneurysm shown in *B* did not change in morphology and maintains the same attenuation as the vasculature outside the ICH (*arrowhead*). Note that there are now spot signs present in this image (*arrows*). (*E*) Delayed axial CTA image at the level of the spot signs shown in *C* demonstrates that they have increased in size and do not have the same attenuation as the vasculature outside the ICH (*arrowhead*), as contrast has pooled within it. (*F*) Coronal reformation of the first-pass CTA demonstrates the aneurysm (*arrowhead*) arising from the small lenticulostriate branch of the left middle cerebral artery (*thick arrow*), as well as the multiple spot signs superiorly within the ICH (*arrows*). The patient died shortly after the CTA was performed.

in the authors' study. However, they were particularly common in patients with arteriovenous fistulae (41.7%) as well as anterior (18.2%) and middle (17.1%) cerebral artery aneurysms with intraparenchymal rupture (**Fig. 10**). Although the presence of a spot sign in this patient population predicted an increased risk of in-hospital mortality (44%, *P* value .027), this was not the case for hematoma expansion (16.7%, *P* value .48). However, the majority of patients in the authors' sample underwent either surgical or endovascular intervention immediately following the CTA and, thus, hematoma expansion could not be adequately assessed in these patients.

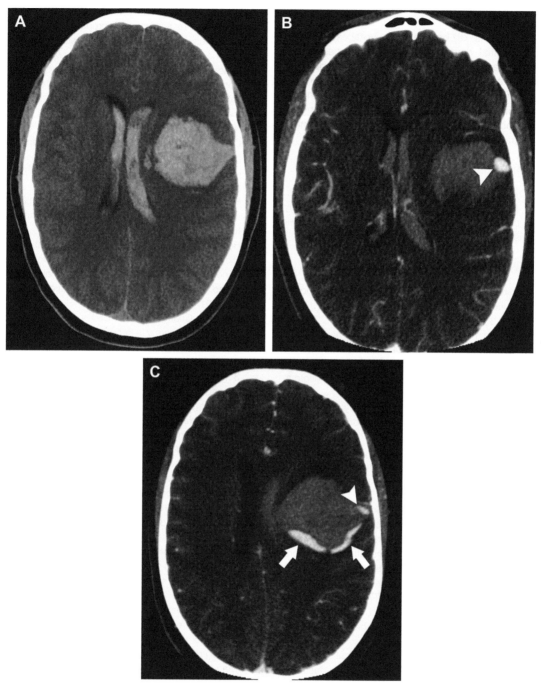

Fig. 10. A 16-year-old man presents with worsening headache and expressive aphasia for 3 hours. (*A*) NCCT demonstrates a left frontal ICH with intraventricular extension. (*B*) Axial CTA source image demonstrates a left middle cerebral artery aneurysm (*arrowhead*). (*C*) Axial CTA source image at a slightly higher level redemonstrates the left middle cerebral artery aneurysm (*arrowhead*) as well as 2 large separate foci of contrast pooling within the ICH, consistent with spot signs (*arrows*). The largest spot sign measured 13 mm and had an attenuation of 184 Hounsfield Units (spot sign score 3). The patient underwent immediate surgical evacuation and aneurysm clipping, and was discharged to a rehabilitation facility after a hospital stay of 13 days.

SUMMARY

MDCTA is rapidly becoming a pivotal examination in the initial diagnostic workup of patients with hemorrhagic stroke, allowing for the prompt and accurate diagnosis of potentially treatable underlying vascular etiologies in the important minority of patients with secondary ICH, and emerging as an important triage tool in the selection of primary ICH patients for novel hemostatic therapies.

ACKNOWLEDGMENTS

The authors would like to thank Eleni K. Balasalle, BA (Massachusetts General Hospital Radiology Educational Media Services, Boston, MA) for her assistance in the artwork for this article.

REFERENCES

1. Qureshi AI, Tuhrim S, Broderick JP, et al. Spontaneous intracerebral hemorrhage. N Engl J Med 2001;344:1450–60.
2. Badjatia N, Rosand J. Intracerebral hemorrhage. Neurologist 2005;11:311–24.
3. Jane JA, Kassell NF, Torner JC, et al. The natural history of aneurysms and arteriovenous malformations. J Neurosurg 1985;62:321–3.
4. The Arteriovenous Malformation Study Group. Arteriovenous malformations of the brain in adults. N Engl J Med 1999;340:1812–8.
5. Ondra SL, Troupp H, George ED, et al. The natural history of symptomatic arteriovenous malformations of the brain: a 24-year follow-up assessment. J Neurosurg 1990;73:387–91.
6. Davis SM, Broderick J, Hennerici M, et al. Recombinant activated factor vii intracerebral hemorrhage trial investigators. hematoma growth is a determinant of mortality and poor outcome after intracerebral hemorrhage. Neurology 2006;66:1175–81.
7. Mayer SA, Brun NC, Begtrup K, et al. Factor Seven for Acute Hemorrhagic Stroke (FAST) Trial Investigators. Efficacy and safety of recombinant activated factor VII for acute intracerebral hemorrhage. N Engl J Med 2008;358:2127–37.
8. Anderson CS, Huang Y, Wang JG, et al. INTERACT Investigators. Intensive blood pressure reduction in acute cerebral haemorrhage trial (INTERACT): a randomised pilot trial. Lancet Neurol 2008;7:391–9.
9. Krol AL, Dzialowski I, Roy J, et al. Incidence of radiocontrast nephropathy in patients undergoing acute stroke computed tomography angiography. Stroke 2007;38:2364–6 Erratum in: Stroke 2007;38:e97.
10. Dittrich R, Akdeniz S, Kloska SP, et al. Low rate of contrast-induced nephropathy after CT perfusion and CT angiography in acute stroke patients. J Neurol 2007;254:1491–7.
11. Langner S, Stumpe S, Kirsch M, et al. No increased risk for contrast-induced nephropathy after multiple CT perfusion studies of the brain with a nonionic, dimeric, iso-osmolal contrast medium. Am J Neuroradiol 2008;29:1525–9.
12. Hopyan JJ, Gladstone DJ, Mallia G, et al. Renal safety of CT angiography and perfusion imaging in the emergency evaluation of acute stroke. Am J Neuroradiol 2008;29:1826–30.
13. Oleinik A, Romero JM, Schwab K, et al. CT angiography for intracerebral hemorrhage does not increase risk of acute nephropathy. Stroke 2009; 40:2393–7.
14. Yeung R, Ahmad T, Aviv RI, et al. Comparison of CTA to DSA in determining the etiology of spontaneous ICH. Can J Neurol Sci 2009;36:176–80.
15. Romero JM, Artunduaga M, Forero NP, et al. Accuracy of CT angiography for the diagnosis of vascular abnormalities causing intraparenchymal hemorrhage in young patients. Emerg Radiol 2009;16: 195–201.
16. Yoon DY, Chang SK, Choi CS, et al. Multidetector row CT angiography in spontaneous lobar intracerebral hemorrhage: a prospective comparison with conventional angiography. Am J Neuroradiol 2009; 30:962–7.
17. Delgado Almandoz JE, Schaefer PW, Forero NP, et al. Diagnostic accuracy and yield of multidetector CT angiography in the evaluation of spontaneous intraparenchymal cerebral hemorrhage. Am J Neuroradiol 2009;30:1213–21.
18. Gazzola S, Aviv RI, Gladstone DJ, et al. Vascular and nonvascular mimics of the CT angiography "spot sign" in patients with secondary intracerebral hemorrhage. Stroke 2008;39:1177–83.
19. Delgado Almandoz JE, Schaefer PW, Goldstein JN, et al. Practical scoring system for the identification of patients with intracerebral hemorrhage at highest risk of harboring an underlying vascular etiology: the secondary ICH score. AJNR Am J Neuroradiol 2010; 31(9):1653–60.
20. Delgado Almandoz JE, Su HS, Schaefer PW, et al. Frequency of adequate contrast opacification of the major intracranial venous structures with CT angiography in the setting of intracerebral hemorrhage: comparison of 16- and 64-slice CT angiography techniques. AJNR Am J Neuroradiol 2011, in press.
21. Becker KJ, Baxter AB, Bybee HM, et al. Extravasation of radiographic contrast is an independent predictor of death in primary intracerebral hemorrhage. Stroke 1999;30:2025–32.
22. Wada R, Aviv RI, Fox AJ, et al. CT angiography "spot sign" predicts hematoma expansion in acute intracerebral hemorrhage. Stroke 2007;38:1257–62.
23. Goldstein JN, Fazen LE, Snider R, et al. Contrast extravasation on CT angiography predicts hematoma

expansion in intracerebral hemorrhage. Neurology 2007;68:889–94.

24. Kim J, Smith A, Hemphill JC III, et al. Contrast extravasation on CT predicts mortality in primary intracerebral hemorrhage. Am J Neuroradiol 2008;29:520–5.

25. Ederies A, Demchuk A, Chia T, et al. Postcontrast CT extravasation is associated with hematoma expansion in CTA spot negative patients. Stroke 2009;40: 1672–6.

26. Thompson AL, Kosior JC, Gladstone DJ, et al, PREDICTS/Sunnybrook ICH CTA Study Group. Defining the CT angiography 'spot sign' in primary intracerebral hemorrhage. Can J Neurol Sci 2009; 36:456–61.

27. Delgado Almandoz JE, Yoo AJ, Stone MJ, et al. Systematic characterization of the computed tomography angiography spot sign in primary intracerebral

hemorrhage identifies patients at highest risk for hematoma expansion. The spot sign score. Stroke 2009;40:2994–3000.

28. Delgado Almandoz JE, Yoo AJ, Stone MJ, et al. The spot sign score in primary intracerebral hemorrhage identifies patients at highest risk of in-hospital mortality and poor outcome among survivors. Stroke 2010;41:54–60.

29. Hallevi H, Abraham AT, Barreto AD, et al. The spot sign in intracerebral hemorrhage: the importance of looking for contrast extravasation. Cerebrovasc Dis 2010;29:217–20.

30. Delgado Almandoz JE, Kelly HR, Brouwers HB, et al. Frequency and predictive value of the CT angiography spot sign in secondary intracerebral hemorrhage. In: Proceedings of the 2010 International Stroke Conference. San Antonio, February 23, 2010.

CT Perfusion Imaging in Acute Stroke

Angelos A. Konstas, MD, PhD[a],*, Max Wintermark, MD[b],
Michael H. Lev, MD[a]

KEYWORDS

- Acute stroke • CT perfusion • Cerebral blood volume
- Cerebral blood flow • Ischemic core • Ischemic penumbra
- CBV/CBF mismatch

The imaging management of acute ischemic stroke remains challenging both diagnostically and therapeutically. Intravenous tissue plasminogen activator (tPA) (to be used within 4.5 hours of stroke onset based on the 2008 European Cooperative Acute Stroke Study [ECASS III][1–3]) and the MERCI clot retrieval device (to be used within 9 hours of stroke onset) are the only treatments currently approved by the Food and Drug Administration (FDA) for acute stroke.[3–10] The only imaging modality currently required before intravenous tPA administration is unenhanced head computed tomography (CT), used to exclude intracranial hemorrhage (an absolute contraindication) and infarct size greater than one-third of the middle cerebral artery (MCA) territory (a relative contraindication, and predictor of increased hemorrhagic risk following tPA administration).[11,12] The limited time window for intravenous (IV) tPA administration (which remains 3 hours on the package insert), delays in transportation and triage, and multiple contraindications to thrombolysis, however, all limit the use of intravenous tPA to typically less than 5% of patients admitted with ischemic stroke.[13]

CT perfusion (CTP) expands the role of CT in the evaluation of acute stroke by providing physiologic insights into cerebral hemodynamics, and in so doing complements the strengths of CT angiography (CTA) by determining the consequences of vessel occlusions and stenoses (**Fig. 1**).[14–17] Acute ischemic stroke is a disorder of blood flow to the brain, and its characterization and management typically require an answer to the following 4 critical questions[18–20]:

- Is there hemorrhage that explains the symptoms or excludes lytic therapies?
- Is there intravascular thrombus that can be targeted for thrombolysis?
- Is there a "core" of critically ischemic infarcted tissue, and if so, how large?
- Is there a "penumbra" of severely ischemic but potentially viable tissue?

CTP can help to address the latter 2 of these questions, whereas unenhanced CT and CTA can address the first and second, respectively.

CTP is fast,[14] increasingly available,[21] safe when performed correctly,[22] and affordable.[23] It typically adds no more than 5 minutes to the time required to perform a standard unenhanced head CT, and does not hinder IV thrombolysis, which can be administered (with appropriate monitoring) directly at the CT scanner table immediately following completion of the unenhanced scan.[24–26] Like diffusion-weighted imaging (DWI) and MR perfusion-weighted imaging (PWI), CTP has the potential to serve as a surrogate marker of stroke severity, likely exceeding the National Institutes of Health Stroke Scale (NIHSS) score or Alberta Stroke Program Early CT Score (ASPECTS) as a predictor of outcome.[27–35] Because of these advantages, advanced CT imaging could have important implications for the management of stroke patients worldwide.[36–39]

Disclosure statement: no disclosures.
[a] Department of Radiology, Massachusetts General Hospital, 55 Fruit Street, Boston, MA 02114, USA
[b] Department of Radiology, University of Virginia, PO Box 800170, Charlottesville, VA 22908, USA
* Corresponding author.
E-mail address: akonstas@partners.org

Neuroimag Clin N Am 21 (2011) 215–238
doi:10.1016/j.nic.2011.01.008

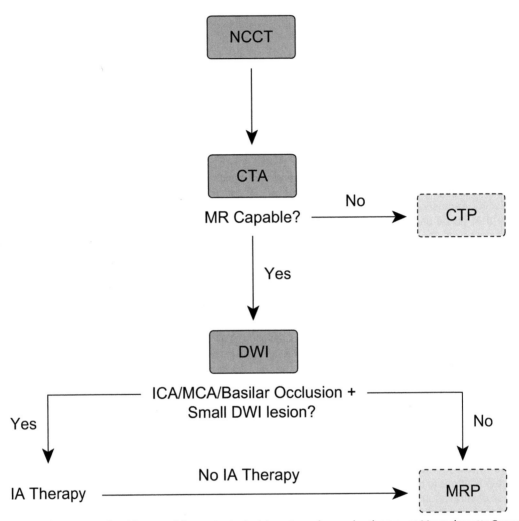

Imaging Algorithm for Acute Stroke/TIA IA Triage **if** *Rapid* DWI Available: the MGH Approach

Fig. 1. Sample imaging algorithms used for acute stroke triage to endovascular therapy at Massachusetts General Hospital (MGH) and at University of Virginia. The choice and order of imaging modalities for stroke varies from patient to patient based on the acuity/severity of the clinical presentation, and from center to center based on the local practice patterns and acute scanner/treatment availability (including intraventricular thrombolysis and endovascular therapies such as urokinase and clot retrieval). At the University of Virginia, for example, the imaging algorithm is to perform CTA/CTP for all suspected stroke on a diagnostic basis—to establish the differential diagnosis, stroke subtype, and extent of ischemia—and to proceed to MR imaging in selected cases where additional workup is clinically justified. CTA, computed tomographic angiography; CTP, computed tomographic perfusion; DWI, diffusion-weighted imaging; IA, intra-arterial; ICA, internal carotid artery; INR, international normalized ratio; MCA, middle cerebral artery; N[C]CT, noncontrast computed tomography; MRI, magnetic resonance imaging; MRP, magnetic resonance perfusion; TIA, transient ischemic attack.

TECHNICAL CONSIDERATIONS OF CTP
Acute Stroke CT Imaging Protocol

At a recent meeting of stroke radiologists, emergency physicians, neurologists, and National Institutes of Health (NIH) administrators in Washington, DC, sponsored by the NIH and the American

Society of Neuroradiology, both the technical and clinical issues regarding advanced acute stroke imaging were discussed. A position paper of the expert consensus achieved was published simultaneously in the *American Journal of Neuroradiology* and *Stroke*.[40,41] In these articles, expert recommendations for minimum required standards of

Imaging Algorithm for Acute Stroke/TIA: the University of Virginia Approach

Suspicion of acute ischemic stroke

Column headers:
- completion of study within 1 hour of ordering & sending the screen form
- completion of study within 1 hour of ordering
- completion of study within 6 hours of ordering & sending the screen form
- completion of study ideally within 12 hours of ordering & sending the screen form no more than 24 hours

anterior circulation

persistent symptoms
- 0-4.5 hours since onset → head NCT
- 4.5-8 hours since onset → stroke CT with perfusion → if indicated & INR ttt considered: stroke MRI → if indicated: dissection MRI
- > 8 hours since onset → head NCT → if indicated: dissection MRI → if indicated: stroke MRI + intracranial MRA (± neck MRA)

resolved symptoms
- head NCT → if indicated: stroke MRI + intracranial MRA (± neck MRA)

posterior circulation / concern for basilar artery disease

- 0-4.5 hours since onset → head NCT → if indicated & INR ttt considered: stroke MRI + intracranial MRA → if indicated: stroke CT without perfusion → if indicated: stroke MRI + intracranial MRA (± neck MRA)
- 4.5-24 hours since onset → stroke CT without perfusion → if indicated & INR ttt considered: stroke MRI + intracranial MRA → if indicated: dissection MRI
- > 24 hours since onset → head NCT → if indicated & INR ttt considered: stroke MRI + intracranial MRA → if indicated: dissection MRI → if indicated: stroke MRI + intracranial MRA (± neck MRA)

Fig. 1. (continued)

CT and MR image acquisition were set forth, although standardization and validation of postprocessing algorithms and, hence, image interpretation, has yet to be reached.

CT-only imaging protocols for complete acute stroke evaluation typically have 3 components: unenhanced CT, an "arch-to-vertex" CTA, and dynamic first-pass cine CTP.

The major role of unenhanced CT in IV thrombolysis triage, as noted previously, is to exclude hemorrhage before treatment.[42] A large, greater than one-third MCA territory hypodensity at presentation is generally considered to reflect irreversible ischemia, portending a poor outcome regardless of treatment, and therefore a contraindication to thrombolysis.[43] Despite advances in resolution, coverage, and reduced radiation dose, unenhanced head CT remains suboptimal in its ability to correctly subtype stroke, localize embolic clot, predict outcome, or assess hemorrhagic risk.[4,6,7,18,44–47] Early ischemic signs of stroke are often absent or subtle, and their interpretation is prone to significant inter- and intraobserver variability.[34,47–51]

When CTA is performed, however, the source images from the CTA vascular acquisition (CTA-SI) offer additional clinically valuable data concerning not only the caliber of the head and neck vessels but also the tissue level perfusion.[52–54] The potential utility of the CTA-SI data in the assessment of brain parenchymal ischemia arises from its visualization of bulk collateral circulation—typically blood *flow* rather than blood *volume* weighted with newer generation multidetector row CT (MDCT) scanners—and is discussed in further detail in the following sections.[55]

CTP Acquisition

The cine acquisition of perfusion data forms the final step in the CT imaging evaluation of acute stroke. With dynamic CTP, a contrast bolus of 35 to 45 mL per imaging volume ("slab") is administered via power injector at a rate of 4 to 7 mL/s, with a saline "chaser" of 20 to 40 mL at the same rate. Typically a more rapid injection rate results in maximal but brief peak enhancement, compatible with cine protocols having a rapid data collection of 1 image per second, whereas a slower injection rate results in a somewhat lower but more prolonged plateau of enhancement, preferable for cine protocols with a lower frequency of data collection, such as "toggle table" or "shuttle mode" protocols acquired at 1 image every 3 seconds.

Acquisition typically begins 5 seconds after the start of contrast administration. With current-generation scan protocols, routine acquisition times have increased from the 45 seconds of early protocols, to greater than 66 to 75 seconds at present.[56,57] The volume of brain tissue included in a first pass cine perfusion CT study is constrained in the craniocaudal direction by the width of the CT detector. Hence, the z-axis coverage of each acquisition depends on the manufacturer and generation of the CT scanner. This limitation arises from the routine rapid cine acquisition rate of 1 image per second performed at a fixed table position (ie, no table movement). The detector configuration can be varied, so that different slice thicknesses can be obtained simultaneously. For example, with a standard 16-detector row scanner, a 2-cm slab can be obtained consisting of either 2 10-mm or 4 5-mm thick slices.[58–60] With a standard 64-detector row scanner, an approximately 3.4- to 4-cm z-direction slab can be acquired, per injection.

The maximum degree of vertical coverage could potentially be doubled for each bolus using a "shuttle-mode" or "toggle table" technique, in which the scanner table moves back and forth, switching between 2 different axial cine views at 2 different levels, separated by the z-direction detector width, albeit at a reduced temporal resolution of data acquisition, so as to permit sufficient time for table motion.[61] Alternatively, 2 boluses can be used to acquire 2 slabs of CTP data at different levels, doubling the overall coverage,[62] but (unlike shuttle mode) requiring twice the contrast and twice the radiation dose. More recently, helical shuttle mode techniques have been developed that permit more frequent temporal sampling per level, with a continuous "ribbon" of acquisition, and hence increased z-direction coverage. For example, a 64-detector row scanner with a 4-cm detector can provide 12 cm of cranial-caudal coverage using helical shuttle mode, with a temporal resolution of less than 3 seconds between serial images at a given z-level. Finally, the newest generation of 256 to 320 or more detector row scanners can provide as much as 16 cm of vertical, high temporal resolution coverage per gantry rotation.

COMPARISON WITH MR-PWI
Advantages

Quantitation and resolution
While CTP and MR-PWI both attempt to evaluate capillary-level hemodynamics, their differences should be considered. Dynamic susceptibility contrast (DSC) MR-PWI techniques rely on the T2* effect induced in adjacent tissues by high concentrations of intravenous gadolinium; CTP relies on direct visualization of intravascular

contrast material. The linear relationship between contrast concentration and CT attenuation more readily lends itself to quantitation, which is not easily achieved with MR-PWI. In addition, CTP has greater spatial (but not contrast) resolution compared with MR-PWI. These factors contribute to the possibility that visual evaluation of core/penumbra mismatch may be more quantitatively reliable with CTP than with MR perfusion (MRP) (**Fig. 2**).[63,64]

Availability and safety

CT also benefits from the practical availability and relative ease of scanning, particularly when dealing with critically ill patients and the attendant monitors or ventilators. CT may also be the only option for a subgroup of patients with an absolute contraindication to MR scanning, such as a pacemaker, and is a safe option when the patient cannot be screened for MR safety. For patients with borderline glomerular filtration rate (GFR 45–60) in whom perfusion data is important to patient management, the risk-to-benefit ratio of administering iodinated contrast is likely less than that of gadolinium.

Disadvantages

Limited coverage

A major disadvantage of some CTP acquisitions is their relatively limited z-direction coverage of 2 to 4 cm, whereas MR-PWI is typically capable of delivering information about the whole brain. Of importance, however, the 8- to 16-cm coverage offered by most newer MDCT scanners, with or without "shuttle mode" capability, is sufficient to image the entire anterior circulation territory (approximately 8 cm cranial-caudal), which is typically the critical region for stroke evaluation.[65,66]

Detection of microbleeds

Another disadvantage of using CT rather than MR imaging for stroke assessment is CT's inability to detect cerebral microbleeds. Microbleeds detected on gradient echo T2*-weighted MR imaging, however, have been shown not to be a contraindication to thrombolysis.[67]

Iodinated contrast

The authors' current protocol employs 35 to 45 mL iodinated contrast material for each CTP cine acquisition, in addition to the contrast required for the CTA. This additional contrast dose could

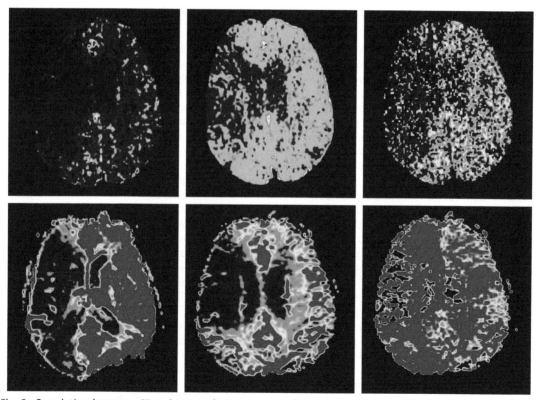

Fig. 2. Correlation between CT and MR perfusion maps, performed approximately 40 minutes apart. Perfusion images in an 88-year-old man who was found unresponsive. CTP images (top row, from left: cerebral blood flow [CBF], cerebral blood volume [CBV], mean transit time [MTT]) and MRP images (bottom row, from left: CBF, CBV, MTT) demonstrate a large perfusion deficit in the right MCA distribution.

be significant in some patients, particularly in the relatively older stroke prone population at risk for hypertension, diabetes, and atheromatous disease. Total dose may be even greater if the patient subsequently requires additional contrast for endovascular intervention. However, nonionic iodinated contrast does not worsen stroke outcome.[68-70]

Complex postprocessing

Postprocessing of CTA and CTP images is more labor intensive than postprocessing of MR angiography (MRA) and MRP images; however, with automation, training, and quality control, 3-dimensional reconstructions of CTA datasets and quantitative CTP maps can be produced rapidly and reliably.[71-73] Automated postprocessing software of CT perfusion data in acute stroke patients is increasingly simplifying the complexity of the postprocessing.[74]

Ionizing radiation

CTA/CTP also requires ionizing radiation, further discussed here.

RADIATION DOSE IN CTP: FACTS, PUBLICITY, AND RESPONSE

On October 8, 2009, the US FDA issued an initial notification regarding a safety investigation of facilities performing CTP scans. Because of incorrect settings on the CT scanner console of a single facility, more than 200 patients over a period of 18 months received radiation doses that were approximately 8 times the expected level. Approximately 40% of the patients lost patches of hair as a result of the overdoses.[75] These incidents followed another unrelated incident in a community hospital in Arcata, California, in 2008, where a CT technologist activated a CT scan 151 times over the same region of the head of a 2-year-old.[76]

These incidences highlight the importance of CT quality assurance programs. Such programs should include regular reviews of CT protocols by a specialized CT physicist, testing protocols on dose phantoms, and monitoring of actual doses received by patients for each type of CT protocol.[75] Radiologists and technologists should be familiar with the dose indices displayed on the CT scanner console and should include the volumetric CT dose index (CTDI$_{vol}$) and the dose-length product (DLP). The CTDI$_{vol}$, represents the average dose delivered within the reconstructed section. The DLP is the CTDI$_{vol}$ multiplied by the scan length expressed in centimeters. DLP can be used to assess the overall radiation burden in a CT study. In response to the Arcata incident, the state of California passed a landmark dose reporting law in November 2010; it mandates the report of CTDI/DLP doses in all CT studies, and that overdoses be reported to the patient, the referring MD, and the state of California. FDA initiatives during 2010 and endorsed by MITA (the Medical Industry and Technology Alliance) will likely result in dose safeguards built into CT scanner designs, dose recording for all CT studies, and tools to track the imaging history of each patient.[77] Moreover, the American College of Radiology Dose Index Registry will monitor the cumulative dose information for each patient.

All CT protocols should respect the ALARA (As Low As Reasonably Achievable) principle. Expert consensus and over a decade of experience suggest that CTP studies should be performed at 80 kVp[60] and no more than 200 mAs. When using such parameters, the effective radiation dose associated with a single slab CTP study is approximately equal to that of an unenhanced head CT, roughly 2 to 3 mSv.[78,79] For comparison, the background radiation for a person living in Boston for a year is approximately 3 mSv. The authors' current shuttle mode CTP scanning protocol at Massachusetts General Hospital results in a radiation exposure, CTDI$_{vol}$, of 0.35 Gy, a value that is substantially below the FDA recommended maximum recommended radiation dose of 0.5 Gy. Note that this kVp setting is lower than that used for standard CT studies (120-140 kVp), and was selected primarily because the conspicuity of the iodine contrast agent is much greater at 80 kVp than at 140 kVp, resulting in improved CTP map image quality at a markedly lower radiation dose.[60]

CTP METHODOLOGY: GENERAL PRINCIPLES

Perfusion-weighted CT and MR, in distinction to those of MR and CTA which detect bulk vessel flow, are sensitive to capillary, tissue-level blood flow.[80] The generic term "cerebral perfusion" refers to tissue level blood flow in the brain. This flow can be described using a variety of parameters, which primarily include cerebral blood flow (CBF), cerebral blood volume (CBV), and mean transit time (MTT). Definitions of these parameters are as follows.

CBV is defined as the total volume of blood in a given unit volume of the brain. This definition includes blood in the tissues, as well as blood in the large capacitance vessels such as arteries, arterioles, capillaries, venules, and veins. CBV has units of milliliters of blood per 100 g of brain tissue (ml/100 g).

CBF is defined as the volume of blood moving through a given unit volume of brain per unit time. CBF has units of ml of blood per 100 g of brain tissue per minute (ml/100 g/min).

MTT is defined as the *average* of the transit time of blood through a given brain region. The transit time of blood through the brain parenchyma varies depending on the distance traveled between arterial inflow and venous outflow, and is measured in seconds. Mathematically, mean transit time is related to both CBV and CBF according to the central volume principle, which states that MTT = CBV/CBF.[81,82]

"Core" is typically operationally defined as brain likely to be irreversibly infarcted at presentation, despite early recanalization (and which indeed may be at increased risk for hemorrhagic transformation with early robust reperfusion), and "penumbra" as the functionally ischemic but potentially salvageable "at-risk" brain parenchyma[83]; the latter is to be distinguished from "benign oligemia" reflecting hypoperfused but functionally viable tissue. "Mismatch" is defined as the difference in volume and location between core and penumbra, although as currently measured in routine practice, "penumbra" often includes regions of benign oligemia as defined by other transit time measures such as TTP or Tmax (time to peak, or maximal, enhancement). A mismatch of greater than 20% is typically, arbitrarily, considered to represent a clinically significant penumbra for both research and clinical management; major trials using this definition include the Diffusion-weighted imaging Evaluation For Understanding Stroke Evolution (DEFUSE) trial and the Echoplanar Imaging Thrombolytic Evaluation Trial (EPITHET).[84,85]

CTP THEORY AND MODELING
Mathematical Models for CBF and MTT Calculation

The two major mathematical approaches involved in calculating CBF and MTT are the deconvolution and nondeconvolution-based methods (for a comprehensive review see Konstas and colleagues[79]). Deconvolution techniques are technically more demanding and involve more complicated and time-consuming processing, whereas nondeconvolution techniques are more straightforward, but depend on simplified assumptions regarding the underlying vascular architecture. As a result, the interpretation of studies based on nondeconvolution methods may be less reliable in some situations.[86–88]

Nondeconvolution-based models
Nondeconvolution methods are based on the application of Fick's principle of conservation of mass to a given Region of Interest (ROI) within the brain parenchyma. After a time-density curve (TDC) is derived for each pixel, CBF can be calculated based on the concept of conservation of flow using the maximal slope method.[89] The ease of the computation of this differential equation, however, is highly dependent on the assumptions made regarding inflow and outflow in the region. The no venous outflow assumption of nondeconvolution methods is clearly an oversimplification, and these methods yield relative, rather than absolute, perfusion measurements, making interpatient or interinstitutional comparison of results difficult. A recent study suggested that the maximal slope method yields the same results with deconvolution methods in terms of therapy decision making in acute stroke.[90]

Deconvolution-based models
When a contrast bolus arrives in an artery supplying a given region of the brain, it undergoes delay and dispersion. Deconvolution attempts to correct for this effect. Deconvolution of the arterial input function and tissue curves can be accomplished using a variety of techniques. Singular value decomposition (SVD) has yielded the most robust results from all the deconvolution methods used to calculate CBF[91] and has gained widespread acceptance. The creation of accurate quantitative maps of CBF, CBV, and MTT using deconvolution methods has been validated in several studies.[58,59,92–96] Once CBF and CBV are known, MTT can be calculated from the ratio of CBV and CBF, using the central volume theorem.[81,97]

Commercial software suppliers use different mathematical methods. In the past, some have incorporated the maximal slope method whereas others have typically used deconvolution techniques. Although deconvolution methods are theoretically superior to nondeconvolution methods, the full clinical implication of using these different models has yet to be established and standardized by the stroke imaging community.

The creation of accurate, quantitative maps of CBV, CBF, and MTT using the deconvolution method has been validated in several studies.[58,59,91–96,98] Specifically, validation has been accomplished by comparison with xenon,[96,99] positron emission tomography (PET),[100] and MRP[101–103] in humans, as well as with microspheres in animals.[58,59,94]

CTP POSTPROCESSING
General Principles

In urgent clinical cases, perfusion changes can often be observed immediately following scanning by direct visual inspection of the axial source images at the CT scanner console. Soft copy review at a workstation using "movie" or "cine" mode can reveal relative perfusion changes over time. It has been suggested that arterial-phase CTP source images (CTP-SI) closely correlate with CTP-CBF and venous-phase CTP-SI with CBV; hence a visual inspection of the CTP-SI can determine penumbra, core, and mismatch.[104] However, advanced postprocessing is required to appreciate subtle changes and to obtain quantification.

Axial source images acquired from a cine CT perfusion study are networked to a free-standing workstation for detailed analysis, including construction of CBF, CBV, and MTT maps. Postprocessing can be manual, semi-automated, or fully automated.

The computation of quantitative first-pass cine cerebral perfusion maps typically requires some combination of the following user inputs (**Fig. 3**).

- *Arterial Input Function (AIF)*: A small ROI is placed over the central portion of a large intracranial artery, preferably an artery orthogonal to the imaging plane to minimize "dilutional" effects from volume averaging. An attempt should be made to select an arterial ROI with maximal peak contrast intensity.
- *Venous Outflow Function (VOF)*: A small venous ROI with similar attributes is selected, most commonly at the superior

sagittal sinus. The purpose of the VOF is to serve as a reference for normalization of the quantitative CTP parameter values, relative to an averaged maximum intravascular contrast measurement. Because veins (particularly the posterior superior sagittal sinus) are typically larger than arteries, the venous TDC is not as subject to partial volume average as is the arterial TDC.
- *Baseline*: The baseline is the "flat" portion of the arterial time density curve, prior to the upward sloping of the curve caused by contrast enhancement. The baseline typically begins to increase after 4 to 6 seconds.
- *Post-Enhancement Cutoff*: This refers to the "tail" portion of the TDC, which may slope upwards toward a second peak value if recirculation effects are present. When such upward sloping at the "tail" of the TDC is noted, the data should be truncated to avoid including the recirculation of contrast. The perfusion analysis program will subsequently ignore data from slices beyond the cutoff.

It is worth noting that major variations in the input values described may not only result in perfusion maps of differing image quality, but potentially in perfusion maps with variation in their quantitative values for CBF, CBV, and MTT.[73,74,105] As previously noted, special care must be taken in choosing

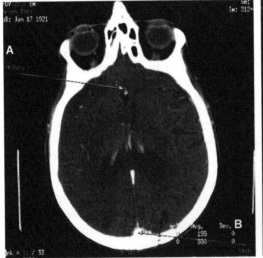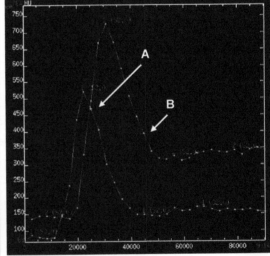

Fig. 3. CTP post processing. (*Left*) Appropriate ROI placement on an artery (anterior cerebral artery, running perpendicular to the plane of section to avoid volume averaging) and on a vein (the superior sagittal sinus, also running perpendicular to the plane of section and placed to avoid the inner table of the skull). (*Right*) the time-density curves (TDC) generated from this artery (A) and vein (B) show the arrival, peak, and passage of the contrast bolus over time. These TDCs serve as the arterial input function and the venous output for the subsequent deconvolution calculation.

an optimal VOF, because that VOF value may be used to normalize the quantitative parameters.

Although the precise choice of CTP scanning level is dependent on both the clinical question being asked and on other available imaging findings, an essential caveat in selecting a CTP slice is that the imaged level must contain a major intracranial artery. This caveat is necessary to assure the availability of an AIF, to be used for the computation of perfusion maps using the deconvolution software.

CORRECTION FOR DELAY AND DISPERSION OF THE AIF: WHY IT MATTERS

Calculation of CBF requires knowledge of the AIF, which in practice is estimated from a major artery, assuming that it represents the exact and only input to the tissue voxel of interest, with neither "delay" nor "dispersion." There are several clinical situations, however, where the AIF TDC will lag, and the tissue TDC will lag behind the AIF curve ("delay"). AIF delay can occur due to extracranial causes (atrial fibrillation, severe carotid stenosis, poor left ventricular ejection fraction) or intracranial causes (proximal intracranial obstructive thrombus with poor collaterals). Moreover, in such cases the contrast bolus forming the AIF can spread out over multiple pathways proximal to the tissue ROI ("dispersion").

Delay and dispersion do not have the same hemodynamic significance or clinical implications in acute versus chronic vascular conditions. In chronic vascular conditions such as an extracranial stenosis, delay and dispersion can result in grossly underestimated CBF and overestimated MTT,[106–108] most notably in regions of nonischemic hypoperfusion (benign oligemia). These changes indicate the hemodynamic significance of the stenosis, but can be misleading clinically in that inexperienced readers may interpret them as the hallmark of an acute ischemic stroke (especially when the distinction between true ischemia and benign oligemia is unclear). As a result, they need to be corrected for. In acute ischemic stroke, however, delay and dispersion are integral to the underlying pathophysiological hemodynamics, and therefore need not necessarily be corrected for so that appropriate clinical interpretation is possible.[109] In practice, many acute stroke patients have associated chronic carotid stenosis, and hence the "truth" lies somewhere in between. Although it can be argued that delay and dispersion should be corrected for so that MTT and CBF maps more accurately reflect physiologic ground truth, such correction can make MTT and CBF maps look too "normal." In any case, commercial

software packages with delay-sensitive deconvolution algorithms can overestimate penumbra (ie, MTT or CBF lesion volume) and consequently final infarct volume, whereas penumbra estimated with delay-insensitive software generally correlates better with final infarct volume.[87,88] Delay-sensitive methods might also overestimate CBV lesion size in some patients with concomitant intra- or extracranial severe hemodynamic delay (Fig. 4).[57]

Several approaches have been used to minimize the effects of delay and dispersion in deconvolution methods.[108,110–112] A detailed description is beyond the scope of this article. (For a review of the methods used for correcting for delay, see Konstas and colleagues.[78])

CLINICAL APPLICATIONS OF CTP

Current indications for performing CTP imaging of acute stroke include: (1) when DWI is unavailable, (2) when the (a) diagnosis, (b) type of stroke, or (c) extent of ischemia is uncertain based on the clinical examination and other imaging, or (3) for postaneurysmal subarachnoid hemorrhage (SAH) vasospasm risk assessment (given cumulative radiation dose issues, performing more than 2 or 3 serial CTPs per admission is ill advised). Although to date there is no high level of evidence to suggest that perfusion scanning has a direct role in the decision to administer IV or intra-arterial (IA) thrombolytic therapy, potential future indications for perfusion imaging in the first 9 to 12 hours after stroke onset include: (1) exclusion of patients most likely to hemorrhage and inclusion of patients most likely to benefit from thrombolysis, (2) extension of the time window beyond 4.5 hours for IV and 6 hours for anterior circulation IA thrombolysis, (3) triage to other available therapies, such as hypertension or hyperoxia administration, (4) disposition decisions regarding neurologic intensive care unit (NICU) admission or emergency department discharge, and (5) rational management of "wake-up" strokes, for which precise time of onset is unknown.[113]

The results of the 2008 ECASS expanded the 3-hour time window for intravenous thrombolysis and revealed that although safe and effective up to 4.5 hours after stroke onset, treatment benefits roughly half as many patients as those treated within 3 hours.[1–3] Hence, the ratio between the hemorrhagic risks of treatment versus the potential clinical benefits becomes a more critical consideration as the time window for therapy is expanded with newer intravenous and IA techniques. It is the mismatch between the size of the infarct core (proportional to hemorrhagic risk) and the size of the ischemic penumbra (proportional to potentially

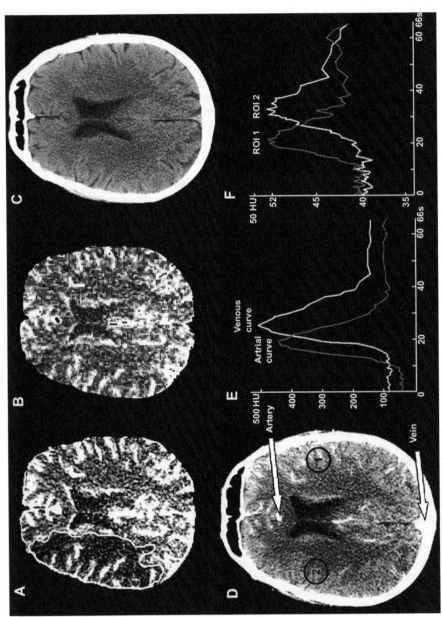

Fig. 4. Example of a false-positive CBV map "core" lesion, which was not present in maps that were postprocessed using newer generation, delay-insensitive software. Patient is a 61-year-old with atrial fibrillation, congestive heart failure, and an ICA thrombus that recanalized following intra-arterial thrombolysis. (A) Admission CT-CBV map processed using "first-generation" delay-sensitive software shows a large right MCA territory low blood volume lesion (white outline). (B) CT-CBV map appears normal when postprocessed using newer generation, delay-insensitive software. (C) Follow-up CT appears normal. (D) ROIs for the TDCs shown in E and F (arrow). (E) Normal arterial input and venous outflow curves. (F) Delay in tissue TDCs on the ischemic compared with the contralateral side, due to proximal vascular obstruction and flow through collateral pathways in the setting of atrial fibrillation and low cardiac output. (Reproduced from Schaefer PW, Mui K, Kamalian S, et al. Avoiding "pseudo-reversibility" of CT-CBV infarct core lesions in acute stroke patients after thrombolytic therapy. The need for algorithmically "delay-corrected" CT perfusion map postprocessing software. Stroke 2009;40(8):2875–8; with permission.)

salvageable tissue), as determined by CTP, that provides an imaging measure of this risk-to-benefit ratio. Evidence suggests that core/penumbra mismatch may persist for up to 24 hours in some patients.[114,115]

Despite this evidence, some large clinical trials that used mismatch as patient selection criteria, such as the Desmoteplase In Acute ischemic Stroke (DIAS)-2 trial, which used both CTP and MRP up to 9 hours after stroke onset, have failed to show a benefit of treatment.[116] The failure of DIAS-2 to demonstrate a role of mismatch imaging for patient selection in IV thrombolysis may have been, in part, related to technical differences between CTP and MRP, and the lack of standardization and validation of these methods (see later discussion).

IMAGE INTERPRETATION: INFARCT DETECTION WITH CTA-SI

Several groups have suggested that CTA source images, like DWI, may sensitively delineate tissue destined to infarct despite successful recanalization.[26,32,117] The superior accuracy of CTA-SI in identifying infarct "core" compared with unenhanced CT has been unequivocally established in multiple studies.[45,117–120] Theoretical modeling indicates that early generation CTA-SI—assuming an approximately steady state of contrast in the brain arteries and parenchyma during image acquisition—are predominantly blood volume weighted rather than blood flow weighted.[52–54,103] However, newer, faster MDCT CTA-SI protocols, such as those used in 64-slice scanners, with injection rates up to 7 mL/s and short preparation delay times of 15 to 20 seconds, change the temporal shape of the "time-density" infusion curve, eliminating a near-steady state during the timing of the CTA-SI acquisition. Hence, with the current generation of CTA protocols on faster state-of-the art MDCT scanners, the CTA-SI maps have become significantly more flow weighted.[55]

With early-generation CTA protocols, in the absence of early recanalization, CTA-SI typically defines minimal final infarct size and, hence, like DWI, can be used to identify "infarct core" in the acute setting (**Fig. 5**).[26] Coregistration and subtraction of the conventional, unenhanced CT brain images from the axial, postcontrast CTA-SI should result in quantitative blood volume maps of the entire brain.[15,53,54] CTA-SI subtraction maps, obtained by coregistration and subtraction of the unenhanced head CT from the CTA-SI, are particularly appealing for clinical use because, unlike quantitative first-pass CT perfusion maps, they provide whole brain coverage. A pilot study from the authors' group, on 22 consecutive patients with MCA stem occlusion who underwent IA thrombolysis following imaging, demonstrated that CTA-SI and CTA-SI subtraction maps improve infarct conspicuity over that of unenhanced CT in patients with hyperacute stroke. Concurrent review of unenhanced CT, CTA-SI, and CTA-SI subtraction images may be indicated for optimal CT assessment of hyperacute MCA stroke.

In another study, CTA-SI preceding DWI imaging was performed in 48 consecutive patients with clinically suspected stroke, presenting within 12 hours of symptom onset.[32] CTA-SI and DWI lesion volumes were independent predictors of final infarct volume, and overall sensitivity and specificity for parenchymal stroke detection were 76% and 90% for CTA-SI, and 100% and 100% for DWI, respectively.

Finally, it is again worth underscoring that with the newer, more flow-weighted CTA protocols, not every acute CTA-SI hypodense ischemic lesion is destined to infarct, and much of the CTA-SI hypodense lesion may reflect "at-risk" ischemic penumbra, or even benign oligemia.[121,122] In the presence of early complete recanalization, sometimes dramatic sparing of regions with reduced blood pool on CTA source images can occur (**Fig. 6**). Recent reports highlight some limitations of CTA-SI as an indicator of infarct "core." A recent study reported that in 28 patients with MCA territory stroke, scanned within 3 hours and recanalized following thrombolytic treatment, the ASPECTS on follow-up DWI strongly correlated with CTP-CBV ($r^2 = 0.91$) and only weakly correlated with CTA-SI ($r^2 = 0.42$), highlighting the flow-weighted nature of CTA-SI maps.[120]

CTP INTERPRETATION: ISCHEMIC PENUMBRA AND INFARCT CORE

CTP maps cannot and should not be interpreted in a vacuum. Accurate CTP image interpretation requires correlation with the clinical presentation, noncontrast CT (NCCT), CTA, CTA-SI, and CT-MTT/CBV/CBF data. A qualitative estimate of the presence and degree of ischemia is typically what is required for guiding clinical management, and this can be accomplished with a variety of vendor platforms, despite the current lack of complete standardization with regard to acquisition, post-processing, and interpretation algorithms.

That said, an important ultimate goal of advanced stroke imaging is to provide an assessment of ischemic tissue viability that transcends an arbitrary "clock time."[123–125] The original theory of penumbra stems from experimental studies in which two thresholds were characterized.[126] One

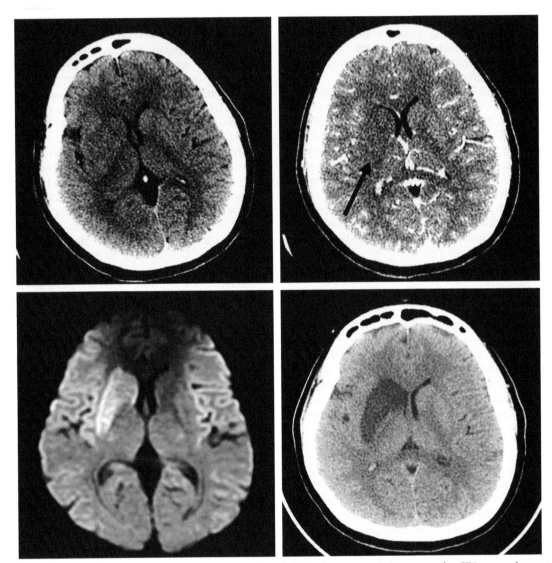

Fig. 5. An acute right MCA distribution basal ganglia infarction is more conspicuous on the CTA source images (CTA-SI, *top right, arrow*) than in the unenhanced CT (*top left*). Subsequent DWI (*bottom left*) and unenhanced CT (*bottom right*) confirm the presence of infarction seen on the CTA-SI. In the setting of a proximal large vessel occlusion without early robust recanalization, low blood pool and poor collateralization on CTA-SI are predictive of infarction. (*From* Schaefer PW, Mui K, Kamalian S, et al. Avoiding "pseudo-reversibility" of CT-CBV Infarct core lesions in acute stroke patients after thrombolytic therapy. The need for algorithmically "delay-corrected" CT perfusion map postprocessing software. Stroke 2009;40(8):2875–8; with permission.)

threshold identified a CBF value below which there was cessation of cortical function, without increase in extracellular potassium or reduction in pH. A second, lower threshold identified a CBF value below which there was disruption of cellular integrity. With the advent of advanced neuroimaging and modern stroke therapy, a more clinically relevant "operationally defined penumbra," which identifies hypoperfused but potentially salvageable tissue, has gained acceptance.[123,127–129]

Ischemic Penumbra

Cine single-slab CT perfusion imaging, which can provide quantitative maps of CBF, CBV, and MTT, has the potential to describe regions of "ischemic penumbra," ischemic but still viable tissue. In the simplest terms, this "operationally defined penumbra" has been described in the early literature as the region of CBF or MTT/CBV mismatch on CTP maps (a *specific, threshold dependent,*

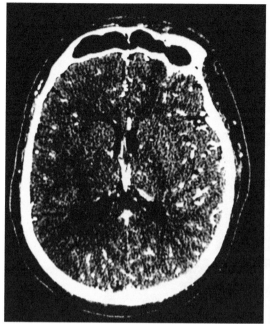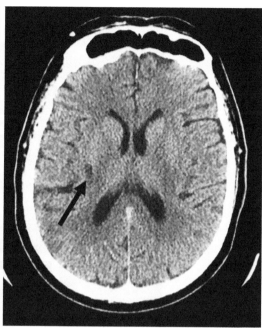

Fig. 6. "Reversal" of CTA-SI lesion in a 57-year-old man with a right M1 thrombus who had complete recanalization 120 minutes following IA thrombolysis. Despite a large right MCA territory lesion on CTA-SI (*left*), there is only a small deep gray lenticular infarct on the postlysis, follow-up unenhanced CT (*right, arrow*). Sparing of the ischemic territory in this case is consistent with the concept that the CTA-SI lesions—especially with newer, faster multidetector row CT scanners—are flow weighted, rather than volume weighted. (*From* Sharma M, Fox AJ, Symons S, et al. CT angiographic source images: flow- or volume-weighted? AJNR Am J Neuroradiol 2011;32:359–64; with permission.)

but not necessarily ideally *sensitive* definition) in which the CBV lesion reflects the infarct "core" and the CBF or MTT lesion reflects the surrounding region of hypoperfused "penumbral" tissue (which typically consists of both benign oligemia and true ischemia, depending on the precise degree of blood flow reduction). Many studies that have investigated the role of CTP in acute stroke triage have assumed predefined threshold values for "core" and "penumbra" based on human and animal studies from the PET, MR, single-photon emission CT (SPECT), or xenon literature, and determined the accuracy of these in predicting outcome.[62]

With regard to these operationally defined thresholds for "core" and "penumbra," however, there is not yet standardization or validation of the quantitative perfusion parameter map values across different vendor platforms for acquisition and postprocessing, or even across different platforms from the same vendor. Some investigators, therefore, favor the use of relative (rather than absolute) CTP values for determining ischemic thresholds for core and penumbra, given this potential for variability in the absolute quantification of CTP map parameters, and the dependence

of these values on an appropriate but often arbitrary VOF scaling factor.

Indeed, in a pilot study of CTP thresholds for infarction, Schaefer and colleagues found that tissue with a CT-CBF reduction of less than 50% (compared with the corresponding, contralateral, uninvolved hemisphere) had a high probability of survival despite the presence or absence of reperfusion, whereas ischemic tissue with greater than 66% reduction from baseline CT-CBF values had a high probability of infarction. No region with absolute CBV of less than 2.2 mL/100 g survived.[56,83] The latter is in close agreement with the CT-CBV threshold of 2.0 mL/100 g selected by Wintermark and colleagues to define core.[62,130]

CT-CBF or MTT/CBV mismatch correlates significantly with lesion enlargement. Untreated or unsuccessfully treated patients with large CBF or MTT/CBV mismatch exhibit substantial lesion growth on follow-up (Fig. 7), whereas those patients without significant mismatch—or those with early, complete recanalization—do not exhibit lesion progression. CTP-defined mismatch might therefore serve as a marker of salvageable tissue, and thus prove useful in patient triage for thrombolysis.[131] This result also clearly has

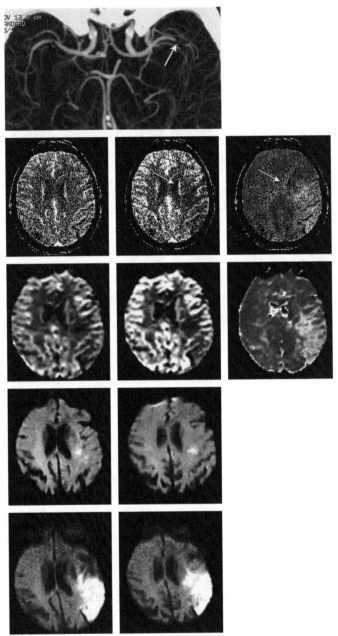

Fig. 7. A 65-year-old man, improving clinically at 5 hours postictus from a left MCA bifurcation embolus, was monitored in the Neurology intensive care unit for management of his labile blood pressure. His 24-hour follow-up DWI showed a small infarction. However, 24 hours after cessation of hypertensive therapy and resumption of his preadmission antihypertensive medications, there was substantial infarct growth into the CT/MR perfusion defined penumbral region. From top: (*row 1*) admission CTA at 4.5 hours shows left MCA bifurcation occlusion (*arrow*); (*row 2*) concurrent CT-CBV, -CBF, and -MTT show normal blood volume without evidence of core infarction, but a moderate flow deficit in the left M2 superior division distribution suggesting benign oligemia rather than true ischemic penumbra (*arrow*); (*row 3*) MR perfusion scan (CBV, CBF, MTT) at 5.25 hours shows development of a possible small left corona radiata infarct on the CBV maps, with similar findings to the CTP on the flow maps; (*row 4*) DWI at 24 hours confirms small corona radiata infarct with sparing of the region with benign oligemia; and (*row 5*) follow-up DWI at 48 hours shows expansion of the infarction into the penumbral region, which—with a possible drop in blood pressure—likely became ischemic.

implications for the utility of a CTP-based model for predicting outcome in patients without robust recanalization. In an earlier pilot study of CTP imaging, ultimate infarct size was most strongly correlated with CT-CBF lesion size in 14 embolic stroke patients without robust recanalization,[132] again demonstrating the importance of considering the mismatch region as tissue at risk for infarction.

Although multiple studies have been published to determine the CTP parameter maps and corresponding threshold values that optimally define infarct core and correlate with DWI, systematic technical differences in both acquisition and postprocessing algorithms between different platforms limit their generalizability and reproducibility, and therefore operators should be familiar with their specific hardware and software. Validation and standardization of CTP methodology will also translate into a stricter definition of "penumbra," hopefully resulting in more accurate selection of patients likely to benefit from treatment. Salvageable "penumbra" is currently overestimated by including brain tissue with "benign oligemia," that is, areas that demonstrate delay in contrast arrival time without sufficient hypoperfusion to result in functional ischemia.[84,133–135] Inclusion of "benign oligemia" in the estimate of "penumbra" may result in selection of patients for treatment who do not have true ischemic "tissue at risk," and are therefore not likely to benefit from recanalization therapy. A particular issue arising from DIAS-2, for example, is the use of the "eyeball technique" in penumbral selection.[136] Absence of standardization and validation of the specific perfusion thresholds for core and penumbra may have resulted in the inclusion of "benign oligemia" in describing the degree of mismatch for some patients; this may also have been exacerbated by the potential variability in quantification across different acquisition and postprocessing platforms.

There is limited literature addressing perfusion thresholds for patients undergoing IA recanalization procedures.[137] One study that showed mean relative CT-CBF (rCBF) thresholds (fractional reduction vs corresponding contralateral uninvolved brain) of 0.19 for core, 0.34 for "at-risk" penumbra, and 0.46 for benign oligemia,[56] is in agreement with the results of a SPECT study in patients with complete recanalization following IA thrombolysis. Regions with prethrombolysis SPECT CBF greater than 55% of normal cerebellar flow never infarcted (benign oligemia), even with delayed (>6 hours) reperfusion.[138] Ischemic tissue with CBF greater than 35% of cerebellar flow was salvageable if recanalization was achieved within 5 hours of stroke onset. Results for mean CT-rCBF thresholds for core and at-risk penumbra

are also consistent with SPECT and MR studies performed in patients who received other stroke treatments.[139–142] Similarly, a recent CTP study of 59 acute stroke patients suggested a CBF threshold of greater than 50% reduction as an indication for recanalization therapy.[143]

Detection of Infarct Core with CTP: Optimal Correlation with DWI?

Most published studies, most notably those using first-generation 45-second CTP acquisitions, have suggested that admission CT-CBV lesion size is highly correlated with infarct core as defined either by DWI or by final infarct size (in patients with early complete recanalization).[15,26,56,83,130] Specifically, studies using these early-generation 45-second duration acquisition protocols and delay-sensitive postprocessing algorithms have reported that no tissue with absolute admission CBV less than 2.2 mL/100 g survived,[56,83] in close agreement with the CBV threshold of 2.0 mL/100 g selected by Wintermark and colleagues to define core.[62,130] A major technical consideration with such studies, however, is that CT-CBV lesion size could be overestimated if there is truncation of the contrast TDCs, especially in cases of marked hemodynamic derangement.[57] In addition, physiologic phenomena such as misery perfusion and luxury perfusion (ie, nonnutritional flow into maximally vasodilated, devitalized tissue) could result in reduced CBF in irreversibly infarcted brain with elevated CBV, and hence greater CBV than CBF variability in critically ischemic regions.[144]

A more recent study comparing various CTP parameter maps to a DWI reference standard (using a longer, more current second-generation 66-second biphasic cine acquisition with both delay-corrected and standard postprocessing software from different vendors[86,145] in 48 acute stroke patients) has suggested that absolute and relative (normalized) thresholded CBF maps may provide a nominally more accurate estimate of infarct core than do CBV maps, owing to less technical and physiologic variability. CBF thresholds varied with the postprocessing software and ranged from 16%, to 32% of the contralateral, uninvolved tissue. These results are in good agreement with several MR imaging studies that reported CBF thresholds of 12% to 26%.[139,142,146]

IMAGING PREDICTORS OF CLINICAL OUTCOME

Predicting outcome is perilous. The penumbra is dynamic, and several factors influence its fate, including time-post ictus, residual and collateral blood flow, admission glucose, temperature, hematocrit, systolic blood pressure, and treatment, including hyperoxia.[147] As already mentioned, CTA/CTP has the potential to serve as a surrogate marker of stroke severity, likely exceeding the NIHSS score or ASPECTS as a predictor of outcome.[27–35]

Infarct Core is Crucial

As noted, measuring the penumbra is technically challenging. Flow thresholds for various states of tissue perfusion vary considerably among studies and techniques applied.[148] Despite this, several consistent messages emerge from a review of the literature regarding imaging outcome prediction in acute ischemic stroke. The most important of these messages is that "core" is crucial. Multiple studies, examining heterogeneous cohorts of patients receiving varied treatments, consistently find that ultimate clinical outcome is strongly correlated with admission "core" lesion volume—be it measured by DWI, CTP-CBV/CBF, xenon CT-CBF, CTA-SI, or unenhanced CT.[149–154]

In one noteworthy study, outcome results were stratified by the degree of recanalization at 24 hours. This study revealed "that 2 factors mainly influenced clinical outcome: (1) recanalization ($P = .0001$) and (2) day-0 DWI lesion volume ($P = .03$)."[155] In a different study of CTP in patients with MCA stem occlusion, those with admission whole brain CT perfusion lesions volumes greater than 100 mL (equal to approximately one-third the volume of the MCA territory) had poor clinical outcome, regardless of recanalization status. Moreover, in those patients from the same cohort who had early complete MCA recanalization, final infarct volume was closely approximated by the size of the admission whole brain CTA source image lesion.[26]

More recent studies have further refined the impact of "core" on clinical outcome. Two studies have demonstrated that in anterior circulation strokes, an acute DWI lesion volume greater than 70 mL has a high specificity for poor outcomes with or without therapy,[156,157] lowering the earlier estimate that 100 mL is a specific core volume cutoff for poor outcome. In acute stroke patients treated with IA thrombolysis between 3 and 6 hours of onset, core size was the best predictor of clinical outcome at 3 months.[158] In particular, any increment of 1 SD (13.2 mL) of the infarct core size increased the modified Rankin Scale (mRS) score by about 1 point, whereas any increment of 1 SD (5.8 points) of admission NIHSS score raised the mRS by approximately 0.5 points.

The interpretation of CTP in the setting of acute stroke is summarized in **Table 1**.

Risk of Hemorrhage

The degree of early CBF reduction in acute stroke also helps predict hemorrhagic risk in patients receiving thrombolytic therapy. Thrombolysis-related intracranial hemorrhage has been classified into 2 types[159]: hemorrhagic infarct (HI), usually without clinical consequence, and parenchymal hemorrhage (PH), which commonly causes clinical deterioration. The latter has been further subclassified into PH1, representing blood clots in 30% or less of the infarcted area with slight space-occupying effect and PH2, representing blood clots in more than 30% of the infarcted area with substantial space-occupying effect.[160] Preliminary results have suggested that severe hypoattenuation, relative to normal tissue on whole brain CTA source images, may also identify ischemic regions more likely to bleed following IA thrombolysis.[161] Other studies have noted that the extent of hypoattenuation on initial head CT and the use of tPA are associated with a higher risk of developing PH-type symptomatic intracranial hemorrhage, highlighting the effect of infarct "core" size on the risk of hemorrhage.[162–164]

Indeed, multiple studies have suggested that severely ischemic regions with early reperfusion are at the highest risk for hemorrhagic transformation.[151,165] In a SPECT study of 30 patients who had complete recanalization within 12 hours of stoke onset, those with less than 35% of normal

Table 1
CTP interpretation guidelines for intra-arterial (IA) thrombolysis triage if MR-DWI is not available

CTP Guidelines for IA Triage if DWI Not Available: "Mismatch"	
Large core, any size transit time map	Poor outcome likely if core >70 mL No treatment
Moderate core, larger transit time map	Possible treatment based on time post ictus, deficit Consider treatment if core <70 mL, time <6–9 h
Small core, larger transit time map	Typically a good candidate for treatment if core <70 mL Consider no treatment if time post ictus >9 h

cerebellar flow at infarct core were at significantly higher risk for hemorrhage.[138] This study did not separate patients into HI- and PH-type bleeds and symptomatic versus asymptomatic hemorrhage. A more recent study of carotid terminus/MCA acute stroke patients receiving IA-lysis and assessed with Xe-CTP reported a threshold of 13 mL/100 g per minute for mean ipsilateral MCA CBF, below which the risk for PH1 and PH2 hemorrhages was too high for IA-lysis to be administered.[166]

An early small study suggested that the presence of punctate microhemorrhage is correlated with the risk of hemorrhagic transformation; these small foci of hemorrhage are seen on gradient echo (susceptibility-weighted) MR sequences and are not visible on unenhanced CT.[167,168] Microbleeds detected on T2*-weighted MR imaging, however, have more recently been shown in large trials not to be a contraindication to thrombolysis.[67] Of note, a recent study compared PH prediction by "very low CBV" (VLCBV) and DWI in patients receiving IV-tPA 3 to 6 hours after symptom onset, using data from the EPITHET study.[169] The median volume of VLCBV was significantly higher in cases with PH. VLCBV predicted PH better than DWI lesion volume and thresholded apparent diffusion coefficient (ADC) lesion volume in receiver operating characteristic (ROC) curve analysis and logistic regression. Prediction was even better in patients with recanalization. These results suggest that addition of VLCBV to prethrombolysis decision making may reduce the incidence of hemorrhagic transformation.

Reperfusion as Predictor of Follow-Up Infarct Volume

Revascularization therapies in acute ischemic stroke aim to rescue the ischemic penumbra by restoring the patency of the occluded artery (recanalization) and the downstream capillary blood flow (reperfusion). Although reperfusion and recanalization have been used interchangeably, the terms describe two distinct concepts.[170] Earlier studies supported the benefit of early recanalization in predicting smaller infarct volumes and clinical outcomes.[3,171,172] However, more recent studies have shown that recanalization does not always lead to reperfusion.[173,174] One explanation is that the main clot may be fragmented and occlude smaller, downstream arterial branches, not allowing capillary reperfusion.[175] A second, distinct, but complementary reason is the "no-reflow" phenomenon: even if recanalization is achieved, tissue edema may not allow blood flow.[176,177]

Reperfusion and recanalization were assessed as markers of clinical outcome after IV thrombolysis in the EPITHET study patients.[85] Reperfusion was defined as greater than 90% reduction in MR-PWI lesion volume and recanalization as improvement of MR Thrombolysis In Myocardial Infarction (TIMI) grading by 2 points or more from baseline to day 3 to 5. Reperfusion was associated with improved clinical outcome independent of whether recanalization occurred. In contrast, recanalization was not associated with clinical outcome when reperfusion was included as a covariate in regression analysis, suggesting that the previously reported impact of recanalization on clinical outcomes was attributable to reperfusion. A more recent study by Soares and colleagues[178] in 22 patients in whom CTP was the imaging modality used reported similar results, using follow-up infarct volume as the outcome measure. Reperfusion (using an MTT reperfusion index >75%) was a more accurate predictor of follow-up infarct volume than was recanalization. These 2 studies emphasize the conceptual distinction between recanalization and reperfusion by demonstrating their difference in predictive values; reperfusion is an outcome predictor, whereas recanalization, in the absence of reperfusion, is not.

SUMMARY

As new treatments are developed for stroke, the potential clinical applications of CTP imaging in the diagnosis, triage, and therapeutic monitoring of these diseases are certain to increase.

Validation and standardization of CTP methodology will be crucial for the widespread acceptance of advanced imaging in patient selection for novel stroke therapies. Expert consensus regarding standardization of CTP image acquisition has already been reached at the "Advanced Neuroimaging for Acute Stroke Treatment" meeting held in the fall of 2007 in Washington, DC.[40,41] Both this group and the Acute Stroke Imaging STandardization group (ASIST) in Japan (http://plaza.umin.ac.jp/index-e.htm), however, have emphasized the continued need for definitive optimization and validation of commercially available CTP acquisition techniques, postprocessing software, and CTP map image interpretation. Once validation is achieved, standardization will minimize interobserver and interhospital variability in selecting patients for novel therapies, including thrombolysis beyond the currently accepted time windows. Level I evidence of improvement in patient outcome using advanced perfusion imaging is, of course, the ultimate goal.

REFERENCES

1. Hacke W, Kaste M, Bluhmki E, et al. Thrombolysis with alteplase 3 to 4.5 hours after acute ischemic stroke. N Engl J Med 2008;359:1317–29.

2. Saver JL, Gornbein J, Grotta J, et al. Number needed to treat to benefit and to harm for intravenous tissue plasminogen activator therapy in the 3- to 4.5-hour window: joint outcome table analysis of the ECASS 3 trial. Stroke 2009;40:2433–7.

3. Ninds G. Tissue plasminogen activator for acute ischemic stroke. N Engl J Med 1995;333:1581–7.

4. Furlan A, Higashida R, Wechsler L, et al. Intra-arterial prourokinase for acute ischemic stroke. JAMA 1999;282:2003–11.

5. Marler JR, Tilley BC, Lu M, et al. Early stroke treatment associated with better outcome: the NINDS rt-PA stroke study. Neurology 2000;55:1649–55.

6. del Zoppo GJ, Poeck K, Pessin MS, et al. Recombinant tissue plasminogen activator in acute thrombotic and embolic stroke. Ann Neurol 1992;32:78–86.

7. Hacke W, Kaste M, Fieschi C, et al. Intravenous thrombolysis with recombinant tissue plasminogen activator for acute hemispheric stroke. The European Cooperative Acute Stroke Study (ECASS). JAMA 1995;274:1017–25.

8. Gobin YP, Starkman S, Duckwiler GR, et al. MERCI 1: a phase 1 study of mechanical embolus removal in cerebral ischemia. Stroke 2004;35:2848–54.

9. Katz JM, Gobin YP. Merci retriever in acute stroke treatment. Expert Rev Med Devices 2006;3:273–80.

10. Smith WS, Sung G, Starkman S, et al. Safety and efficacy of mechanical embolectomy in acute ischemic stroke: results of the MERCI trial. Stroke 2005;36:1432–8.

11. Phan TG, Donnan GA, Koga M, et al. The ASPECTS template is weighted in favor of the striatocapsular region. Neuroimage 2006;31:477–81.

12. Phan TG, Donnan GA, Koga M, et al. Assessment of suitability of thrombolysis in middle cerebral artery infarction: a proof of concept study of a stereologically-based technique. Cerebrovasc Dis 2007;24:321–7.

13. Fang MC, Cutler DM, Rosen AB. Trends in thrombolytic use for ischemic stroke in the United States. J Hosp Med 2010;5:406–9.

14. Lev MH, Farkas J, Rodriguez VR, et al. CT angiography in the rapid triage of patients with hyperacute stroke to intraarterial thrombolysis: accuracy in the detection of large vessel thrombus. J Comput Assist Tomogr 2001;25:520–8.

15. Lev MH, Gonzalez RG. CT angiography and CT perfusion imaging. In: Toga AW, Mazziotta JC, editors. Brain mapping: the methods. 2nd edition. San Diego (CA): Academic Press; 2002. p. 427–84.

16. Wildermuth S, Knauth M, Brandt T, et al. Role of CT angiography in patient selection for thrombolytic therapy in acute hemispheric stroke. Stroke 1998;29:935–8.

17. Knauth M, vonKummer R, Jansen O, et al. Potential of CT angiography in acute ischemic stroke [see comments]. AJNR Am J Neuroradiol 1997;18:1001–10.

18. Lev MH, Nichols SJ. Computed tomographic angiography and computed tomographic perfusion imaging of hyperacute stroke. Top Magn Reson Imaging 2000;11:273–87.

19. Schellinger PD, Fiebach JB, Hacke W. Imaging-based decision making in thrombolytic therapy for ischemic stroke: present status. Stroke 2003;34:575–83.

20. Warach S. Tissue viability thresholds in acute stroke: the 4-factor model. Stroke 2001;32:2460–1.

21. Fox SH, Tanenbaum LN, Ackelsberg S, et al. Future directions in CT technology. Neuroimaging Clin N Am 1998;8:497–513.

22. Smith WS, Roberts HC, Chuang NA, et al. Safety and feasibility of a CT protocol for acute stroke: combined CT, CT angiography, and CT perfusion imaging in 53 consecutive patients. AJNR Am J Neuroradiol 2003;24:688–90.

23. Gleason S, Furie KL, Lev MH, et al. Potential influence of acute CT on inpatient costs in patients with ischemic stroke. Acad Radiol 2001;8:955–64.

24. Lee KH, Lee SJ, Cho SJ, et al. Usefulness of triphasic perfusion computed tomography for intravenous thrombolysis with tissue-type plasminogen activator in acute ischemic stroke. Arch Neurol 2000;57:1000–8.

25. Lee KH, Cho SJ, Byun HS, et al. Triphasic perfusion computed tomography in acute middle cerebral artery stroke: a correlation with angiographic findings. Arch Neurol 2000;57:990–9.

26. Lev MH, Segal AZ, Farkas J, et al. Utility of perfusion-weighted CT imaging in acute middle cerebral artery stroke treated with intra-arterial thrombolysis: prediction of final infarct volume and clinical outcome. Stroke 2001;32:2021–8.

27. Albers GW. Expanding the window for thrombolytic therapy in acute stroke. The potential role of acute MRI for patient selection. Stroke 1999;30:2230–7.

28. Barber PA, Demchuk AM, Zhang J, et al. Validity and reliability of a quantitative computed tomography score in predicting outcome of hyperacute stroke before thrombolytic therapy. ASPECTS Study Group. Alberta Stroke Programme Early CT Score. Lancet 2000;355:1670–4.

29. Broderick JP, Lu M, Kothari R, et al. Finding the most powerful measures of the effectiveness of tissue plasminogen activator in the NINDS tPA stroke trial. Stroke 2000;31:2335–41.

30. Schellinger PD, Jansen O, Fiebach JB, et al. Monitoring intravenous recombinant tissue plasminogen activator thrombolysis for acute ischemic stroke with diffusion and perfusion MRI. Stroke 2000;31: 1318–28.

31. Tong D, Yenari M, Albers G, et al. Correlation of perfusion- and diffusion weighted MRI with NIHSS Score in acute (<6.5 hour) ischemic stroke. Stroke 1998;29:2673.

32. Berzin T, Lev M, Goodman D, et al. CT perfusion imaging versus MR diffusion weighted imaging: prediction of final infarct size in hyperacute stroke [abstract]. Stroke 2001;32:317.

33. Warach S. New imaging strategies for patient selection for thrombolytic and neuroprotective therapies. Neurology 2001;57:S48–52.

34. von Kummer R, Holle R, Grzyska U, et al. Interobserver agreement in assessing early CT signs of middle cerebral artery infarction. AJNR Am J Neuroradiol 1996;17:1743–8.

35. Grotta JC, Chiu D, Lu M, et al. Agreement and variability in the interpretation of early CT changes in stroke patients qualifying for intravenous rtPA therapy [see comments]. Stroke 1999;30:1528–33.

36. Koroshetz WJ, Gonzales RG. Imaging stroke in progress: magnetic resonance advances but computed tomography is poised for counterattack. Ann Neurol 1999;46:556–8.

37. Koroshetz WJ, Lev MH. Contrast computed tomography scan in acute stroke: "you can't always get what you want but you get what you need". Ann Neurol 2002;51:415–6.

38. Lev MH. CT versus MR for acute stroke imaging: is the "obvious" choice necessarily the correct one? AJNR Am J Neuroradiol 2003;24:1930–1.

39. Lev MH, Koroshetz WJ, Schwamm LH, et al. CT or MRI for imaging patients with acute stroke: visualization of "Tissue at Risk"? Stroke 2002;33:2736–7.

40. Wintermark M, Albers GW, Alexandrov AV, et al. Acute stroke imaging research roadmap. Stroke 2008;39:1621–8.

41. Wintermark M, Albers GW, Alexandrov AV, et al. Acute stroke imaging research roadmap. AJNR Am J Neuroradiol 2008;29:e23–30.

42. von Kummer R, Allen KL, Holle R, et al. Acute stroke: usefulness of early CT findings before thrombolytic therapy [see comments]. Radiology 1997;205:327–33.

43. von Kummer R. Early major ischemic changes on computed tomography should preclude use of tissue plasminogen activator. Stroke 2003;34: 820–1.

44. Madden KP, Karanjia PN, Adams HP Jr, et al. Accuracy of initial stroke subtype diagnosis in the TOAST study. Trial of ORG 10172 in acute stroke treatment. Neurology 1995;45:1975–9.

45. Ezzeddine MA, Lev MH, McDonald CT, et al. CT angiography with whole brain perfused blood volume imaging: added clinical value in the assessment of acute stroke. Stroke 2002;33:959–66.

46. Dubey N, Bakshi R, Wasay M, et al. Early computed tomography hypodensity predicts hemorrhage after intravenous tissue plasminogen activator in acute ischemic stroke. J Neuroimaging 2001;11:184–8.

47. Wardlaw J, Dorman P, Lewis S, et al. Can stroke physicians and neuroradiologists identify signs of early cerebral infarction on CT? J Neurol Neurosurg Psychiatry 1999;67:651–3.

48. Fiorelli M, von Kummer R. Early ischemic changes on computed tomography in patients with acute stroke. JAMA 2002;287:2361–2 [author reply: 2362].

49. Mullins ME, Lev MH, Schellingerhout D, et al. Influence of availability of clinical history on detection of early stroke using unenhanced CT and diffusion-weighted MR imaging. AJR Am J Roentgenol 2002;179:223–8.

50. Lev M, Farkas J, Gemmete J, et al. Acute stroke: improved nonenhanced CT detection—benefits of soft-copy interpretation by using variable window width and center level settings. Radiology 1999; 213:150–5.

51. Fiorelli M, Toni D, Bastianello S, et al. Computed tomography findings in the first few hours of ischemic stroke: implications for the clinician. J Neurol Sci 2000;173:10–7.

52. Axel L. Cerebral blood flow determination by rapid-sequence computed tomography. Radiology 1980; 137:679–86.

53. Hunter GJ, Hamberg LM, Ponzo JA, et al. Assessment of cerebral perfusion and arterial anatomy in hyperacute stroke with three-dimensional functional CT: early clinical results. AJNR Am J Neuroradiol 1998;19:29–37.

54. Hamberg LM, Hunter GJ, Kierstead D, et al. Measurement of cerebral blood volume with subtraction three-dimensional functional CT. AJNR Am J Neuroradiol 1996;17:1861–9.

55. Sharma M, Fox AJ, Symons S, et al. CT angiographic source images: flow- or volume-weighted? AJNR Am J Neuroradiol 2010. [Epub ahead of print].

56. Schaefer PW, Roccatagliata L, Ledezma C, et al. First-pass quantitative CT perfusion identifies thresholds for salvageable penumbra in acute stroke patients treated with intra-arterial therapy [see comment]. AJNR Am J Neuroradiol 2006;27: 20–5.

57. Schaefer PW, Mui K, Kamalian S, et al. Avoiding "pseudo-reversibility" of CT-CBV infarct core lesions in acute stroke patients after thrombolytic therapy. The need for algorithmically "delay-corrected" CT perfusion map postprocessing software. Stroke 2009;40(8):2875–8.

58. Cenic A, Nabavi DG, Craen RA, et al. Dynamic CT measurement of cerebral blood flow: a validation study. AJNR Am J Neuroradiol 1999;20:63–73.

59. Nabavi DG, Cenic A, Craen RA, et al. CT assessment of cerebral perfusion: experimental validation and initial clinical experience. Radiology 1999;213: 141–9.

60. Wintermark M, Maeder P, Verdun FR, et al. Using 80 kVp versus 120 kVp in perfusion CT measurement of regional cerebral blood flow. AJNR Am J Neuroradiol 2000;21:1881–4.

61. Roberts HC, Roberts TP, Smith WS, et al. Multisection dynamic CT perfusion for acute cerebral ischemia: the "toggling-table" technique. AJNR Am J Neuroradiol 2001;22:1077–80.

62. Wintermark M, Reichhart M, Thiran JP, et al. Prognostic accuracy of cerebral blood flow measurement by perfusion computed tomography, at the time of emergency room admission, in acute stroke patients. Ann Neurol 2002;51:417–32.

63. Coutts SB, Simon JE, Tomanek AI, et al. Reliability of assessing percentage of diffusion-perfusion mismatch. Stroke 2003;34:1681–3.

64. Roccatagliata L, Lev MH, Mehta N, et al. Estimating the size of ischemic regions on CT perfusion maps in acute stroke: is freehand visual segmentation sufficient? In: Proceedings of the 89th Scientific Assembly and Annual Meeting of the Radiological Society of North America. Chicago (IL); 2003. p. 1292.

65. Siebert E, Bohner G, Dewey M, et al. 320-slice CT neuroimaging: initial clinical experience and image quality evaluation. Br J Radiol 2009;82:561–70.

66. Klingebiel R, Siebert E, Diekmann S, et al. 4-D Imaging in cerebrovascular disorders by using 320-slice CT: feasibility and preliminary clinical experience. Acad Radiol 2009;16:123–9.

67. Fiehler J, Albers GW, Boulanger JM, et al. Bleeding Risk Analysis in Stroke Imaging before thromboLysis (BRASIL): pooled analysis of T2*-weighted magnetic resonance imaging data from 570 patients. Stroke 2007;38:2738–44.

68. Kendell B, Pullicono P. Intravascular contrast injection in ischemic lesions, II. Effect on prognosis. Neuroradiology 1980;19:241–3.

69. Doerfler A, Engelhorn T, von Kommer R, et al. Are iodinated contrast agents detrimental in acute cerebral ischemia? An experimental study in rats. Radiology 1998;206:211–7.

70. Palomaki H, Muuronen A, Raininko R, et al. Administration of nonionic iodinated contrast medium does not influence the outcome of patients with ischemic brain infarction. Cerebrovasc Dis 2003; 15:45–50.

71. Fiorella D, Heiserman J, Prenger E, et al. Assessment of the reproducibility of postprocessing dynamic CT perfusion data. AJNR Am J Neuroradiol 2004;25:97–107.

72. Kealey SM, Loving VA, Delong DM, et al. User-defined vascular input function curves: influence on mean perfusion parameter values and signal-to-noise ratio. Radiology 2004;231:587–93.

73. Sanelli PC, Lev MH, Eastwood JD, et al. The effect of varying user-selected input parameters on quantitative values in CT perfusion maps. Acad Radiol 2004;11(10):1085–92.

74. Soares BP, Dankbaar JW, Bredno J, et al. Automated versus manual post-processing of perfusion-CT data in patients with acute cerebral ischemia: influence on interobserver variability. Neuroradiology 2009;51:445–51.

75. Wintermark M, Lev MH. FDA investigates the safety of brain perfusion CT. AJNR Am J Neuroradiol 2010;31:2–3.

76. Bogdanovich W. Radiation overdoses point up dangers of CT scans. New York Times. October 15, 2009.

77. Smith-Bindman R. Is computed tomography safe? N Engl J Med 2010;363:1–4.

78. Konstas AA, Goldmakher GV, Lee TY, et al. Theoretic basis and technical implementations of CT perfusion in acute ischemic stroke, part 2: technical implementations. AJNR Am J Neuroradiol 2009;30:885–92.

79. Konstas AA, Goldmakher GV, Lee TY, et al. Theoretic basis and technical implementations of CT perfusion in acute ischemic stroke, part 1: theoretic basis. AJNR Am J Neuroradiol 2009;30:662–8.

80. Villringer A, Rosen BR, Belliveau JW, et al. Dynamic imaging with lanthanide chelates in normal brain: contrast due to magnetic susceptibility effects. Magn Reson Med 1988;6:164–74.

81. Meier P, Zieler K. On the theory of the indicator-dilution method for measurement of blood flow and volume. J Appl Physiol 1954;6:731–44.

82. Roberts G, Larson K. The interpretation of mean transit time measurements for multi-phase tissue systems. J Theor Biol 1973;39:447–75.

83. Shetty SK, Lev MH. CT perfusion in acute stroke. Neuroimaging Clin N Am 2005;15:481–501, ix.

84. Olivot JM, Mlynash M, Thijs VN, et al. Optimal Tmax threshold for predicting penumbral tissue in acute stroke. Stroke 2009;40:469–75.

85. De Silva DA, Fink JN, Christensen S, et al. Assessing reperfusion and recanalization as markers of clinical outcomes after intravenous thrombolysis in the echoplanar imaging thrombolytic evaluation trial (EPITHET). Stroke 2009;40:2872–4.

86. Konstas AA, Lev MH. CT perfusion imaging of acute stroke: the need for arrival time, delay insensitive, and standardized postprocessing algorithms? Radiology 2010;254:22–5.

87. Kudo K, Sasaki M, Yamada K, et al, Acute Stroke Imaging Standardization Group Japan (ASIST-Japan) Investigators. Differences in CT perfusion maps generated by different commercially

available software: quantitative analysis using identical source data of acute stroke patients. Radiology 2010;254(1):200–9.

88. Kudo K, Sasaki M, Ogasawara K, et al. Difference in tracer delay-induced effect among deconvolution algorithms in CT perfusion analysis: quantitative evaluation with digital phantoms. Radiology 2009;251:241–9.

89. Mullani NA, Gould KL. First-pass measurements of regional blood flow with external detectors. J Nucl Med 1983;24:577–81.

90. Abels B, Klotz E, Tomandl BF, et al. Perfusion CT in acute ischemic stroke: a qualitative and quantitative comparison of deconvolution and maximum slope approach. AJNR Am J Neuroradiol 2010; 31:1690–8.

91. Ostergaard L, Weisskoff RM, Chesler DA, et al. High resolution of cerebral blood flow using intravascular tracer bolus passages. Part I: mathematical approach ad statistical analysis. Magn Reson Med 1996;36(5):715–25.

92. Wirestam R, Andersson L, Ostergaard L, et al. Assessment of regional cerebral blood flow by dynamic susceptibility contrast MRI using different deconvolution techniques. Magn Reson Med 2000; 43:691–700.

93. Cenic A, Nabavi DG, Craen RA, et al. A CT method to measure hemodynamics in brain tumors: validation and application of cerebral blood flow maps. AJNR Am J Neuroradiol 2000;21:462–70.

94. Nabavi DG, Cenic A, Dool J, et al. Quantitative assessment of cerebral hemodynamics using CT: stability, accuracy, and precision studies in dogs. J Comput Assist Tomogr 1999;23:506–15.

95. Nabavi DG, Cenic A, Henderson S, et al. Perfusion mapping using computed tomography allows accurate prediction of cerebral infarction in experimental brain ischemia. Stroke 2001;32:175–83.

96. Wintermark M, Thiran JP, Maeder P, et al. Simultaneous measurement of regional cerebral blood flow by perfusion CT and stable xenon CT: a validation study. AJNR Am J Neuroradiol 2001;22:905–14.

97. Stewart GN. Researches on the circulation time in organs and on the influences which affect it. J Physiol 1894;15:1.

98. Ostergaard L, Chesler DA, Weisskoff RM, et al. Modeling cerebral blood flow and flow heterogeneity from magnetic resonance residue data. J Cereb Blood Flow Metab 1999;19:690–9.

99. Furukawa M, Kashiwagi S, Matsunaga N, et al. Evaluation of cerebral perfusion parameters measured by perfusion CT in chronic cerebral ischemia: comparison with xenon CT. J Comput Assist Tomogr 2002;26:272–8.

100. Gillard JH, Antoun NM, Burnet NG, et al. Reproducibility of quantitative CT perfusion imaging. Br J Radiol 2001;74:552–5.

101. Eastwood JD, Lev MH, Wintermark M, et al. Correlation of early dynamic CT perfusion imaging with whole-brain MR diffusion and perfusion imaging in acute hemispheric stroke. AJNR Am J Neuroradiol 2003;24:1869–75.

102. Wintermark M, Reichhart M, Cuisenaire O, et al. Comparison of admission perfusion computed tomography and qualitative diffusion- and perfusion-weighted magnetic resonance imaging in acute stroke patients. Stroke 2002;33:2025–31.

103. Schramm P, Schellinger PD, Klotz E, et al. Comparison of perfusion computed tomography and computed tomography angiography source images with perfusion-weighted imaging and diffusion-weighted imaging in patients with acute stroke of less than 6 hours' duration. Stroke 2004; 35(7):1652–8.

104. Wang XC, Gao PY, Xue J, et al. Identification of infarct core and penumbra in acute stroke using CT perfusion source images. AJNR Am J Neuroradiol 2010;31(1):34–9.

105. van der Schaaf I, Vonken EJ, Waaijer A, et al. Influence of partial volume on venous output and arterial input function. AJNR Am J Neuroradiol 2006; 27:46–50.

106. Calamante F, Gadian DG, Connelly A. Delay and dispersion effects in dynamic susceptibility contrast MRI: simulations using singular value decomposition. Magn Reson Med 2000;44: 466–73.

107. Calamante F, Yim PJ, Cebral JR. Estimation of bolus dispersion effects in perfusion MRI using image-based computational fluid dynamics. Neuroimage 2003;19:341–53.

108. Wu O, Ostergaard L, Weisskoff RM, et al. Tracer arrival timing-insensitive technique for estimating flow in MR perfusion-weighted imaging using singular value decomposition with a block-circulant deconvolution matrix. Magn Reson Med 2003;50:164–74.

109. Knash M, Tsang A, Hameed B, et al. Low cerebral blood volume is predictive of diffusion restriction only in hyperacute stroke. Stroke 2010;41: 2795–800.

110. Wittsack HJ, Wohlschlager AM, Ritzl EK, et al. CT-perfusion imaging of the human brain: advanced deconvolution analysis using circulant singular value decomposition. Comput Med Imaging Graph 2008;32:67–77.

111. Calamante F, Morup M, Hansen LK. Defining a local arterial input function for perfusion MRI using independent component analysis. Magn Reson Med 2004;52:789–97.

112. Ibaraki M, Shimosegawa E, Toyoshima H, et al. Tracer delay correction of cerebral blood flow with dynamic susceptibility contrast-enhanced MRI. J Cereb Blood Flow Metab 2005;25:378–90.

113. Serena J, Davalos A, Segura T, et al. Stroke on awakening: looking for a more rational management. Cerebrovasc Dis 2003;16:128–33.

114. Darby DG, Barber PA, Gerraty RP, et al. Pathophysiological topography of acute ischemia by combined diffusion-weighted and perfusion MRI. Stroke 1999;30:2043–52.

115. Neumann-Haefelin T, Wittsack HJ, Wenserski F, et al. Diffusion- and perfusion-weighted MRI. The DWI/PWI mismatch region in acute stroke. Stroke 1999;30:1591–7.

116. Hacke W, Furlan AJ, Al-Rawi Y, et al. Intravenous desmoteplase in patients with acute ischaemic stroke selected by MRI perfusion-diffusion weighted imaging or perfusion CT (DIAS-2): a prospective, randomised, double-blind, placebo-controlled study. Lancet Neurol 2009;8: 141–50.

117. Schramm P, Schellinger PD, Fiebach JB, et al. Comparison of CT and CT angiography source images with diffusion-weighted imaging in patients with acute stroke within 6 hours after onset. Stroke 2002;33:2426–32.

118. Aviv RI, Shelef I, Malam S, et al. Early stroke detection and extent: impact of experience and the role of computed tomography angiography source images. Clin Radiol 2007;62:447–52.

119. Coutts SB, Lev MH, Eliasziw M, et al. ASPECTS on CTA source images versus unenhanced CT: added value in predicting final infarct extent and clinical outcome. Stroke 2004;35:2472–6.

120. Lin K, Rapalino O, Law M, et al. Accuracy of the Alberta Stroke Program Early CT Score during the first 3 hours of middle cerebral artery stroke: comparison of noncontrast CT, CT angiography source images, and CT perfusion. AJNR Am J Neuroradiol 2008;29:931–6.

121. Kidwell CS, Saver JL, Mattiello J, et al. Thrombolytic reversal of acute human cerebral ischemic injury shown by diffusion/perfusion magnetic resonance imaging. Ann Neurol 2000;47:462–9.

122. Kidwell CS, Saver JL, Starkman S, et al. Late secondary ischemic injury in patients receiving intra-arterial thrombolysis. Ann Neurol 2002;52:698–703.

123. Warach S. Measurement of the ischemic penumbra with MRI: it's about time. Stroke 2003;34:2533–4.

124. Wu O, Koroshetz WJ, Ostergaard L, et al. Predicting tissue outcome in acute human cerebral ischemia using combined diffusion- and perfusion-weighted MR imaging. Stroke 2001;32:933–42.

125. Barber PA, Darby DG, Desmond PM, et al. Prediction of stroke outcome with echoplanar perfusion- and diffusion-weighted MRI. Neurology 1998;51: 418–26.

126. Astrup J, Siesjo BK, Symon L. Thresholds in cerebral ischemia—the ischemic penumbra. Stroke 1981;12: 723–5.

127. Sorensen AG, Buonanno FS, Gonzalez RG, et al. Hyperacute stroke: evaluation with combined multisection diffusion-weighted and hemodynamically weighted echo-planar MR imaging. Radiology 1996;199:391–401.

128. Sunshine JL, Tarr RW, Lanzieri CF, et al. Hyperacute stroke: ultrafast MR imaging to triage patients prior to therapy. Radiology 1999;212: 325–32.

129. Schlaug G, Benfield A, Baird AE, et al. The ischemic penumbra: operationally defined by diffusion and perfusion MRI. Neurology 1999;53:1528–37.

130. Wintermark M, Flanders AE, Velthuis B, et al. Perfusion-CT assessment of infarct core and penumbra: receiver operating characteristic curve analysis in 130 patients suspected of acute hemispheric stroke. Stroke 2006;37:979–85.

131. Mehta N, Lev MH, Mullins ME, et al. Prediction of final infarct size in acute stroke using cerebral blood flow/cerebral blood volume mismatch: added value of quantitative first pass CT perfusion imaging in successfully treated versus unsuccessfully treated/untreated patients. In: Proceedings of the 41st Annual Meeting of the American Society of Neuroradiology. Washington, DC, April 27 to May 2, 2003.

132. Aksoy FG, Lev MH, Eskey CJ, et al. CT perfusion imaging of acute stroke: how well do CBV, CBF, and MTT maps predict final infarct size? In: Proceedings of the 86th Scientific Assembly and Annual Meeting of the Radiological Society of North America. Chicago (IL), November 26 to December 1, 2000.

133. Donnan GA, Baron JC, Ma H, et al. Penumbral selection of patients for trials of acute stroke therapy. Lancet Neurol 2009;8:261–9.

134. Albers GW, Thijs VN, Wechsler L, et al. Magnetic resonance imaging profiles predict clinical response to early reperfusion: the diffusion and perfusion imaging evaluation for understanding stroke evolution (DEFUSE) study. Ann Neurol 2006;60:508–17.

135. Sobesky J, Weber OZ, Lehnhardt FG, et al. Which time-to-peak threshold best identifies penumbral flow? A comparison of perfusion-weighted magnetic resonance imaging and positron emission tomography in acute ischemic stroke. Stroke 2004;35:2843–7.

136. Davis SM, Donnan GA. MR mismatch and thrombolysis: appealing but validation required. Stroke 2009;40:2910.

137. Sasaki O, Takeuchi S, Koizumi T, et al. Complete recanalization via fibrinolytic therapy can reduce the number of ischemic territories that progress to infarction. AJNR Am J Neuroradiol 1996;17:1661–8.

138. Ueda T, Sakaki S, Yuh W, et al. Outcome in acute stroke with successful intra-arterial thrombolysis procedure and predictive value of initial single-photon

emission-computed tomography. J Cereb Blood Flow Metab 1999;19:99–108.

139. Liu Y, Karonen JO, Vanninen RL, et al. Cerebral hemodynamics in human acute ischemic stroke: a study with diffusion- and perfusion-weighted magnetic resonance imaging and SPECT. J Cereb Blood Flow Metab 2000;20:910–20.

140. Hatazawa J, Shimosegawa E, Toyoshima H, et al. Cerebral blood volume in acute brain infarction: a combined study with dynamic susceptibility contrast MRI and 99mTc-HMPAO-SPECT. Stroke 1999;30:800–6.

141. Shimosegawa E, Hatazawa J, Inugami A, et al. Cerebral infarction within six hours of onset: prediction of completed infarction with technetium-99m-HMPAO SPECT. J Nucl Med 1994;35:1097–103.

142. Rohl L, Ostergaard L, Simonsen CZ, et al. Viability thresholds of ischemic penumbra of hyperacute stroke defined by perfusion-weighted MRI and apparent diffusion coefficient. Stroke 2001;32:1140–6.

143. Suzuki Y, Nakajima M, Ikeda H, et al. Perfusion computed tomography for the indication of percutaneous transluminal reconstruction for acute stroke. J Stroke Cerebrovasc Dis 2006;15:18–25.

144. Marchal G, Young AR, Baron JC. Early postischemic hyperperfusion: pathophysiologic insights from positron emission tomography. J Cereb Blood Flow Metab 1999;19:467–82.

145. Kudo K, Sasaki M, Yamada K, et al. Differences in CT perfusion maps generated by different commercial software: quantitative analysis by using identical source data of acute stroke patients. Radiology 2010;254:200–9.

146. Sorensen AG, Copen WA, Ostergaard L, et al. Hyperacute stroke: simultaneous measurement of relative cerebral blood volume, relative cerebral blood flow, and mean tissue transit time. Radiology 1999;210:519–27.

147. Koennecke HC. Editorial comment—Challenging the concept of a dynamic penumbra in acute ischemic stroke. Stroke 2003;34:2434–5.

148. Heiss WD. Ischemic penumbra: evidence from functional imaging in man. J Cereb Blood Flow Metab 2000;20:1276–93.

149. Jovin TG, Yonas H, Gebel JM, et al. The cortical ischemic core and not the consistently present penumbra is a determinant of clinical outcome in acute middle cerebral artery occlusion. Stroke 2003;34:2426–33.

150. Lev MH, Roccatagliata L, Murphy EK, et al. A CTA based, multivariable, "benefit of recanalization" model for acute stroke triage: core infarct size on CTA source images independently predicts outcome. In: Proceedings of the 42nd Annual Meeting of the American Society of Neuroradiology. Seattle (WA), June 5–11, 2004.

151. Suarez J, Sunshine J, Tarr R, et al. Predictors of clinical improvement, angiographic recanalization, and intracranial hemorrhage after intra-arterial thrombolysis for acute ischemic stroke. Stroke 1999;30:2094–100.

152. Molina CA, Alexandrov AV, Demchuk AM, et al. Improving the predictive accuracy of recanalization on stroke outcome in patients treated with tissue plasminogen activator. Stroke 2004;35:151–6.

153. Baird AE, Dambrosia J, Janket S, et al. A three-item scale for the early prediction of stroke recovery. Lancet 2001;357:2095–9.

154. Rosenthal ES, Schwamm LH, Roccatagliata L, et al. Role of recanalization in acute stroke outcome: rationale for a CT angiogram-based "benefit of recanalization" model. AJNR Am J Neuroradiol 2008;29:1471–5.

155. Nighoghossian N, Hermier M, Adeleine P, et al. Baseline magnetic resonance imaging parameters and stroke outcome in patients treated by intravenous tissue plasminogen activator. Stroke 2003;34:458–63.

156. Sanak D, Nosal V, Horak D, et al. Impact of diffusion-weighted MRI-measured initial cerebral infarction volume on clinical outcome in acute stroke patients with middle cerebral artery occlusion treated by thrombolysis. Neuroradiology 2006;48:632–9.

157. Yoo AJ, Verduzco LA, Schaefer PW, et al. MRI-based selection for intra-arterial stroke therapy: value of pretreatment diffusion-weighted imaging lesion volume in selecting patients with acute stroke who will benefit from early recanalization. Stroke 2009;40:2046–54.

158. Gasparotti R, Grassi M, Mardighian D, et al. Perfusion CT in patients with acute ischemic stroke treated with intra-arterial thrombolysis: predictive value of infarct core size on clinical outcome. AJNR Am J Neuroradiol 2009;30:722–7.

159. Pessin MS, Del Zoppo GJ, Estol CJ. Thrombolytic agents in the treatment of stroke. Clin Neuropharmacol 1990;13:271–89.

160. Hacke W, Kaste M, Fieschi C, et al. Randomised double-blind placebo-controlled trial of thrombolytic therapy with intravenous alteplase in acute ischaemic stroke (ECASS II). Second European-Australasian Acute Stroke Study Investigators. Lancet 1998;352:1245–51.

161. Swap C, Lev M, McDonald C, et al. Degree of oligemia by perfusion-weighted CT and risk of hemorrhage after IA thrombolysis. In: Stroke—Proceedings of the 27th International Conference on Stroke and Cerebral Circulation. San Antonio (TX), February 7–9, 2002.

162. Dzialowski I, Hill MD, Coutts SB, et al. Extent of early ischemic changes on computed tomography (CT) before thrombolysis: prognostic value of the

Alberta Stroke Program Early CT Score in ECASS II. Stroke 2006;37:973–8.

163. Larrue V, von Kummer RR, Muller A, et al. Risk factors for severe hemorrhagic transformation in ischemic stroke patients treated with recombinant tissue plasminogen activator: a secondary analysis of the European-Australasian Acute Stroke Study (ECASS II). Stroke 2001;32:438–41.

164. Hacke W, Donnan G, Fieschi C, et al. Association of outcome with early stroke treatment: pooled analysis of ATLANTIS, ECASS, and NINDS rt-PA stroke trials. Lancet 2004;363:768–74.

165. Ogasawara K, Ogawa A, Ezura M, et al. Brain single-photon emission CT studies using 99mTc-HMPAO and 99mTc-ECD early after recanalization by local intraarterial thrombolysis in patients with acute embolic middle cerebral artery occlusion. AJNR Am J Neuroradiol 2001;22:48–53.

166. Gupta R, Yonas H, Gebel J, et al. Reduced pretreatment ipsilateral middle cerebral artery cerebral blood flow is predictive of symptomatic hemorrhage post-intra-arterial thrombolysis in patients with middle cerebral artery occlusion. Stroke 2006;37:2526–30.

167. Kidwell CS, Chalela JA, Saver JL, et al. Hemorrhage early MRI evaluation (HEME) study [abstract]. Stroke 2003;34:239.

168. Kidwell CS, Chalela JA, Saver JL, et al. Comparison of MRI and CT for detection of acute intracerebral hemorrhage. JAMA 2004;292:1823–30.

169. Campbell BC, Christensen S, Butcher KS, et al. Regional very low cerebral blood volume predicts hemorrhagic transformation better than diffusion-weighted imaging volume and thresholded apparent diffusion coefficient in acute ischemic stroke. Stroke 2010;41(1):82–8.

170. Tomsick T. Timi, TIBI, TICI: I came, I saw, I got confused. AJNR Am J Neuroradiol 2007;28:382–4.

171. Zaidat OO, Suarez JI, Sunshine JL, et al. Thrombolytic therapy of acute ischemic stroke: correlation of angiographic recanalization with clinical outcome. AJNR Am J Neuroradiol 2005;26:880–4.

172. Rha JH, Saver JL. The impact of recanalization on ischemic stroke outcome: a meta-analysis. Stroke 2007;38:967–73.

173. Tomsick T, Broderick J, Carrozella J, et al. Revascularization results in the interventional management of stroke II trial. AJNR Am J Neuroradiol 2008;29:582–7.

174. Soares BP, Chien JD, Wintermark M. MR and CT monitoring of recanalization, reperfusion, and penumbra salvage: everything that recanalizes does not necessarily reperfuse! Stroke 2009;40:S24–7.

175. Janjua N, Alkawi A, Suri MF, et al. Impact of arterial reocclusion and distal fragmentation during thrombolysis among patients with acute ischemic stroke. AJNR Am J Neuroradiol 2008;29:253–8.

176. Ames A 3rd, Wright RL, Kowada M, et al. Cerebral ischemia. II. The no-reflow phenomenon. Am J Pathol 1968;52:437–53.

177. del Zoppo GJ. Virchow's triad: the vascular basis of cerebral injury. Rev Neurol Dis 2008;5(Suppl 1):S12–21.

178. Soares BP, Tong E, Hom J, et al. Reperfusion is a more accurate predictor of follow-up infarct volume than recanalization. a proof of concept using ct in acute ischemic stroke patients. Stroke 2010;41(1):e34–40.

Stroke Imaging Research Road Map

Carlos Leiva-Salinas, MD[a,b], Jason Hom, MD[c],
Steven Warach, MD, PhD[d], Max Wintermark, MD[a,*]

KEYWORDS

- Stroke • MR imaging • CT • DWI • Perfusion
- Thrombolysis

THE NEED FOR STANDARDIZATION AND VALIDATION

Since the approval of intravenous tissue plasminogen activator (IV tPA) in 1996, the number of acute stroke patients receiving this agent has remained less than 5%, mainly because of delayed presentation to care.[1] A recent study suggested that the time window for tPA administration could be extended from 3 to 4.5 hours in certain patients.[2] Although this extension might slightly increase the rate of tPA administration, it does not change the fundamental limitation, which lies in the fact that currently the decision to initiate thrombolytic therapy depends on a generalized statistical rule regarding time to presentation rather than on an individualized pathophysiologic assessment of the ischemic penumbra, the target of tPA treatment. Several studies[3–5] have suggested and validated the concept that the ischemic penumbra can be imaged and quantified, and an optimal therapeutic decision regarding thrombolytic agents can be based on such imaging, within an extended time window of up to 9 hours. Such an approach would not only increase the fraction of acute stroke patients amenable to thrombolytic treatment, possibly up to 40%, but also might allow more precise patient selection, thereby improving overall clinical outcomes.[6]

However, this concept of penumbral image-guided thrombolytic therapy has not yet been validated in a large phase 3 trial[7,8] and as a result, has not become part of the clinical standard of care in tPA treatment decisions. One of the reasons for this delay in validation is the lack of standardization in penumbral imaging, which can result in different treatment decisions in the same patient when different penumbral imaging methods are applied to the same perfusion imaging data set.[9] Current methods available for defining the penumbra vary for several reasons. The mathematical algorithms that calculate variables such as cerebral blood volume (CBV), cerebral blood flow (CBF), and mean transit time (MTT) differ. The variables that are used to define the infarct core and penumbra (eg, MTT vs CBF vs CBV in perfusion computed tomographic [CT] imaging) and their corresponding thresholds also differ (Figs. 1–3).[10]

The differences between the imaging methods that identify the ischemic penumbra are not irreconcilable. Rather, they just need some refining to give concordant results, which is one of the goals pursued by the Stroke Imaging Repository (STIR) consortium.[11]

The authors have nothing to disclose.

[a] Neuroradiology Division, Department of Radiology, University of Virginia, 1215 Lee Street-New Hospital, PO Box 800170, Charlottesville, VA 22908, USA

[b] Departamento de Medicina, Universidad Autónoma de Barcelona. Carretera de Bellaterra, 08290, Cerdañola del Vallés, Spain

[c] Neuroradiology Section, Department of Radiology, University of California, 505 Parnassus Avenue, Box 0628, San Francisco, CA 94143, USA

[d] Section on Stroke Diagnostics and Therapeutics, National Institute of Neurological Disorders and Stroke, National Institutes of Health, 10 Center Drive, Room B1D733, MSC 1063, Bethesda, MD 20892, USA

* Corresponding author.
E-mail address: Max.Wintermark@virginia.edu

Neuroimag Clin N Am 21 (2011) 239–245
doi:10.1016/j.nic.2011.01.009

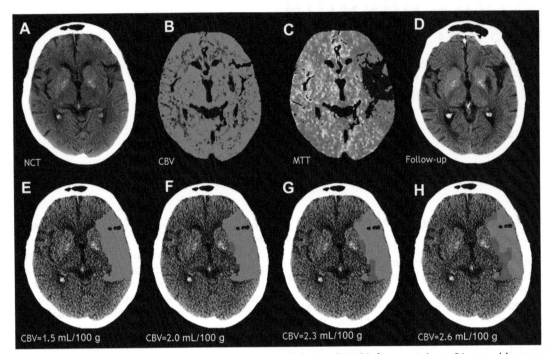

Fig. 1. Effect of varying the threshold based on the size of the predicted infarct core in an 81-year-old woman with acute left MCA territory infarct, who was treated successfully with tPA. (A) NCT of the head obtained 2.5 hours after symptom onset shows no definite abnormality. (B, C) Perfusion CT parametric maps show a mismatch between the region with prolonged MTT (involving the anterior superficial left MCA territory) and the region of decreased CBV (limited to the left putamen), which represents the predicted infarct core. (D) Follow-up NCT performed 36 hours later shows that the final infarct corresponds to the area of the predicted infarct core as represented by the area of decreased CBV. (E–H) Perfusion CT prognostic maps generated using different CBV thresholds (1.5, 2.0, 2.3, and 2.6 mL/100 g) show that the volume of the predicted infarct core (red) in case of recanalization varies depending on the chosen value. The CBV that best predicts the size of the final infarct is 2.0 mL/100 g, as published in the literature. The threshold for the delineation of the ischemic penumbra (green) was set at a relative 145%. MCA, middle cerebral artery; NCT, noncontrast CT.

THE STIR

History

In September 2007, the National Institutes of Health, in conjunction with the American Society of Neuroradiology and the Neuroradiology Education and Research Foundation, sponsored a research symposium entitled "Advanced Neuroimaging for Acute Stroke Treatment." This meeting brought together stroke neurologists, neuroradiologists, emergency physicians, and neuroimaging research scientists to discuss the role of advanced neuroimaging in acute stroke treatment. In particular, the goals of the meeting were to discuss unresolved issues regarding (1) the standardization of perfusion and penumbral imaging techniques, (2) the validation of the accuracy and clinical utility of imaging biomarkers of the ischemic penumbra, and (3) the validation of imaging biomarkers relevant to clinical outcome.[12]

One of the recommendations was the creation of an international consortium of investigators, the STIR, to combine efforts and promote excellence in stroke care and stroke trial design and more specifically to overcome the issues faced by advanced stroke imaging, as mentioned earlier.[12]

This central repository was designed to work in collaboration with 2 other collaborative groups, namely, Virtual International Stroke Trials Archive (VISTA) and MR Stroke. VISTA is an international collaborative venture that was established to facilitate the planning of randomized clinical trials and collects and gathers data sets from multiple institutions. The VISTA database provides the possibility to access a large volume of patient data on which original analyses can be performed, which would ultimately aid clinical trial design and development.[13,14] MR Stroke is a collaborative effort between leading clinicians and clinical scientists around the world with a common interest in Magnetic Resonance Imaging in Stroke.[15] MR Stroke is intended to facilitate the sharing and exchange of information and ideas, to provide

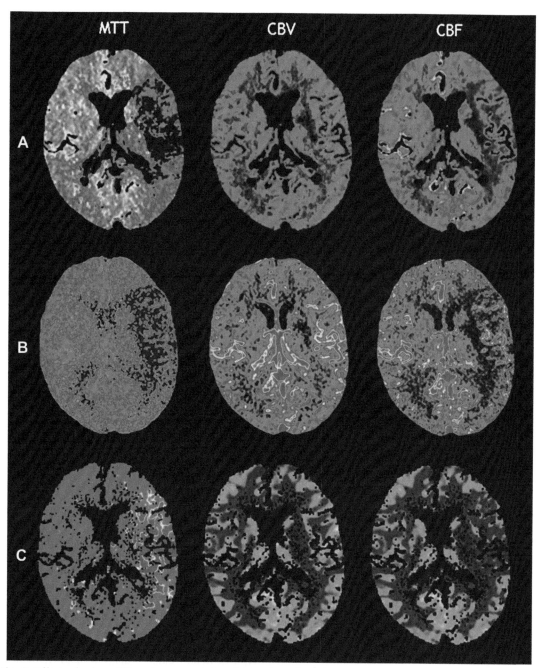

Fig. 2. Effect of using different commercial perfusion CT software packages (*A–C*) on the MTT, CBV, and CBF parametric maps in the same patient from Fig. 1. Even if the discordance is not major or incongruous, the area of predicted ischemic penumbra as represented by the area of prolonged MTT differs slightly depending on the software used to process the source images. The area of predicted infarct core as represented by the area of decreased CBV is very similar for all the 3 software packages. Note that parametric maps from software packages *A* and *C* are displayed with vessels removed.

access to a range of Web-based MR imaging tools and resources relevant to stroke, and to establish a forum for the exchange of information relevant to research using MR imaging in stroke.

Overall Goals

The overall purpose of the STIR is to create a repository of source MR images and CT images that could be used toward the objectives of

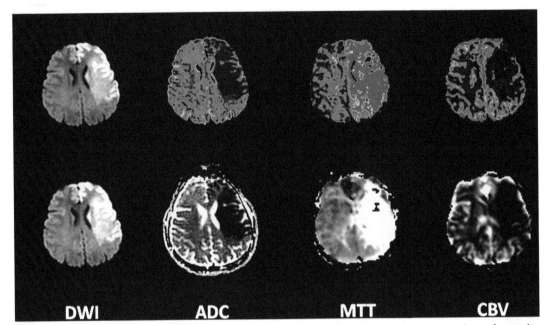

DWI   ADC   MTT   CBV

Fig. 3. Comparison of acute diffusion and perfusion maps generated by commercial postprocessing software (*top row*) and MR imaging scanner tools (*bottom row*). Images were obtained 1 hour and 20 minutes after a sudden onset of right-sided hemiparesis and aphasia, as well as a left middle cerebral artery occlusion in a 59-year-old woman. The perfusion maps generated from the commercial software were based on an arterial input function model, whereas the scanner-generated maps were not. Different programs and algorithms produce different results for parameters that are nominally the same (eg, MTT). ADC, apparent diffusion coefficient; DWI, diffusion-weighted MR imaging.

standardization and validation of image acquisition, of image analysis, and of clinical research methods for image-based stroke research. More specifically, the consortium was originally established to collect and provide a rich resource of patient data sets to contribute meaningful information regarding the goals listed earlier: (1) the standardization of perfusion and penumbral imaging techniques, (2) the validation of the accuracy and clinical utility of imaging biomarkers of the ischemic penumbra, and (3) the validation of imaging biomarkers relevant to clinical outcomes.[16]

Main Ongoing Tasks

To achieve these goals, the STIR consortium is focusing its initial efforts and resources on 3 main tasks.[17]

Task 1: review of the literature

A systematic review of the stroke perfusion literature is needed to assess the different parameters and thresholds that have been used to define the infarct core and penumbra in acute stroke patients imaged with CT and/or MR perfusion imaging in prior studies or clinical trials. This systematic review will provide an approximation of the

accuracy of each of these methods and the modifications required to optimize and standardize these methods.

Task 2: mathematical models and processing algorithms

This task involves establishing a list of the key postprocessing components typically implemented in perfusion software (motion correction, deconvolution, selection of the arterial input function, types of maps produced, and methods to calculate infarct core and penumbra), describing the types/values of each of these components in the different perfusion software packages (eg, type of deconvolution, delay sensitivity, number of arterial input functions), and finally, assessing the acceptable deviations for the different perfusion software components.

Ideally, the resultant standard perfusion software would fulfill the following premises: (1) the perfusion postprocessing would be completely automated and available either on the scanner console or on a remote workstation, (2) the perfusion software would generate an automated delineation of the infarct core and penumbra and produce an automated calculation of their volumes, (3) image processing and generation of the maps and volumes would take less than 5 minutes, and (4) processing would be robust, despite the use of slightly different image acquisition protocols and different degrees of image quality and noise.

Task 3: clinical validation of MR imaging and CT
The different perfusion software packages available, both academic and commercial ones, should be systematically compared and their results harmonized. In order to achieve this goal, a large data set of cases for each modality (MR imaging and CT) is collected. These cases are randomly divided into 2 groups. The first set of cases (training set) is analyzed separately from the second set (validation set). The training set is used to compare each software package to the same gold standard data set and to determine the required modifications specific to each software package. After this initial phase of refining, the software packages are "locked," and the improved version is used to analyze the validation data set. The results of this analysis are collected and interpreted centrally, in an independent fashion, to validate the improved locked version of the different perfusion software packages and to show that all the software packages lead to concordant standardized results, appropriate to use in a stroke treatment trial.

Next Steps and Other Needs in the Field

Single institutions contributing to the central repository create a network that will apply standardized image acquisition protocols, allowing the constitution of a large homogenous data set.[12] This image data set facilitates sample size calculations when planning a trial. In addition, studies to determine the optimal imaging modality and the optimal timing to perform imaging to predict clinical outcomes are made possible. If shorter follow-up periods are validated to assess outcome and if imaging is demonstrated as an accurate diagnostic method, the feasibility of stroke treatment clinical trials will be greatly enhanced and their cost will be decreased.

All these steps will facilitate and, hopefully, contribute to a successful phase 3 clinical trial of stroke thrombolytic therapy in an extended time window. This development will, in turn, allow a significantly increased number of acute stroke patients to benefit from thrombolytic therapy and will reduce the burden associated with stroke in the society.

Individual Projects

Analyses and/or research projects taking advantage of the STIR data set can be proposed by any STIR member through a written application sent to the Steering Committee.

Current individual projects or study proposals to the consortium that are related to imaging techniques, models, standardization, and validation include the follwing.[11]

Tissue Infarction Risk Maps Applied to Multicenter Stroke Data (Project Leader: Ona Wu, PhD, Boston, MA)

This study proposes the application of a voxel-wise approach, to define the infarct core and the potentially salvageable tissue, to a large multicenter acute stroke series for model development and validation. Preliminary results based on single center data have shown that these algorithms can be used for tissue characterization.[18,19] Traditionally, the presence of mismatch between diffusion-weighted MR imaging (DWI) and perfusion-weighted MR imaging (PWI) lesion volumes has been considered as the hallmark of potentially salvageable tissue. The use of the PWI-DWI mismatch, however, has been criticized as being suboptimal because of the lesion heterogeneity in both DWI and PWI that can possibly confound accurate assessment of tissue viability within regions of ischemic tissue.[20] In comparison, voxel-wise methods, such as tissue risk maps, may provide a more sensitive and specific approach for identifying potentially salvageable tissue.

Improved Assessment of Infarct Size on Diffusion Magnetic Resonance Imaging; Use of the Graph-Cut Algorithm (Project Leader: Peter J. Yim, PhD, New Brunswick, NJ)

This study proposes the use of a novel approach to medical image segmentation, a graph-cut algorithm, for estimation of the infarct size by diffusion MR imaging to overcome the subtle but potential meaningful differences obtained from manual methods.[21] The main hypotheses to be tested are (1) this method can reduce interobserver variability in the segmentation of cerebral infarct size obtained from diffusion-weighted MR images and (2) the infarct size estimated by this algorithm from DWI is predictive of final infarct size as assessed at follow-up imaging.

Predicting Final Extent of Ischemic Infarction Using Artificial Neural Network Analysis of Multi-parametric MR imaging in Patients With Stroke (Project Leader: Hassan Bagher-Ebadian, PhD, Detroit, MI)

In ischemic stroke, the final size of the ischemic lesion is the most important correlate of clinical functional outcome. This study proposes the application of an artificial neural network, to predict the final infarct volume, to a large data set of treated acute stroke patients. Preliminary results on stroke patients from a single center, who did not receive thrombolytic therapy have shown that this approach, using baseline MR images, produced a map that correlated well with the T2-weighted abnormality at 3 months. Because this model was trained to predict tissue fate in the absence of any treatment, its performance in treated patient populations remains to be assessed. The proposed study is intended to apply the trained artificial neural network to treated patients (preferably tPA-treated patients) and validate its results in a large patient population.

SUMMARY

The establishment of the STIR consortisum will facilitate the validation and widespread use of imaging for acute stroke patients' care. At present, the consortium is creating a central repository of imaging studies and clinical data obtained from acute stroke patients and is developing a standardized image analysis toolbox. Contributions to the central repository from academic institutions is crucial not only to obtain a large and diverse data set but also to constitute a broad network of international stroke care centers that will, with the collaboration of the National Institutes of Health, Food and Drug Administration, and industry, form the basis for future acute stroke trials, including, but not limited to, treatment of stroke patients with intravenous thrombolytic therapy in an extended time window. This development would result in more acute stroke patients being appropriately treated and in an overall improvement of their outcome, as well as in reduced societal costs related to stroke.

REFERENCES

1. Bambauer KZ, Johnston SC, Bambauer DE, et al. Reasons why few patients with acute stroke receive tissue plasminogen activator. Arch Neurol 2006; 63(5):661–4.
2. Hacke W, Kaste M, Bluhmki E, et al. Thrombolysis with alteplase 3 to 4.5 hours after acute ischemic stroke. N Engl J Med 2008;359(13):1317–29.
3. Albers GW, Thijs VN, Wechsler L, et al. Magnetic resonance imaging profiles predict clinical response to early reperfusion: the diffusion and perfusion imaging evaluation for understanding stroke evolution (DEFUSE) study. Ann Neurol 2006;60(5):508–17.
4. Furlan AJ, Eyding D, Albers GW, et al. Dose Escalation of Desmoteplase for Acute Ischemic Stroke (DEDAS): evidence of safety and efficacy 3 to 9 hours after stroke onset. Stroke 2006; 37(5):1227–31.
5. Hacke W, Albers G, Al-Rawi Y, et al. The Desmoteplase in Acute Ischemic Stroke Trial (DIAS): a phase II MRI-based 9-hour window acute stroke thrombolysis trial with intravenous desmoteplase. Stroke 2005;36(1):66–73.
6. Schellinger PD, Warach S. Therapeutic time window of thrombolytic therapy following stroke. Curr Atheroscler Rep 2004;6(4):288–94.
7. Davis SM, Donnan GA, Parsons MW, et al. Effects of alteplase beyond 3 h after stroke in the Echoplanar Imaging Thrombolytic Evaluation Trial (EPITHET): a placebo-controlled randomised trial. Lancet Neurol 2008;7(4):299–309.
8. Hacke W, Furlan AJ, Al-Rawi Y, et al. Intravenous desmoteplase in patients with acute ischaemic stroke selected by MRI perfusion-diffusion weighted imaging or perfusion CT (DIAS-2): a prospective, randomised, double-blind, placebo-controlled study. Lancet Neurol 2009;8(2):141–50.
9. Leiva-Salinas C, Wintermark M. The future of stroke imaging: what we need and how to get to it. AJNR Am J Neuroradiol 2010;41(Suppl 1):S152–3.
10. Provenzale JM, Wintermark M. Optimization of perfusion imaging for acute cerebral ischemia: review of recent clinical trials and recommendations for future studies. AJR Am J Roentgenol 2008; 191(4):1263–70.
11. Stroke Imaging Repository home. Available at: https://stir.ninds.nih.gov/html/index.html. Accessed September 27, 2010.
12. Wintermark M, Albers GW, Alexandrov AV, et al. Acute stroke imaging research roadmap. AJNR Am J Neuroradiol 2008;29(5):e23–e30.
13. Ali M, Bath PM, Curram J, et al. The virtual international stroke trials archive. Stroke 2007;38(6):1905–10.
14. Virtual International Stroke Trials Archive home. Available at: http://www.vista.gla.ac.uk/. Accessed September 27, 2010.
15. M.R Stroke home. Available at: http://www.mrstroke.com/. Accessed September 27, 2010.
16. Stroke Imaging Repository charter. Available at: https://stir.ninds.nih.gov/html/charter.html. Accessed September 27, 2010.
17. Stroke Imaging Repository projects. Available at: https://stir.ninds.nih.gov/html/projects.html. Accessed September 27, 2010.
18. Wu O, Christensen S, Hjort N, et al. Characterizing physiological heterogeneity of infarction risk in acute human ischaemic stroke using MRI. Brain 2006; 129(Pt 9):2384–93.

19. Wu O, Koroshetz WJ, Ostergaard L, et al. Predicting tissue outcome in acute human cerebral ischemia using combined diffusion- and perfusion-weighted MR imaging. Stroke 2001;32(4):933–42.

20. Ostergaard L, Sorensen AG, Chesler DA, et al. Combined diffusion-weighted and perfusion-weighted flow heterogeneity magnetic resonance imaging in acute stroke. Stroke 2000;31(5):1097–103.

21. Ay H, Arsava EM, Vangel M, et al. Interexaminer difference in infarct volume measurements on MRI: a source of variance in stroke research. Stroke 2008;39(4):1171–6.

Role of Diffusion and Perfusion MRI in Selecting Patients for Reperfusion Therapies

Mikayel Grigoryan, MD*, Christie E. Tung, MD,
Gregory W. Albers, MD

KEYWORDS

• MRI • Diffusion • Perfusion • Mismatch • Penumbra

Stroke remains a major health care challenge worldwide and is the second leading cause of death and the leading cause of disability in Western countries. Ischemic stroke represents the most common subtype of stroke. An occlusion of a cerebral vessel in acute ischemic stroke may lead to a dramatic reduction of blood flow followed by death of brain cells within minutes. Several acute interventions to improve outcomes after stroke have been introduced recently, and others are still being investigated.[1]

The only acute intervention in ischemic stroke that is proven to be effective is intravenous alteplase (rt-PA) given within first the 4.5 hours after the onset of symptoms.[2,3] The eligibility of patients undergoing thrombolytic therapy within the current time window is determined using clinical and laboratory criteria and a noncontrast head CT scan (to rule out intracranial hemorrhage). Unfortunately, only approximately 2% to 5% of patients with acute ischemic stroke receive this treatment.[4,5] Therefore, to increase the number of individuals treated, either more patients must present within the 4.5-hour therapeutic window, or the time window itself must be extended.

An ischemic brain lesion consists of an area of irreversibly injured cells referred to as the *ischemic core*, intertwined with potentially salvageable ischemic tissue at risk, commonly referred to as an *ischemic penumbra*.[6] The penumbra consists of ischemic tissue that is functionally impaired and at risk of infarction but that has the potential to be salvaged through reperfusion or other strategies. Imaging studies have shown that salvage of this tissue is consistently linked to clinical recovery and that if not salvaged, it is progressively recruited into the infarct core, thereby worsening the clinical outcome.[6,7] Several markers of the ischemic penumbra have been studied in animals and humans and several imaging techniques, such as positron emission tomography (PET),[8,9] Xenon CT (Xe-CT),[10] diffusion-weighted (DWI) and perfusion-weighted (PWI) MRI,[11,12] and perfusion CT,[13] have been used to estimate penumbral volume. Of these, DWI/PWI and CT perfusion are the most practical and commonly used in selecting patients with acute stroke for reperfusion therapies.

Multimodal MRI offers several important advantages over CT, particularly in the extent of information provided that pertains to the diagnosis, management, and prognosis of an acute stroke.[14] DWI can confirm the diagnosis of acute ischemic stroke within minutes after the onset and can estimate the volume and location of the infarct core.[15,16] PWI assesses cerebral hemodynamics.[17] The mismatch between the infarct core on DWI and the hypoperfusion region on PWI has been hypothesized to represent an imaging surrogate for the ischemic penumbra.[12] In addition, MR

Stanford Stroke Center, Department of Neurology and Neurological Sciences, Stanford University Medical Center, 780 Welch Road, Palo Alto, CA 94304, USA
* Corresponding author.
E-mail address: mikayel@gmail.com

Neuroimag Clin N Am 21 (2011) 247–257
doi:10.1016/j.nic.2011.01.002
1052-5149/11/$ – see front matter © 2011 Published by Elsevier Inc.

angiography (MRA) provides information on major vessel patency, and gradient echo (GRE) and fluid-attenuated inversion recovery (FLAIR) imaging detect intracranial hemorrhage, as does CT.[18] All of these attractive features have inspired several clinical trials to investigate the ability of MRI to improve the selection of patients most likely to respond to treatment in delayed time windows. This article discusses the discoveries and insights gained from these trials and ongoing investigations to improve the ability of MRI to select patients for reperfusion therapies.

DIFFUSION MRI

In a normal state random diffusion of water molecules occurs across cell membranes. Tissue damage and ischemia begin to occur at a cerebral blood flow value of approximately 30 mL per 100 g per minute. Severe ischemia of brain tissue induces the rapid dysfunction of cellular metabolism and ion exchange pumps responsible for adenosine triphosphate (ATP) metabolism. This dysfunction causes a massive shift of water from the extracellular to the intracellular compartment, leading to cytotoxic edema that is associated with restricted diffusion of water molecules. This reduction in water diffusion can be quantified by a decrease in the apparent diffusion coefficient (ADC) and can be visualized as an increased signal on DWI.[19] In contrast to CT, in which brain ischemia is typically not visualized for several hours, diffusion signal increases within minutes of stroke onset.[15] Several studies have confirmed the greater sensitivity of DWI for detecting stroke compared with CT scanning or conventional MRI during the acute period (**Fig. 1**).[20–22] Thus, in the evaluation of acute stroke, DWI increases diagnostic confidence and may help identify candidates for reperfusion therapies.

DWI may also yield important prognostic information in the evaluation of acute stroke. Large-volume hemispheric ischemic strokes that cause severe space-occupying edema with the risk of resultant brain herniation are called *malignant infarctions* (**Fig. 2**). Early DWI lesion volumes larger

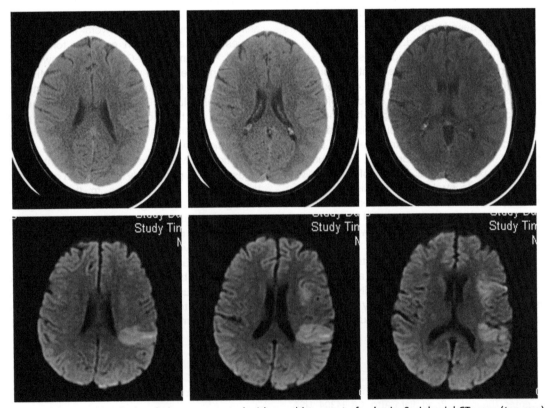

Fig. 1. A 53-year-old right-handed man presented with a sudden onset of aphasia. Serial axial CT scans (*top row*) at 1 hour after the symptom onset showed no obvious abnormalities. The patient received intravenous alteplase. Serial diffusion-weighted imaging scans at the same levels as the CT (*bottom row*) obtained approximately 1 hour later show no definite ischemia in the left middle cerebral artery territory.

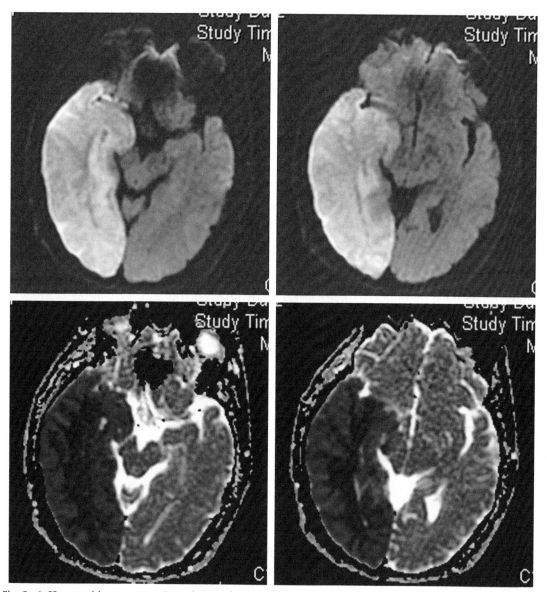

Fig. 2. A 62-year-old man presenting 5 hours after the onset of left-sided weakness and hemianopia. Diffusion-weighted imaging (*top row*) and apparent diffusion coefficient (*bottom row*) maps show a malignant right middle cerebral artery/posterior cerebral artery territory infarct (approximately 200 mL).

than 145 mL predict malignant infarction.[23] Despite medical treatments to reduce intracranial pressure, their prognosis is poor, with fatality rates of nearly 80%.[24,25] A life-saving emergent surgical decompression (hemicraniectomy), if performed early, reduces mortality and increases the chance for favorable functional outcome in patients with malignant infarction.[26] DWI lesion volume larger than 145 mL is now a validated criterion for emergent hemicraniectomy.[26]

In addition to providing information regarding which patients may benefit from emergent surgical decompression, DWI lesions may also predict the risk of hemorrhagic transformation after thrombolysis. The risk for symptomatic intracerebral hemorrhage after thrombolysis has been associated with pretreatment DWI lesion size.[27] Additionally, areas of severe ADC reduction have been reported to predict subsequent hemorrhagic transformation.[28] In the Diffusion and Perfusion Imaging Evaluation For Understanding Stroke Evolution (DEFUSE) study,[29] patients with a "malignant MRI profile" characterized by a DWI lesion larger than 100 mL and/or a PWI lesion larger than 100 mL with longer than 8 seconds of T_{max} delay had a high risk of symptomatic hemorrhagic transformation and death after rt-PA therapy. Furthermore, in a more recent study, patients with a DWI lesion larger than 70 mL before intra-arterial thrombolysis had a poor prognosis and high mortality rate despite a 50% recanalization rate.[30] The large volume of severe ischemic brain and microvascular injury in these malignant infarcts may increase the risk for reperfusion-related hemorrhage. Excluding patients with unfavorable imaging profiles from recanalization therapies may improve the safety and efficacy of these therapies.

The degree of reduction in ADC values may also predict DWI lesion reversal after recanalization/reperfusion. Several studies have shown that, for patients who do not have a malignant stroke profile, acute DWI lesions can be partially reversed through recanalization/reperfusion. These findings indicate that an acute DWI lesion does not necessarily represent irreversible injury, and may contain a portion of the ischemic penumbra.[31] ADC values typically decrease sharply soon after stroke onset. In animal studies, the reduction in ADC in acute stroke has been shown to occur before irreversible failure of energy metabolism.[32] Other supportive data have emerged from voxel-based comparisons between MRI and PET. Portions of acute DWI lesions show PET scan characteristics of penumbra.[33,34] Higher ADC values and successful early reperfusion are factors associated with DWI reversal.[35] In the DEFUSE study, an ADC threshold of 615×10^{-6} mm^2/s or less provided a sensitivity of 80% and specificity of 77% for identifying the infarct core. Thus, ADC thresholds may be useful to help distinguish ischemic core from penumbra.

PERFUSION MRI

Bolus tracking perfusion imaging using a paramagnetic contrast agent (eg, gadolinium) is the most commonly used MRI technique for assessing cerebral perfusion. The delay in gadolinium arrival to the vascular bed and the intensity of the signal change induced by its passage within capillaries can be used to generate a time/concentration curve. Various maps and parameters can be generated from these data, including cerebral blood flow (CBF), cerebral blood volume (CBV), and time-based factors such as T_{max}, mean transit time (MTT), and time to peak (TTP) (**Fig. 3**).[36]

The concept of the perfusion-diffusion (PWI/DWI) mismatch for selecting patients for thrombolysis was introduced with several small case series approximately 10 years ago,[37] followed by larger series by several international groups over the past few years. Studies have used multiple different perfusion parameters and thresholds to define critical hypoperfusion as the PWI lesion that will predict the extent of final infarction if the tissue does not experience early reperfusion.[38,39] T_{max}, the time to peak of the residue function, indicating a delay in bolus arrival between the site of selection of the arterial input function and the tissue, was used to define critical hypoperfusion in both the DEFUSE trial[29] and the Echoplanar Imaging Thrombolytic Evaluation Trial

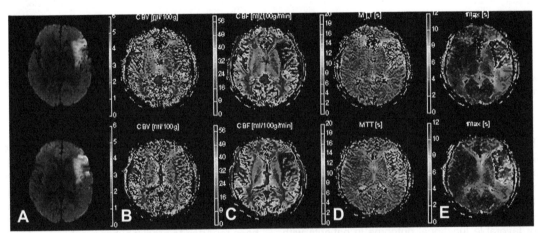

Fig. 3. A 55-year-old man approximately 4 hours after the onset of expressive aphasia. (*A*) Diffusion-weighted imaging (DWI) of the left frontal infarct. Hemodynamic maps from the MR perfusion study are obtained at the same time: (*B*) cerebral blood flow (CBF), (*C*) cerebral blood volume (CBV), (*D*) mean transit time (MTT), and (*E*) T_{max}. Within the infarct core, a markedly reduced CBV and CBF and markedly elevated MTT and T_{max} are seen. Posterior to the infarct core (the DWI lesion), in the left temporal parietal region, a region with less severely reduced CBF and less severely prolonged MTT and T_{max} is seen, consistent with the penumbra.

(EPITHET).[40] These studies selected a T_{max} value of greater than 2 seconds to threshold the PWI lesions in an attempt to exclude benign oligemia. However, retrospective analyses of these studies showed that higher T_{max} thresholds provide a more accurate assessment of critical hypoperfusion. For instance, a post hoc analysis of DEFUSE showed that a PWI lesion with a T_{max} delay between 4 and 6 seconds provides a better estimation of final infarct volume in patients who did not reperfuse compared with the threshold of greater than 2 second threshold.[41] These findings are supported by the results of direct voxel-to-voxel comparisons between MRI PWI and either PET[42] or Xe-CT scans[10] that suggest that 4- to 6-second T_{max} delays correspond most closely with penumbral cerebral blood flow values on PET or Xe-CT. A pooled analysis of both DEFUSE and EPITHET datasets presented at the International Stroke Conference in February 2010 showed that PWI lesions larger than 125 mL defined by a T_{max} threshold of greater than 8 seconds were associated with significantly worse clinical outcomes in patients treated with rt-PA versus placebo.[43]

Overall, the refinement of PWI techniques for acute stroke is ongoing. PWI does not provide an accurate quantitative estimate of cerebral blood flow in individual stroke patients compared with Xe-CT or PET gold standards. Corrections for contrast delay and dispersion seem to improve PWI performance. Although penumbral imaging algorithms are part of several guidelines, including those of the American Heart Association[44] and European Stroke Organization,[45] the ability of DWI/PWI mismatch to detect penumbra requires further validation using quantitative methods.

EVOLUTION OF MISMATCH DEFINITIONS AND CONCEPTS

The initial MRI concept of an acute ischemic brain lesion involved a central core outlined by DWI surrounded by a single circumferential region of hypoperfusion defined by PWI. However, recent studies have shown that this is rarely present in patients with untreated acute stroke imaged within 3 to 6 hours after symptom onset. In most of the patients enrolled in DEFUSE, more than 50% of the acute DWI volume did not have a superimposed PWI lesion, suggesting that partial reperfusion had occurred before thrombolysis. These regions of presumed spontaneous early reperfusion had the highest rate of DWI reversal, and reperfusion of these areas was associated with clinical recovery, suggesting that part of the penumbra extended into this portion of the early DWI lesion (**Fig. 4**). This region was termed *RADAR* (Reversible Acute DWI Already Reperfused).[35]

The MRI mismatch is usually calculated by the PWI/DWI volume ratio or the difference between the total PWI and total DWI lesion volumes. When this concept was originally introduced, the proportion of mismatch volume was arbitrarily set at 20%, and both DEFUSE and EPITHET used this threshold. However, when visualized with standard imaging techniques, the difference between DWI and PWI lesion volumes is more modest, because of the cubed root relation of radius with volume.[1] A recent analysis of the DEFUSE dataset suggested that a 2:1 mismatch ratio is a better predictor of clinical outcomes, and therefore is a more realistic target for therapy.[46] Also, because the calculation of the mismatch volume is based on the classical centripetal mismatch geography, which is frequently not observed, many patients will have a larger mismatch volume if the PWI and DWI lesions are coregistered, and mismatch is defined as the portion of the acute PWI lesion that does not show a superimposed DWI lesion.[47–49] These findings suggest that coregistration of acute DWI and PWI may improve the identification of tissue at risk.

TRIALS THAT TESTED AND USED THE DWI/PWI MISMATCH HYPOTHESIS
DEFUSE

In this trial, the investigators used open-label intravenous rt-PA to treat 74 patients with ischemic stroke who presented between 3 and 6 hours after the onset of symptoms.[29] MRI was performed immediately before treatment and then repeated 3 to 6 hours after treatment and again at 3 months. Patients were not selected based on the MRI findings, but the primary hypothesis postulated that prespecified MRI profiles would identify patients with a robust clinical response (National Institutes of Health Stroke Scale [NIHSS] = 0–1 or improvement ≥8 points between baseline and 30 days) after reperfusion. Mismatch was defined as a baseline PWI lesion ($T_{max}>2$ s) more than 20% larger than the baseline DWI lesion. Among the patients, 54% had a mismatch, and the key findings were that reperfusion or recanalization was associated with favorable clinical outcome in this group ($P<.05$) and even better outcome ($P = .005$) in patients with a target mismatch profile, which were those who did not have the malignant profile defined as a baseline DWI lesion greater than 100 mL or a baseline PWI lesion ($T_{max} >8$ s) greater than

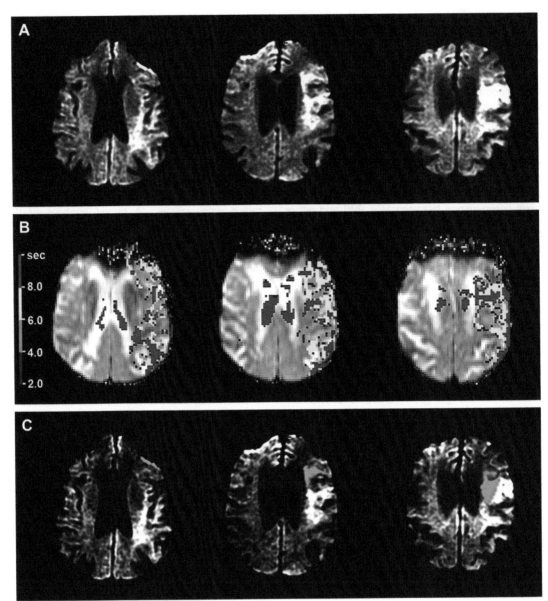

Fig. 4. An example of diffusion-weighted imaging (DWI) reversal. An 88-year-old man with a baseline National Institutes of Health Stroke Scale (NIHSS) of 24 had a baseline MRI performed 270 minutes after symptom onset. After the baseline MRI, he was treated with intravenous alteplase, and a follow-up MRI was obtained 270 minutes after the start of treatment. The follow-up MRI scan (not shown) revealed reperfusion (perfusion-weighted imaging lesion volume was reduced from 79 to 12 mL) and reversal of the DWI lesion (DWI lesion volume was reduced from 42 to 12 mL). The final MRI was performed 27 days after symptom onset. The 30-day NIHSS was 2. T_{max} color scale: T_{max} 2 to 4 seconds (blue); T_{max} 4 to 6 seconds (green); T_{max} 6 to 8 seconds (yellow); T_{max} greater than 8 seconds (red). (A) Baseline DWI: lesion volume 42 mL (normal perfusion 39%; mild-moderately hypoperfused 29% and severely hypoperfused 42%). (B) Baseline PWI: lesion volumes according to T_{max} delay: T_{max} greater than 2 seconds = 79 mL; greater than 4 seconds = 71 mL; greater than 6 seconds = 59 mL; and greater than 8 seconds = 34 mL. (C) Baseline DWI with the final infarct volume from the 27-day FLAIR superimposed in pink; final infarct volume: 13 mL.

100 mL. Patients without a mismatch did not seem to benefit from early reperfusion; however, the sample size in this group was too small for any definitive conclusions. Of the six patients with the malignant profile, three had a fatal intracerebral hemorrhage. Additional analyses showed that clinical improvement among mismatch cases was associated with reduced infarct growth when comparing the baseline DWI lesion and final infarct on 30-day FLAIR.[50]

EPITHET

EPITHET was a randomized double-blind placebo-controlled phase II clinical trial that randomized 101 patients with acute hemispheric ischemic stroke to receive rt-PA or placebo within 3 to 6 hours of onset.[40] As in DEFUSE, MRI was not used to select patients but was used to determine the effect of rt-PA on reperfusion, lesion growth, and clinical outcomes in patients with a PWI/DWI mismatch in the 3- to 6-hour time window. Follow-up MRIs were performed later than in DEFUSE (at 3–5 days and again 90 days after the onset), but the mismatch definition was the same. The primary efficacy end point was a reduction in infarct growth between the baseline DWI and the 90-day T2 lesion volume among mismatch patients. The prevalence of a mismatch was 86%. In patients with a mismatch, the rt-PA group showed attenuation of infarct growth compared with the placebo group. This difference was not statistically significant in the primary analysis but did reach significance in several secondary analyses. Reperfusion was strongly associated a good clinical outcome and reduced infarct growth among mismatch patients ($P = .01$). The study was not powered to adequately assess clinical recovery among the mismatch cases; however, trends favoring rt-PA were observed in mismatch patients.

Both of these studies provided strong biologic support for the associations among reperfusion, clinical recovery, and decreased infarct growth in mismatch patients. However, some potentially important differences were seen. The percentage of patients considered to have a mismatch was substantiality greater in EPITHET than in DEFUSE, and the malignant profile was much more common in EPITHET. In addition, the association between reperfusion and intracranial hemorrhage seen in DEFUSE was not confirmed in EPITHET. Post hoc analyses showed that the T_{max} threshold of greater than 2 seconds overestimated the extent of critical hypoperfusion in both studies. A pooled analysis has been performed with DWI and PWI scans from both studies using the same software program, and a preliminary report indicates that some of the key differences between the studies are no longer present. This finding emphasizes the importance of developing standardized processing methods for MRI studies. In addition, both DEFUSE and EPITHET results are based on lesion volumes that were not obtained at the time of the stroke. Cumbersome software was used to define the DWI and PWI lesion volumes, and post-processing typically required more than 40 minutes to generate these volumes. New automated software is now available and can process both DWI and PWI images within a matter of minutes. Clinical trials using this approach are awaited.

Desmoteplase Trials (DIAS and DEDAS)

Desmoteplase has several theoretical advantages over alteplase: it is more fibrin-specific, more likely to lyse recently formed clots, and less likely to cause direct neuronal damage.[51,52] The main hypothesis studied in the desmoteplase clinical trials was that intravenous administration of desmoteplase within 3 to 9 hours after onset will provide clinical benefits for patients with a DWI/PWI mismatch of at least 20%. The decision regarding presence or absence of a mismatch was based on visual judgment, without using any perfusion thresholds or quantification of volumes. The Desmoteplase in Acute Stroke (DIAS) trial[52] showed a dose–response effect on reperfusion rates seen on PWI and an acceptable hemorrhage rate of 7%. These results were replicated in the Dose Escalation of Desmoteplase for Acute Ischemic Stroke (DEDAS) trial.[51]

Based on these encouraging phase II results, a multicenter, placebo-controlled, double-blind phase III trial randomized patients believed to have a 20% visual mismatch (based on either DWI/PWI or perfusion CT) to one of two doses of desmoteplase (90 or 125 µg/kg) or placebo at 3 to 9 hours after symptom onset.[53] The rate of clinical recovery in the 90 µg/kg desmoteplase group was no different from placebo. The group receiving 125 µg/kg of desmoteplase had a higher mortality rate (21% vs 6%) and a lower rate of spontaneous recovery (36% vs 46%) compared with the placebo group. Various explanations have been proposed to explain the negative results of this study. Unfortunately, the mismatch status of patients in this trial was not uniformly confirmed by an expert panel; 15% of the patients were eventually assessed as not having a mismatch. Perhaps the penumbral selection of patients with perfusion CT was more difficult and less accurate than with MRI because it allowed only four slices of brain in the area of interest. In addition, the baseline median NIHSS of 9 was particularly low (11.5 in DEFUSE and

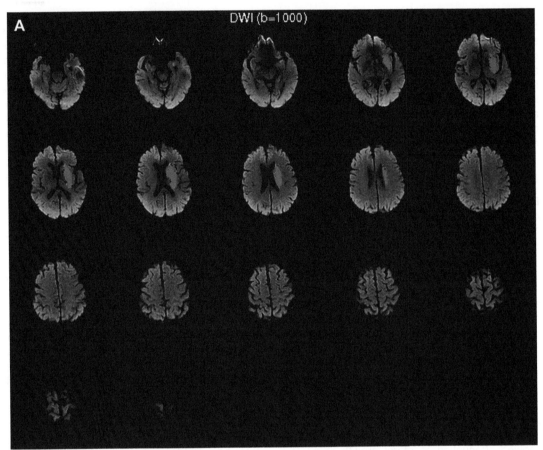

DWI (b=1000)

Fig. 5A. An 88 year-old woman presented with aphasia and right hemiplegia (NIHSS = 18). MRI was obtained approximately 2.5 hours after the onset. RAPID maps demonstrate a large mismatch between the infarct core of 16 ccm (*A*) and critical hypoperfusion of 130 ccm defined as Tmax >6 sec (*B*). The patient underwent successful mechanical thrombectomy of the left M1 clot with complete neurological recovery (NIHSS = 0).

12 in EPITHET), which may have led to the high spontaneous clinical recovery rate in the placebo group (46%). Furthermore, most deaths in the trial were nonneurologic and occurred late.

Regardless of the reasons, however, the failure of this study emphasizes the challenges in establishing the efficacy of a delayed therapy using mismatch criteria. A quantitative assessment of mismatch, which can be automatically generated in real time, will likely be essential. In addition, quantitative evaluation should account for recent refinements in the estimation of penumbra with imaging techniques, such as the use of appropriate perfusion and ADC thresholds.

FUTURE DIRECTIONS

Ongoing studies are investigating the use of automated MRI software to identify patients who benefit from various reperfusion strategies. Two of these studies involve endovascular recanalization techniques: MR and Recanalization of Stroke Clots Using Embolectomy (MR RESCUE) uses an algorithm that takes multiple DWI and PWI parameters into account to identify a penumbral pattern before randomization to treatment with one of the Merci clot retrieval devices (Concentric Medical, Mountain View, CA, USA) versus no recanalization therapy. DEFUSE 2 uses an automated software package called RAPID (Rapid Software Corporation, Grapevine, TX, USA) to perform quantitative evaluation of the ADC to estimate the ischemic core, and a PWI threshold of T_{max} greater than 6 seconds to define critical hypoperfusion before open-label intra-arterial therapy (**Fig. 5**). The upcoming Extending the Time for Thrombolysis in Emergency Neurologic Deficits (EXTEND) phase III trial will also use the RAPID software to select patients for rt-PA versus placebo beyond 4.5 hours.

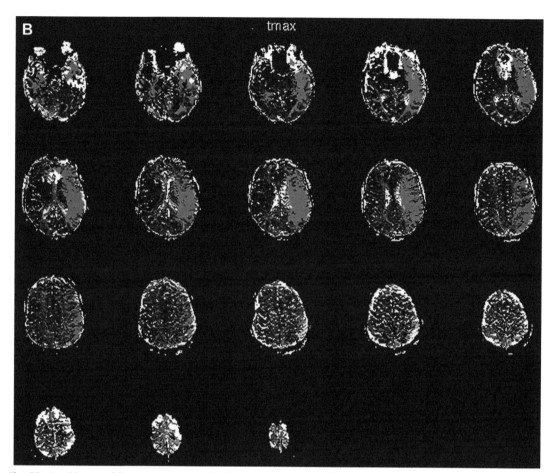

Fig. 5B. An 88 year-old woman presented with aphasia and right hemiplegia (NIHSS = 18). MRI was obtained approximately 2.5 hours after the onset. RAPID maps demonstrate a large mismatch between the infarct core of 16 ccm (*A*) and critical hypoperfusion of 130 ccm defined as Tmax >6 sec (*B*). The patient underwent successful mechanical thrombectomy of the left M1 clot with complete neurological recovery (NIHSS = 0).

SUMMARY

Results of several recent trials support the role of acute MRI for guiding emergency management of stroke. Patients with a malignant MRI pattern may be poor candidates for reperfusion therapies, yet may benefit from hemicraniectomy. Post hoc analyses of recent studies suggest that PWI techniques that use a threshold to exclude benign oligemia from penumbra, and DWI techniques that use ADC thresholds to exclude reversible DWI lesions to distinguish the ischemic core form penumbra, seem to provide more accurate determinations of the volume of salvageable tissue. New automated software programs are now implementing these techniques to generate quick quantitative PWI and DWI maps. Prospective trials investigating these new techniques are in progress and their results will further refine the application of MRI to select optimal patients for acute recanalization therapies. Successful phase III trials are required to verify the usefulness of imaging-based algorithms for extending the therapeutic time window before these techniques can be incorporated into routine clinical practice.

REFERENCES

1. Donnan GA, Baron JC, Ma H, et al. Penumbral selection of patients for trials of acute stroke therapy. Lancet Neurol 2009;8(3):261–9.
2. Hacke W, Kaste M, Bluhmki E, et al. Thrombolysis with alteplase 3 to 4.5 hours after acute ischemic stroke. N Engl J Med 2008;359(13):1317–29.
3. Marler JR, Brott T, Broderick J, et al. Tissue-Plasminogen activator for acute ischemic stroke. N Engl J Med 1995;333(24):1581–7.
4. Kleindorfer D, Lindsell CJ, Brass L, et al. National US estimates of recombinant tissue plasminogen activator use—ICD-9 codes substantially underestimate. Stroke 2008;39(3):924–8.

5. Nadeau JO, Shi S, Fang JM, et al. TPA use for stroke in the Registry of the Canadian Stroke Network. Can J Neurol Sci 2005;32(4):433–9.

6. Astrup J, Siesjo BK, Symon L. Thresholds in cerebral-ischemia—the ischemic penumbra. Stroke 1981;12(6):723–5.

7. Furlan M, Marchal G, Viader F, et al. Spontaneous neurological recovery after stroke and the fate of the ischemic penumbra. Ann Neurol 1996;40(2):216–26.

8. Baron JC. Mapping the ischaemic penumbra with PET: implications for acute stroke treatment. Cerebrovasc Dis 1999;9(4):193–201.

9. Read SJ, Hirano T, Abbott DF, et al. The fate of hypoxic tissue on F-18-fluoromisonidazole positron emission tomography after ischemic stroke. Ann Neurol 2000;48(2):228–35.

10. Olivot JM, Mlynash M, Zaharchuk G, et al. Perfusion MRI (Tmax and MTT) correlation with xenon CT cerebral blood flow in stroke patients. Neurology 2009; 72(13):1140–5.

11. Albers GW, Lansberg MG, Norbash AM, et al. Yield of diffusion-weighted MRI for detection of potentially relevant findings in stroke patients. Neurology 2000; 54(8):1562–7.

12. Kidwell CS, Alger JR, Saver JL. Evolving paradigms in imaging the ischemic penumbra with multimodal magnetic resonance imaging. Stroke 2003;34(11):2729–35.

13. Wintermark M, Flanders AE, Velthuis B, et al. Perfusion-CT assessment of infarct core and penumbra: receiver operating characteristic curve analysis in 130 patients suspected of acute hemispheric stroke. Stroke 2006;37(4):979–85.

14. Chalela JA, Kidwell CS, Nentwich LM, et al. Magnetic resonance imaging and computed tomography in emergency assessment of patients with suspected acute stroke: a prospective comparison. Lancet 2007;369(9558):293–8.

15. Hjort N, Christensen S, Solling C, et al. Ischemic injury detected by diffusion imaging 11 minutes after stroke. Ann Neurol 2005;58(3):462–5.

16. Moseley ME, Kucharczyk J, Mintorovitch J, et al. Diffusion-weighted MR imaging of acute stroke-correlation with T2-weighted and magnetic susceptibility-enhanced MR imaging in cats. AJNR Am J Neuroradiol 1990;11(3):423–9.

17. Baird AE, Warach S. Magnetic resonance imaging of acute stroke. J Cereb Blood Flow Metab 1998;18(6):583–609.

18. Kidwell CS, Wintermark M. Imaging of intracranial haemorrhage. Lancet Neurol 2008;7(3):256–67.

19. Hossmann KA, Fischer M, Bockhorst K, et al. NMR imaging of the apparent diffusion-coefficient (ADC) for the evaluation of metabolic suppression and recovery after prolonged cerebral-ischemia. J Cereb Blood Flow Metab 1994;14(5):723–31.

20. Fiebach JB, Schellinger PD, Jansen O, et al. CT and diffusion-weighted MR imaging in randomized order: diffusion-weighted imaging results in higher accuracy and lower interrater variability in the diagnosis of hyperacute ischemic stroke. Stroke 2002; 33(9):2206–10.

21. Kucinski T, Vaterlein O, Fiehler J, et al. Correlation of apparent diffusion coefficient and computed tomography density in acute ischemic stroke. Stroke 2003; 34(5):E17–8.

22. Mullins ME, Schaefer PW, Sorensen AG, et al. CT and conventional and diffusion-weighted MR imaging in acute stroke: study in 691 patients at presentation to the emergency department. Radiology 2002;224(2):353–60.

23. Oppenheim C, Samson Y, Manai R, et al. Prediction of malignant middle cerebral artery infarction by diffusion-weighted imaging. Stroke 2000;31(9):2175–81.

24. Berrouschot J, Sterker M, Bettin S, et al. Mortality of space-occupying ('malignant') middle cerebral artery infarction under conservative intensive care. Intensive Care Med 1998;24(6):620–3.

25. Hacke W, Schwab S, Horn M, et al. 'Malignant' middle cerebral artery territory infarction-Clinical course and prognostic signs. Arch Neurol 1996; 53(4):309–15.

26. Vahedi K, Hofmeijer J, Juettler E, et al. Early decompressive surgery in malignant infarction of the middle cerebral artery: a pooled analysis of three randomised controlled trials. Lancet Neurol 2007; 6(3):215–22.

27. Singer OC, Kurre W, Humpich MC, et al. Risk assessment of symptomatic intracerebral hemorrhage after thrombolysis using DWI-ASPECTS. Stroke 2009;40(8):2743–8.

28. Singer OC, Humpich MC, Fiehler J, et al. Risk for symptomatic intracerebral hemorrhage after thrombolysis assessed by diffusion-weighted magnetic resonance imaging. Ann Neurol 2008;63(1):52–60.

29. Albers GW, Thijs VN, Wechsle L, et al. Magnetic resonance imaging profiles predict clinical response to early reperfusion: the diffusion and perfusion imaging evaluation for understanding stroke evolution (DEFUSE) study. Ann Neurol 2006;60(5):508–17.

30. Yoo AJ, Verduzco LA, Schaefer PW, et al. MRI-based selection for intra-arterial stroke therapy value of pretreatment diffusion-weighted imaging lesion volume in selecting patients with acute stroke who will benefit from early recanalization. Stroke 2009; 40(6):2046–54.

31. Kidwell CS, Saver JL, Mattiello J, et al. Thrombolytic reversal of acute human cerebral ischemic injury shown by diffusion/perfusion magnetic resonance imaging. Ann Neurol 2000;47(4):462–9.

32. Kohno K, Hoehnberlage M, Mies G, et al. Relationship between diffusion-weighted MR-Images, Cerebral

Blood-Flow, and Energy-State in experimental brain infarction. Magn Reson Imaging 1995;13(1):73–80.

33. Guadagno JV, Jones PS, Fryer TD, et al. Local relationships between restricted water diffusion and oxygen consumption in the ischemic human brain. Stroke 2006;37(7):1741–8.

34. Guadagno JV, Warburton EA, Jones PS, et al. How affected is oxygen metabolism in DWI lesions? A combined acute stroke PET-MR study. Neurology 2006;67(5):824–9.

35. Olivot JM, Mlynash M, Thijs VN, et al. Relationships between cerebral perfusion and reversibility of acute diffusion lesions in DEFUSE insights from RADAR. Stroke 2009;40(5):1692–7.

36. Belliveau JW, Rosen BR, Kantor HL, et al. Functional cerebral imaging by susceptibility-contrast NMR. Magn Reson Med 1990;14(3):538–46.

37. Schellinger PD, Jansen O, Fiebach JB, et al. Monitoring intravenous recombinant tissue plasminogen activator thrombolysis for acute ischemic stroke with diffusion and perfusion MRI. Stroke 2000;31(6):1318–28.

38. Christensen S, Mouridsen K, Wu O, et al. Comparison of 10 perfusion MRI parameters in 97 sub-6-hour stroke patients using voxel-based receiver operating characteristics analysis. Stroke 2009;40(6):2055–61.

39. Kane I, Carpenter T, Chappell F, et al. Comparison of 10 different magnetic resonance perfusion imaging processing methods in acute ischemic stroke: effect on lesion size, proportion of patients with diffusion/perfusion mismatch, clinical scores, and radiologic outcomes. Stroke 2007;38(12):3158–64.

40. Davis SM, Donnan GA, Parsons MW, et al. Effects of alteplase beyond 3 h after stroke in the Echoplanar Imaging Thrombolytic Evaluation Trial (EPITHET): a placebo-controlled randomised trial. Lancet Neurol 2008;7(4):299–309.

41. Olivot JM, Mlynash M, Thijs VN, et al. Optimal Tmax threshold for predicting penumbral tissue in acute stroke. Stroke 2009;40(2):469–75.

42. Takasawa M, Jones PS, Guadagno JV, et al. How reliable is perfusion MR in acute stroke? Validation and determination of the penumbra threshold against quantitative PET. Stroke 2008;39(3):870–7.

43. Mlynash M, De Silva DA, Lansberg MG, et al. Optimal definition of the malignant profile in the DEFUSE-EPITHET pooled database. Stroke 2010;41(4):e8.

44. Culebras A, Kase CS, Masdeu JC, et al. Practice guidelines for the use of imaging in transient ischemic attacks and acute stroke. A report of the stroke council, American heart association. Stroke 1997;28(7):1480–97.

45. Ringleb P, Schellinger PD, Hacke W. European Stroke Organisation 2008 guidelines for managing acute cerebral infarction or transient ischemic attack. Part 1. Nervenarzt 2008;79(8):936–57.

46. Kakuda W, Lansberg MG, Thijs VN, et al. Optimal definition for PWI/DWI mismatch in acute ischemic stroke patients. J Cereb Blood Flow Metab 2008; 28(6):1272.

47. Albers GW, Mlynash M, Lansberg MG, et al. The geography of the ischemic core and penumbra: fried egg or Archipelago? Stroke 2009;40(4): E162.

48. Ma H, Zavala JA, Teoh H, et al. Penumbral mismatch is underestimated using standard volumetric methods and this is exacerbated with time. J Neurol Neurosurg Psychiatry 2009;80(9):991–6.

49. Olivot JM, Mlynash M, Thijs VN, et al. Geography, structure, and evolution of diffusion and perfusion lesions in diffusion and perfusion imaging evaluation for understanding stroke evolution (DEFUSE). Stroke 2009;40(10):3245–51.

50. Olivot JM, Mlynash M, Thijs VN, et al. Relationships between infarct growth, clinical outcome, and early recanalization in diffusion and perfusion imaging for understanding stroke evolution (DEFUSE). Stroke 2008;39(8):2257–63.

51. Furlan AJ, Eyding D, Albers GW, et al. Dose escalation of desmoteplase for acute ischemic stroke (DEDAS): evidence of safety and efficacy 3 to 9 hours after stroke onset. Stroke 2006;37(5):1227–31.

52. Hacke W, Albers G, Al-Rawi Y, et al. The Desmoteplase In Acute Ischemic Stroke Trial (DIAS): a phase II MRI-based 9-hour window acute stroke thrombolysis trial with intravenous desmoteplase. Stroke 2005;36(1):66–73.

53. Hacke W, Furlan AJ, Al-Rawi Y, et al. Intravenous desmoteplase in patients with acute ischaemic stroke selected by MRI perfusion-diffusion weighted imaging or perfusion CT (DIAS-2): a prospective, randomised, double-blind, placebo-controlled study. Lancet Neurol 2009;8(2):141–50.

MR Perfusion Imaging in Acute Ischemic Stroke

William A. Copen, MD[a,b,]*, Pamela W. Schaefer, MD[a,c],
Ona Wu, PhD[b,c]

KEYWORDS

- Stroke • Brain ischemia • Magnetic resonance imaging
- Cerebrovascular circulation

When magnetic resonance (MR) imaging–based techniques for studying brain perfusion were developed in the 1980s and 1990s,[1] one of the first pathologic conditions to which they were applied was ischemic stroke, a disease that is caused fundamentally by impaired perfusion. Like the positron emission tomography (PET) and single-photon emission computed tomography (SPECT)-based methods that preceded it, MR perfusion imaging of acute stroke patients offered a window into a rapidly evolving disease process, in which changes in tissue perfusion may have dramatic effects on patient outcomes. MR-based perfusion-weighted imaging allowed perfusion measurements to be obtained more quickly than with PET or SPECT, and with scanners that were more widely available.

Interest in imaging perfusion rapidly was spurred by the US Food and Drug Administration's 1996 approval of intravenous tissue plasminogen activator (tPA), a thrombolytic drug whose purpose is restore brain perfusion, but which was approved for use only in those very few acute stroke patients who can be treated within 3 hours of symptom onset. Because tPA offers both the potential for life-saving rescue of underperfused tissue and the risk of catastrophic intracranial hemorrhage, the most active focus of research on MR perfusion imaging in acute stroke has been its potential application in refining the selection of patients for thrombolysis. However, perfusion imaging also has other potential roles in ischemic cerebrovascular disease, including establishing diagnosis, predicting prognosis, and guiding nonthrombolytic therapies designed to maintain cerebral perfusion.

Before addressing MR perfusion imaging's potential uses in these roles, this review first discusses the ways in which the various perfusion parameters that can be measured by perfusion imaging vary under different hemodynamic conditions. The following section presents the computational techniques that are used to create the various kinds of clinically used MR perfusion images. Although the details of these techniques and the artifacts that they may create are often overlooked in discussions of perfusion imaging, understanding them is essential to integrating the results of past research on MR perfusion imaging, and to using perfusion imaging in patient care.

Drs Copen and Schaefer have no disclosures. Ona Wu has a patent on "Delay-compensated calculation of tissue blood flow," US Patent 7,512,435. March 31, 2009, and the patent has been licensed to General Electric, Siemens, and Olea Medical.

This work was supported in part by grant R01 NS059775 from the National Institutes of Health.

[a] Department of Radiology, Division of Neuroradiology, Massachusetts General Hospital, GRB-273A, 55 Fruit Street, Boston, MA 02114, USA

[b] MGH/MIT/HMS Athinoula A. Martinos Center for Biomedical Imaging, 149 Thirteenth Street, Suite 2301, Charlestown, MA 02129, USA

[c] Department of Radiology, Harvard Medical School, 25 Shattuck Street, Boston, MA 02115, USA

* Corresponding author. Department of Radiology, Division of Neuroradiology, Massachusetts General Hospital, GRB-273A, 55 Fruit Street, Boston, MA 02114.

E-mail address: wcopen@partners.org

THE HEMODYNAMICS OF ISCHEMIC STROKE

The changes in perfusion that occur in acute stroke are driven fundamentally by global and/or regional changes in cerebral perfusion pressure (CPP).[2] CPP is the difference between mean arterial pressure and venous pressure, the latter of which is usually equal to intracranial pressure. The cerebral vasculature responds to small reductions in CPP by dilating small arteries, thereby reducing cerebrovascular resistance, and successfully maintaining normal cerebral blood flow (CBF) over a wide range of perfusion pressures.[3] This vasodilatory response results in an increase in cerebral blood volume (CBV),[4] which is the volume of the intravascular space within a particular volume of brain tissue, such as that within a single image voxel. The increase in CBV may be subtle and difficult to detect in MR perfusion images. Vasodilation also results in an increase in mean transit time (MTT), which is the average amount of time that red blood cells spend within a particular volume of tissue. CBF, CBV, and MTT are related via the central volume theorem[5]:

$$MTT = \frac{CBV}{CBF}$$

When CPP drops below the threshold at which the brain maintains autoregulation, the compensatory vasodilatory response is overwhelmed. CBF begins to decrease, and becomes pressure-dependent, that is, further reductions in CPP lead to worsening decreases in CBF. Although this reflects a decrease in the rate of oxygen delivery to the capillary bed, metabolic compromise can be avoided if CBF is only mildly reduced, because of the effect of MTT prolongation on oxygen extraction. When MTT is increased, red blood cells spend a longer time within oxygen-permeable capillaries, and this allows for an increase in the proportion of the available oxygen that can be extracted from the blood by the brain (oxygen extraction fraction, or OEF). If the CBF reduction is mild, the increase in OEF is sufficient to maintain oxygen metabolism (cerebral metabolic rate of oxygen consumption, CMRO2), and neither the brain's electrical function nor its viability is threatened.[6] This level of hypoperfusion has been called "benign oligemia,"[7] although that term has also been used to refer less specifically to any underperfused state that does not threaten tissue viability, regardless of whether electrical function is preserved.[8]

With even further reductions in CPP, CBF falls so low that increased oxygen extraction is unable to maintain normal oxygen metabolism, and CMRO2 falls. With a sufficient reduction in CMRO2, neurons cease their electrical transmission, and the patient may experience a neurologic deficit. If the CMRO2 reduction is mild enough, the survival of the tissue is not threatened, despite its electrical silence, and this situation can persist indefinitely without permanent damage. If there is an even more severe reduction in CPP, and therefore an even greater reduction in CBF, CMRO2 falls to such a low level that the survival of the affected tissue is threatened. One of the most important principles of ischemic pathophysiology is that the time that it takes for ischemic damage to become irreversible is inversely related to the severity of the ischemia.[9] Brain tissue dies after just a few minutes without any blood flow, but moderately ischemic tissue may remain potentially viable for hours before becoming irreversibly injured. A primary goal of perfusion imaging in acute stroke is the identification of tissue that may be a target for thrombolytic therapy, in that it is threatened by ischemia, but still may be potentially salvageable. Tissue that is still structurally intact and hence viable but electrically dysfunctional has been called the "ischemic penumbra,"[10] with the word "penumbra" chosen because the mildly ischemic tissue sometimes forms a ring-like shape, surrounding a central area ("infarct core") where more severe ischemia has resulted in irreversible injury. It has been suggested that the term can be more usefully redefined to describe tissue that is potentially therapeutically treatable.[11]

It has been proposed[2] that, in conditions of extremely low CPP, low CBV may occur despite maximal vascular relaxation, perhaps because perfusion pressure is so low that the patency of blood vessels cannot be maintained. However, the early studies on which current understanding of cerebral hemodynamics is based offer little direct evidence of the occurrence of decreased CBV. These studies focused more often on the CBV/CBF ratio (ie, MTT), rather than CBV itself.[2] When early studies did measure CBV within infarcts, they often found that CBV was elevated, although these measurements were usually made in subacute infarcts that were days to weeks in age.[12–14] One study found that in an experimental model, macrovascular and microvascular CBV became uncoupled in response to severe hypotension, with macrovascular CBV increasing in some anatomic regions while microvascular CBV decreased.[15]

If the arterial lesion that caused ischemia resolves, either spontaneously or as a result of treatment, the affected tissue is reperfused. Reperfusion can occur in both viable and nonviable tissue, and therefore the absence of any apparent hypoperfusion does not preclude the existence of completed infarction. Reperfusion is the goal of thrombolytic therapy, and it also has been seen spontaneously within

8 hours of stroke onset in 16% of patients,[16] within 48 hours of onset in 33% of patients,[17] and within 1 week of onset in 42% to 60% of patients.[18,19] When reperfusion occurs, either spontaneously or as a result of therapeutic intervention, resistance vessels within the previously ischemic tissue sometimes remain inappropriately dilated for hours to days, despite reestablishment of normal CPP.[20] In this situation, CBV remains high, and CBF is elevated to above-normal levels. Various studies have reported that this state of postischemic hyperperfusion may occur in tissue that both has and has not undergone irreversible infarction.[21,22] In either case, blood flow is greater than required for the tissue's metabolic needs, a situation that has been called "luxury perfusion."[23]

Table 1 lists the effects of different hemodynamic conditions on the 3 physiologic parameters that are most often measured with perfusion imaging: CBV, CBF, and MTT. **Table 1** also includes the changes that are most often seen in various nonphysiologic "timing parameters" that can be measured with perfusion imaging. In acute stroke, perfusion imaging is capable of defining perfusion conditions in different parts of the brain as apparently normal, or assigning them to one of the four abnormal categories listed in **Table 1**: delayed bolus arrival with preserved CPP, compensated low CPP, underperfused, or postischemic hyperperfusion. Of note, irreversibly injured tissue can exist in any of these four categories, and can also exhibit apparently normal perfusion.

DYNAMIC SUSCEPTIBILITY CONTRAST IMAGING: BASIC PHYSICS AND IMAGE ACQUISITION

Because currently available techniques quantify the passage of blood through vessels that are too small to visualize directly with standard clinical MR imaging scanners, MR perfusion imaging must rely on detection of tracer agents within blood, rather than direct visualization of the vessels. This review focuses on dynamic susceptibility contrast (DSC) imaging, the technique that is used for MR perfusion imaging of acute stroke in most clinical centers. Arterial spin labeling (ASL)[24] is another technique for measuring perfusion without requiring exogenous contrast agents, which currently is rarely used in acute stroke imaging, because of its low signal-to-noise ratio, relatively long imaging times, and its difficulty in distinguishing between reduced blood flow and delayed transit times. Ongoing research seeks to eliminate artifacts, and ASL offers great potential for the future.

DSC uses a gadolinium chelate as an exogenous contrast agent. Although conventional contrast-enhanced MR imaging relies on the T1 effects of gadolinium to detect increased permeability of the blood-brain barrier, in DSC image contrast is based instead on gadolinium's susceptibility effect,[25] because the T1 relaxivity effect of gadolinium extends over extremely short distances. If the blood-brain barrier is intact, as is usually the case in acute stroke, only the approximately 1% to 7% of water spins that are also within blood vessels[26] would experience an appreciable change in T1 relaxation, and the pulse sequence's ability to detect small changes in local concentrations of gadolinium would be limited. However, the susceptibility effect of gadolinium ions inside of blood vessels extends over a range that is comparable in magnitude to the radius of the blood vessel, which is many orders of magnitude larger than gadolinium's T1 effects. Therefore, all water spins within a voxel may be affected by the presence of the gadolinium, and the resulting signal change is much larger than the signal change that would have been caused by T1 effects.

In DSC, susceptibility-sensitive images are acquired dynamically during the passage of a gadolinium-based contrast agent through the brain. As the contrast agent arrives in the brain and then washes out again, first the large arteries demonstrate a transient loss in signal intensity, followed by transient parenchymal signal loss as the contrast agent moves through smaller vessels, and then finally signal loss in the large intracranial veins (**Fig. 1**). To create high-quality perfusion maps, the passage of contrast agent in each part of the brain must be measured with high temporal resolution. Ideally, images should be obtained no less frequently than one every 1.5 seconds for human stroke imaging, assuming a normal MTT

Table 1
Distinguishing abnormal perfusion states using perfusion imaging

	CBV	CBF	MTT	Timing Parameters (eg, Tmax)
Delayed arrival, preserved CPP	—	—	—	↑
Compensated low CPP	↑	—	↑	↑
Underperfused	↑↓	↓	↑↓	↑
Postischemic hyperperfusion	↑	↑	↑↓	↑↓ (usually ↓)

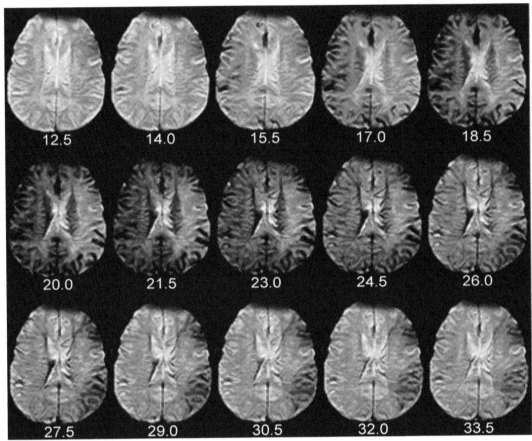

Fig. 1. Dynamic susceptibility contrast (DSC) perfusion imaging. The number of seconds elapsed since the beginning of contrast injection appears beneath each image. Note the appearance of contrast in some large arteries, which become hypointense and "bloom" slightly, at 14.0 and 15.5 seconds postinjection (ie, 24.0 and 25.5 seconds after the beginning of the scan). By 20.0 seconds postinjection, the presence of gadolinium in small vessels causes loss of parenchymal signal intensity in the normally perfused right hemisphere. Arrival of contrast is delayed and prolonged in the left hemisphere. These perfusion source images were used to create the graph and CBV maps in **Figs. 8** and **9**, respectively.

of approximately 3 to 4 seconds.[27] This is generally accomplished using an echo planar imaging (EPI) pulse sequence, which permits acquisition of an entire image slice with only a single radiofrequency excitation. Either spin-echo (SE) or gradient-echo (GRE) EPI images can be used. However, because SE EPI images are less sensitive to gadolinium's susceptibility effects, using a SE EPI pulse sequence at 1.5 T requires injecting a larger dose of the contrast agent, typically 0.2 mmol/kg, while a standard dose of 0.1 mmol/kg is usually sufficient for GRE EPI imaging. However, because susceptibility effects are more pronounced at higher field strengths, the standard dose of 0.1 mmol/kg may be sufficient for SE EPI perfusion imaging at field strengths of 3 T or higher. Nevertheless, GRE imaging is performed more often than SE imaging at all field strengths. The pulse sequence parameters used at the authors' institution are listed in **Table 2**. All of the examples depicted in this review were generated using these parameters.

The physical basis of image contrast in DSC results in several noteworthy properties of the perfusion maps produced by DSC. First, DSC's sensitivity to changes in precession frequency of all of the spins within each brain voxel gives the technique far greater sensitivity for detecting changes in contrast agent concentration than computed tomography (CT) perfusion imaging, which relies on the x-ray attenuation of an iodine-based contrast agent that remains within the intravascular space (**Fig. 2**). CT perfusion postprocessing algorithms usually compensate for the far greater noise level within their source images by performing spatial and temporal

Table 2
Sample imaging parameters for MR perfusion imaging

Pulse sequence	Gradient echo, echo-planar
Orientation	Axial
Phase-encoding direction	Anterior-posterior
Repetition time/echo time/flip angle	1500 ms/40 ms/60 degrees
Field of view	22 cm
Matrix size	128×128
Slice thickness/ interslice gap	5 mm/1 mm
Number of slices	As many as permitted by scanner at TR = 1500 milliseconds (approximately 14)
Number of acquisitions	80
Pulse sequence duration:	2 minutes
Contrast material	Gadopentatate dimeglumine, 20 mL, injected intravenously at 5 mL/s, beginning 10 seconds after initiation of the scan. Following the contrast agent injection, 20 mL of normal saline is injected at the same rate.

blurring, which is not usually done in DSC post-processing. Second, unlike CT perfusion imaging, which is equally sensitive to the presence of the contrast agent within vessels of all sizes, DSC produces different degrees of signal change for similar quantities of gadolinium in blood vessels of different sizes.[28] GRE EPI is more sensitive to contrast agent in larger vessels, whereas SE EPI demonstrates greater sensitivity to contrast agent in smaller vessels. Some DSC pulse sequences exploit this vessel-size sensitivity by acquiring both SE and GRE images during the same contrast injection, enabling elementary measurements of the relative proportions of smaller and larger blood vessels. Although this interleaved technique has shown promise in assessing neo-vascularity within brain tumors,[29] it is not generally used in acute stroke imaging. However, findings in animal models suggest that combining GRE-based and SE-based perfusion imaging may provide improved insight into tissue status after stroke.[15]

DYNAMIC SUSCEPTIBILITY CONTRAST IMAGING: MEASUREMENT OF PERFUSION PARAMETERS
Overview

Direct inspection of DSC images can yield rudimentary information about regional brain perfusion, and this approach is sometimes useful when severe patient motion precludes additional postprocessing. However, under most circumstances, individual DSC images like those in **Fig. 1** undergo additional postprocessing to produce maps of various perfusion-related parameters, in which each pixel's value reflects a single scalar measurement that is derived from the signal intensity-versus-time function for the corresponding voxel. It is these maps that are interpreted in the clinical setting. Many different perfusion measurements can be derived from DSC images, but five are most commonly used: time to peak contrast concentration (TTP), CBV, CBF, MTT, and time at which the deconvolved residue function reaches its maximum value (Tmax).

Examples of these five perfusion maps, illustrating each of the 4 abnormal perfusion conditions listed in **Table 1**, are presented in **Figs. 3–6**. As is evident from these examples, the various kinds of perfusion maps vary greatly in appearance, and they provide vastly different information about brain perfusion.[30] Nevertheless, it has become commonplace for published stroke imaging articles to refer to these maps generically as "perfusion imaging," and this has led to considerable confusion and inconsistency. Confusion surrounding the different types of perfusion maps is exacerbated by the fact that although most of these perfusion maps (specifically CBV, CBF, and MTT) ostensibly depict well-defined fundamental physiologic parameters, detailed examination of the algorithms that are used to compute them reveals several major technique-dependent artifacts. To best understand the use of perfusion imaging in the care of stroke patients, it is important to understand in some detail the postprocessing techniques that are used to create each kind of perfusion map, and the artifacts that they may introduce.

Time to Peak Concentration

Of the five parameters that are discussed here, TTP is the simplest to calculate and provides the least specific information about brain perfusion. In each voxel, TTP is the time at which signal intensity reaches its minimum, and therefore contrast concentration reaches its maximum. For example, for a particular DSC acquisition in which images are acquired every 1.5 seconds, possible TTP

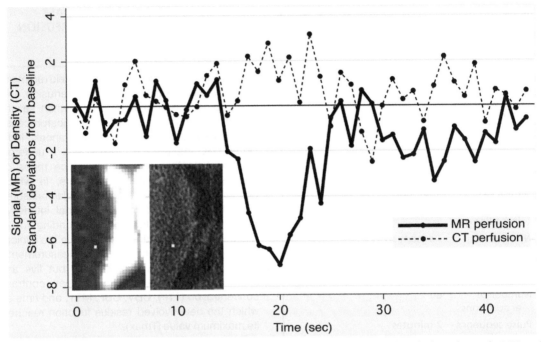

Fig. 2. Comparison of MR and CT perfusion imaging. A 59-year-old man presented with slurred speech. DWI and CT angiography were normal, and the patient was subsequently diagnosed with ethanol intoxication. MR perfusion imaging (MRP) was performed 17 minutes after CT perfusion imaging (CTP). Identically sized regions of interest were placed on MRP (left inset, 1 × 1 pixel) and CTP (right inset, 4 × 4 pixels) source images in a randomly selected location in the right corona radiata. The graph shows MR signal intensity and CT density as a function of time, with both expressed in terms of standard deviations above or below the mean value obtained from baseline images acquired before the arrival of the contrast bolus. Note the much larger signal change observed with MRP compared with the changes observed with CTP, which are barely discernible from random noise fluctuations.

values could include 20.0 seconds, 21.5 seconds, 23.0 seconds, and so forth.

Numerous studies have used increases in regional TTP for putative identification of brain tissue that is threatened by ischemia,[31–38] including one clinical trial that used diffusion-weighted imaging (DWI)-TTP mismatch to select patients for intravenous thrombolytic therapy outside of the usual 3-hour time window.[39] The advantages of TTP in this role are that lesions in TTP maps are conspicuous and usually well defined, and that TTP is a reproducible technique, in that measurements obtained by different centers from a single data set are similar, with fewer technique-dependent artifacts to complicate interpretation. TTP is very sensitive to motion artifacts and noise, so some algorithms that perform motion correction and prefiltering will produce differing results. Some algorithms also perform curve fitting to obtain TTP. A primary disadvantage of using TTP is that TTP can be prolonged in a wide variety of acute and chronic hemodynamic conditions, in which tissue viability may or may not be threatened. As shown in **Figs. 3–5** and **Fig. 7**, TTP prolongation may be caused by reduced blood flow, but also occurs when the arrival of the injected contrast bolus is delayed, but CBF is normal. In some circumstances, TTP may even be prolonged in reperfused tissue whose CBF is higher than normal, tissue whose survival clearly is no longer threatened by ischemia.

Converting Signal Changes to Concentration Measurements

Calculation of all of the four remaining perfusion parameters that are discussed here relies on a common first step: conversion of each voxel's signal intensity-versus-time curve into a contrast agent concentration-versus-time curve. To accomplish this conversion, the signal intensity-versus-time curve must be divided into two portions, reflecting signal intensity before and after arrival of the injected contrast bolus, respectively. Before bolus arrival, signal intensity fluctuates slightly, due to random noise, around a baseline value that is determined by time-invariant properties of the tissue within the voxel and the pulse sequence that is used. Preinjection points are typically averaged to produce an estimate of baseline signal

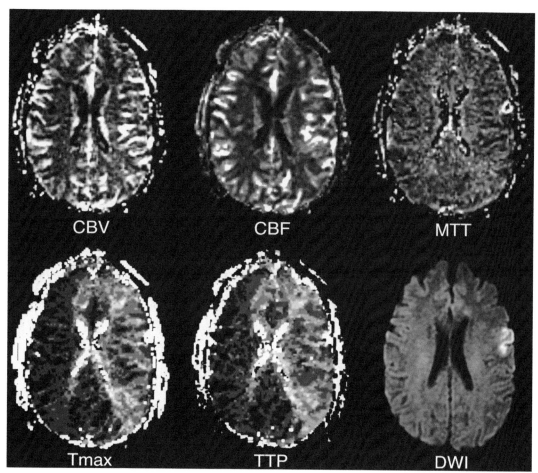

Fig. 3. Delayed bolus arrival with preserved CPP. Tmax and TTP maps reflect delayed bolus arrival in most of the left cerebral hemisphere. Although there is the suggestion of slightly elevated CBF in some of the involved tissue, which could represent postischemic hyperperfusion, CBV, CBF, and MTT otherwise appear normal. A corresponding DWI image is presented for reference.

intensity, S_0. Following the arrival of the bolus, the concentration of gadolinium in a voxel can be derived from signal intensity by the equation

$$C(t) = -k\ln\left(\frac{S_t}{S_0}\right)$$

in which $C(t)$ is the contrast agent concentration at a particular time t, S_t is the signal intensity at that time, S_0 is the baseline signal intensity before the arrival of the contrast agent, and k is a constant whose value depends on the pulse sequence used, the manner in which the contrast is injected, and complex characteristics of the patient's circulatory system that are difficult to model.[28] Because the value of k is difficult to estimate, absolute perfusion measurements are difficult to obtain, and most perfusion maps provide only relative quantification of perfusion parameters. Although techniques have been proposed for computing absolute measurements of CBF with MR perfusion

imaging, these measurements, like those obtained from CT perfusion imaging, typically vary by as much as a factor of 2 or 3, compared with those obtained by gold-standard methods such as xenon CT and PET.[40–51]

Cerebral Blood Volume

Of the remaining four perfusion parameters (CBV, CBF, MTT, and Tmax), calculation of CBV is the simplest, requiring the fewest additional computational steps. Although CBV was one of the first perfusion parameters to be derived from MR perfusion imaging in human stroke,[52] MR CBV maps historically have had little utility in acute stroke imaging, because the role that was presumptively assigned to them is better filled by DWI. The lesion seen on DWI is generally accepted to be the best available indicator of the irreversibly injured tissue in the infarct core. Several studies found that CBV

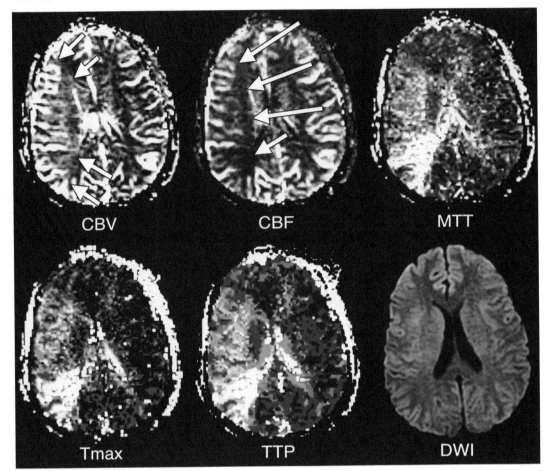

Fig. 4. Compensated low CPP. Elevated CBV (*arrows*) in the right middle cerebral artery territory reflects vasodi-lation in response to decreased CPP. The CBF map shows that this response has been successfully in maintaining apparently normal CBF (*arrows*). MTT is elevated in the affected tissue. The Tmax map shows delayed bolus arrival. TTP is prolonged, probably as a result of both delayed bolus arrival and increased MTT. A corresponding DWI image is presented for reference.

maps often demonstrated a low-CBV lesion whose volume was small, like that of the DWI lesion, and that the volumes of both lesions served well as a lower limit of the volume of the infarct that was ulti-mately seen in later follow-up images.[53–57] Because of these observations, it was suggested that CBV maps, like DWI, could be used to identify the infarct core. However, CBV maps were rarely used for this purpose in practice, because lesions in DWI images are far more conspicuous and clearly delineated than those in CBV maps. In addition, many of these studies used SE EPI for the data acquisition, which is more sensitive to smaller vessels that may manifest injury earlier than larger vessels, whereas currently the majority of clinical MR imaging centers use GRE EPI.

Interest in using CBV maps to define the infarct core increased greatly with the emergence of CT perfusion imaging. Although CT-based and MR-based techniques can provide similar perfu-sion maps, there is no CT equivalent for DWI, and so there is no accepted way to identify the infarct core without MR imaging. Some investigators have suggested that the core can be identified by CT-derived CBV maps, thereby obviating the need for DWI.[58] This practice implicitly accepts that the significant proportion of core tissue that experiences spontaneous reperfusion will not be identifiable as such, and that the diagnosis of stroke may be missed if the entire infarct has reperfused.[59] Even without reperfusion, the notion that CBV is reduced in the infarct core contradicts the physio-logic principle that blood vessels dilate in underper-fused tissue, in order to recruit additional blood flow. Although it has been hypothesized that CBV may drop when extremely low perfusion pressures cause vascular collapse, this phenomenon is poorly documented and its prevalence is unclear.

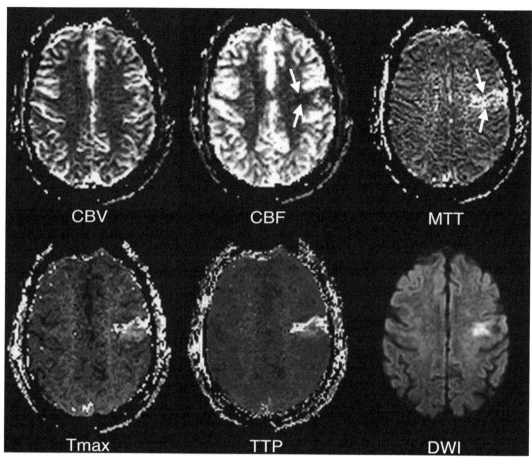

Fig. 5. Hypoperfusion. CBF is decreased within a small wedge-shaped region in the left middle cerebral artery territory (*arrows*). There is a corresponding region of MTT prolongation (*arrows*). Tmax and TTP maps, as well as a DWI image, also show corresponding abnormalities.

The apparent contradiction between MR-based and CT-based findings of reduced CBV in the infarct core, and theoretical and empirical predictions of elevated CBV, may be explained by artifactual flow-weighting and delay-weighting that are introduced by the algorithms used to calculate CBV. CBV theoretically can be calculated by integrating the area under the contrast agent concentration-versus-time curve, $C(t)$, for the first pass of the injected contrast bolus through each voxel. However, measuring just the first pass is difficult, because recirculation usually results in the arrival of the second pass before the first pass is complete, and the two passes therefore are summed together in the measured $C(t)$. Some researchers have attempted to extract the first pass of the contrast bolus by fitting gamma variates[60] or other functions[61] to the first portion of $C(t)$. However, no particular model has been shown to reflect the first pass reliably.

Because of these challenges, CBV is usually calculated by numerically integrating the area under the entire $C(t)$. This method produces truly accurate CBV measurements only for infinitely long scan durations because, as the time postinjection approaches infinity, contrast agent concentration in all parts of the brain approaches steady state. However, actual MR perfusion scans have finite durations, typically on the order of 60 seconds. During that time, the contrast agent concentration-versus-time curves in different parts of the brain may reflect different numbers of passes of the contrast agent. Specifically, in regions where the arrival of the contrast bolus is delayed, and/or low regional CBF results in a slower rate of arrival of the contrast bolus, $C(t)$ is effectively truncated. Fewer passes of the contrast bolus will be recorded in a particular finite time period, and CBV will be underestimated, in comparison to other parts of the brain. In effect, CBV maps produced by this method are flow-weighted and delay-weighted.

Unfortunately, bolus arrival delay and decreased blood flow are common phenomena in acute stroke. When an injected contrast agent bolus

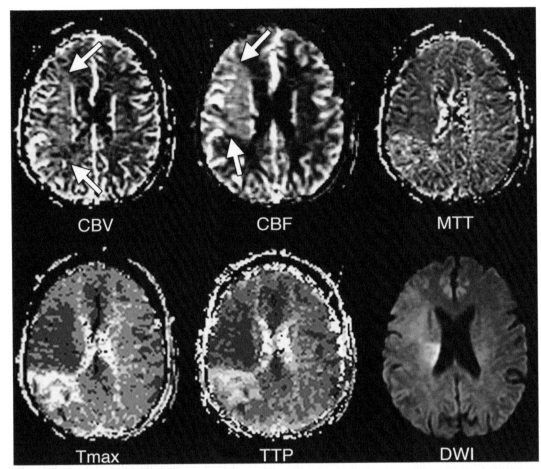

Fig. 6. Postischemic hyperperfusion. CBV is slightly elevated (*arrows*) in most of the right middle cerebral artery territory, reflecting vasodilation. In most of this tissue, CBF is higher than normal (*arrows*), demonstrating the vasodilation has persisted following an ischemic insult. MTT in this tissue may be minimally decreased in the hyperperfused tissue, although normal or elevated MTT are sometimes seen in such conditions. The Tmax map shows that bolus arrival is early in the hyperperfused tissue, although normal or (rarely) delayed arrival also can be seen in postischemic hyperperfusion. Postischemic hyperperfusion can occur in tissue that did or did not experience irreversible injury, as shown by the DWI image, in which some but not all of the hyperperfused tissue appears abnormal. Note that there is a persistently underperfused region posterior to the hyperperfused area.

reaches brain tissue via a pathologically narrowed artery, or via long collateral perfusion pathways, its arrival is delayed, and CBV is therefore underestimated. If the arterial lesion is severe enough to cause a CBF reduction, this too will cause underestimation of CBV. This artifact is mitigated by longer scan durations, and is exacerbated by shorter scan durations (**Fig. 8**). Some centers have employed scans as short as 40 seconds, which usually is not long enough even to completely sample the first pass of the bolus in tissue with low CBF.

Truncation of $C(t)$ by short scan durations can produce artifactually large low-CBV lesions (**Fig. 9**), and may produce apparent low-CBV lesions

where low CBV does not actually exist (**Fig. 10**). One recent study[62] found that within DWI-delineated infarct cores, calculated CBV increased with increasing duration of the perfusion scan. When the longest scan duration of 110 seconds following contrast injection was used, the majority of infarcts demonstrated above-normal CBV. This study demonstrated that CBV measurements are technique-dependent, producing lesions whose presence and size are dependent on scan duration and postprocessing algorithms. When low CBV is truly present, this is likely to reflect microvascular collapse that indicates ischemia so severe that tissue viability is unlikely. However, it appears that many apparent low-CBV lesions in acute stroke

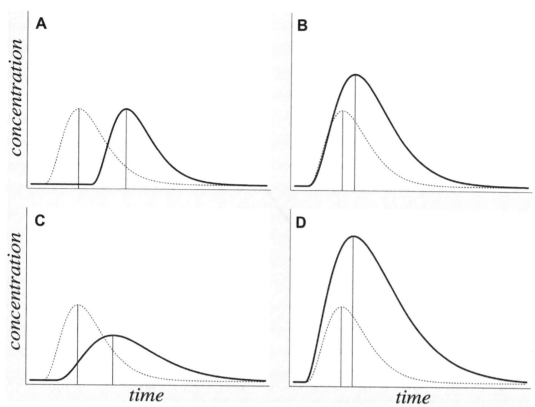

Fig. 7. TTP delay in varying hemodynamic conditions. Theoretical concentration-versus-time curves (*solid lines*) reflect the four different abnormal hemodynamic conditions listed in Table 1: (*A*) delayed bolus arrival with preserved CPP, (*B*) compensated low CPP, (*C*) hypoperfusion, and (*D*) postischemic hyperperfusion. In each case, a concentration-versus-time curve for normal tissue is presented for comparison (*dotted lines*). TTP (*vertical lines*) can be delayed (ie, farther to the right) in all 4 conditions.

may be artifactual, so that CBV cannot substitute for DWI in identifying the infarct core.

Cerebral Blood Flow

Of the major parameters derived from MR perfusion images, CBF is the most directly connected to tissue viability, because CBF measures the rate of delivery of oxygen and glucose to ischemic brain tissue. Seminal animal experiments demonstrated that CBF thresholds for tissue viability exist, with threatened tissue surviving for longer periods of time when CBF is more mildly reduced.[9] Furthermore, from a qualitative perspective, examination of Table 1 shows that of the major perfusion parameters, CBF is the only one that can reliably identify underperfused brain tissue, and distinguish it from tissue with normal or elevated blood flow. Nevertheless, CBF maps are seldom used to identify threatened brain tissue, and no major clinical trial to date has used CBF maps to select patients for experimental thrombolytic therapy.

The preference for using the less physiologically relevant TTP, MTT, and Tmax maps may be attributable to greater lesion conspicuity on these maps as compared with CBF maps. Like CBV maps, CBF maps demonstrate considerable heterogeneity in normal tissue, because CBV and CBF values are several times greater in gray matter than in white matter.[26] Consequently, it can be difficult to distinguish underperfused gray matter from normally perfused white matter. Lesions may also be difficult to detect in CBF and CBV maps because brain parenchyma must be distinguished from large blood vessels, which "bloom" in GRE perfusion maps, and appear larger than they actually are. By contrast, when TTP, MTT, and Tmax maps are used, gray matter–white matter differences are greatly reduced, and macroscopic blood vessels are reduced in conspicuity, resulting in lesions that are easier to detect and delineate.

Calculation of CBF is more complex than calculation of TTP and CBV. Roughly speaking, CBF in any voxel is related to the slope of increase of $C(t)$ as the contrast agent bolus arrives. Indeed, if

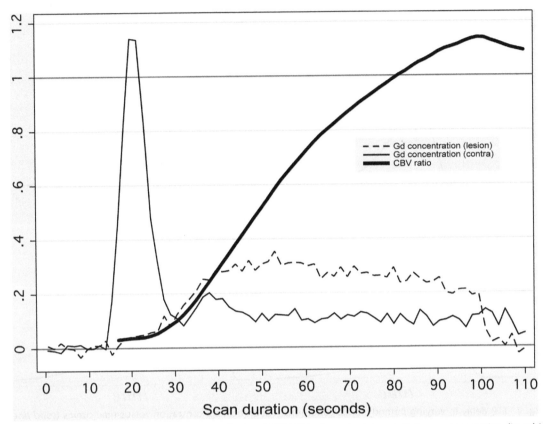

Fig. 8. Effect of perfusion scan duration on calculated CBV. Thin lines depict gadolinium concentration (in arbitrary units) versus time following contrast injection, within small regions of interest (ROIs) placed in an acute stroke patient's low-CBF lesion (*thin dashed line*), and in the corresponding location in the unaffected contralateral hemisphere (*thin solid line*). ROI locations are shown in **Fig. 9**. Because of low blood flow, the curve rises much more slowly in the low-CBF lesion. CBV in each ROI (not shown) is calculated as the area under the concentration-versus-time curve. Therefore, for simulated short scan durations, the ratio of CBV in the lesion to normal CBV (*thick solid line*) is far below unity. However, when longer, more accurate scan durations are used, the ratio rises above unity, showing that CBV is actually elevated in the low-CBF ROI.

images are acquired with greater temporal resolution than is currently feasible in most clinical settings, CBF can be calculated by measuring this slope.[63] However, in current practice, quantitative computation of CBF requires incorporation of the concentration-versus-time curve not just in the voxel but also in the arteries that supply blood to that voxel. In an idealized experiment, the contrast agent would be injected directly into a small artery supplying a tissue voxel, such that the concentration of contrast agent in the artery is a unit value for a single instant in time, and zero otherwise. If this could be achieved, then the observed $C(t)$ in the voxel would be a so-called residue function that reaches its maximum instantly, and decays gradually, reflecting the proportion of the contrast agent remaining in the vessel over time.

However, in reality the contrast agent is injected over several seconds, into a peripheral vein. The injected bolus must then pass through systemic veins, the heart, the pulmonary circulation, and systemic arteries before it arrives in the brain.[64,65] In the process, the duration of the bolus is further increased, and its $C(t)$ profile is reshaped in complex ways that are difficult to model. This bolus reshaping changes the concentration-versus-time function in the voxel, which is observable, but it does not change the residue function, which cannot be observed directly. Mathematically, the observed $C(t)$ is the *convolution* of the arterial input function (AIF), which describes the contrast agent concentration versus time in the artery supplying the voxel, and a multiple of the residue function in the voxel that has been scaled by the value of CBF (**Fig. 11**).

To compute CBF, an AIF is calculated by measuring $C(t)$ in voxels near an artery or arteries, and averaging those $C(t)$ functions. This process may be accomplished manually or automatically.[45,66–68]

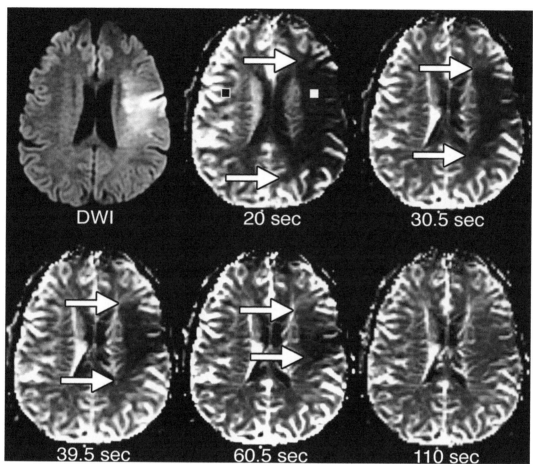

Fig. 9. Effect of perfusion scan duration on CBV maps. CBV maps were made from the perfusion data shown in Figs. 1 and 8. Maps were made using the entire scan, which lasted 110 seconds after contrast injection, as well as truncated data sets simulating the effects of shorter scan durations lasting 20, 30.5, 39.5, and 60.5 seconds after contrast injection. With the shortest scan duration of 20 seconds, there is a region of very low apparent CBV, which is much larger than the DWI lesion. With progressively longer scan durations, the size of the apparent CBV lesion shrinks. With the full 110-second scan duration, there is only a poorly delineated region of slightly reduced CBV that is considerably smaller than the DWI lesion.

After an AIF has been generated, *deconvolution* can be used to derive the scaled residue function in each voxel from the AIF and the voxel's C(t) function. The amplitude of the deconvolved signal is measured as the CBF, and the time at which this maximum value is reached, is called Tmax (see later discussion). From this description, it is apparent that a single MR perfusion data set could be processed by different centers to yield different CBF maps, depending on two factors: the deconvolution algorithm that is used and the AIF that is chosen. The deconvolution algorithm generally used for MR perfusion imaging is singular value decomposition (SVD), an algorithm that is model independent, in that it makes no assumptions regarding the shape of the AIF, residue function, or voxel concentration function.[69–71]

If scan duration is very short, and/or bolus arrival is highly delayed, the passage of the bolus may be inadequately sampled, and calculated CBF values will be artifactually low. Artifactual underestimation of CBF with short scan durations is less severe than underestimation of CBV, and occurs only at very short scan durations (see **Fig. 11**). However, the versions of the SVD algorithm that were used in the great majority of published research on stroke suffer from a different artifact: they artifactually underestimate CBF in regions where the arrival of the contrast bolus is delayed, relative to its arrival in the AIF.[72–74] One simulation found that bolus arrival delays of 1.5 to 2.0 seconds may result in underestimation of CBF by approximately 35%, with even greater underestimation also possible due to bolus dispersion.[72]

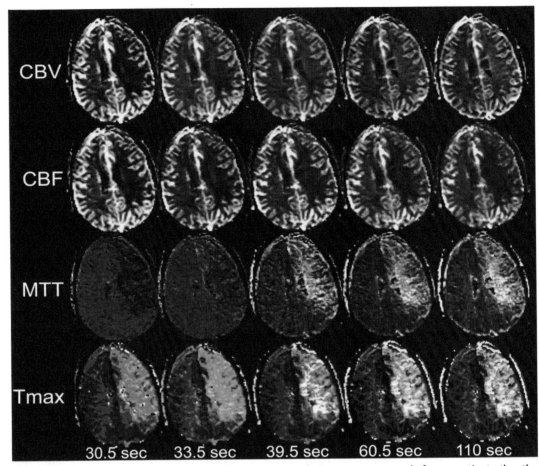

Fig. 10. Effects of scan duration on various perfusion maps. Perfusion maps were made from a patient other than those depicted in previous figures, using data from the entire scan lasting 110 seconds after contrast injection, as well as temporally truncated subsets of the data simulating shorter scan durations. With the shortest scan duration of 30.5 seconds, there is a large low-CBV lesion occupying most of the left cerebral hemisphere. The apparent severity of CBV reduction is decreased with the 33.5-second scan, and no CBV lesion is apparent with the 39.5-second scan. With the 60.5- and 110-second scans, it is apparent that CBV is mildly elevated in the left hemisphere. CBF is artifactually reduced with the 30.5-second scan, but does not change significantly in the longer scans. Because MTT is calculated as the quotient of CBV divided by CBF, the effect of scan duration on CBV results in apparently reduced MTT with the shortest scan duration, and no obvious MTT lesion at 33.5 seconds, although a large region of prolonged MTT is clearly evident with longer scan durations. Tmax is not significantly changed by scan duration. DWI (not shown) was normal in this part of the brain.

Unfortunately, delays of at least this magnitude are typical in tissue that is supplied by stenotic arteries. Therefore, such tissue will appear underperfused on CBF maps, even if CBF is actually preserved at a normal level by vasodilation and/or collateral circulation.

Several methods have been employed to overcome the delay artifact. One approach is to define the AIF by sampling arteries that are as close as possible to the infarct, distal to any proximal arterial lesions, in order to minimize delay between bolus arrival in the AIF and arrival in the tissue of interest.[75] A second approach is to use numerous "local AIFs" instead of a single global AIF. In the local AIF approach, the AIF for each voxel is constructed by searching in its immediate vicinity for other voxels whose concentration-versus-time curves seem most artery-like.[76–80] In theory, these local AIFs better approximate not only bolus arrival times, but the varying shapes of the actual AIFs in each voxel. However, in practice most voxels do not have a macroscopic artery that can be sampled within their immediate vicinity, so that generating a local AIF that truly

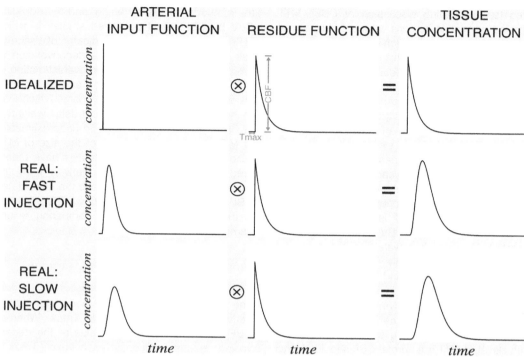

ARTERIAL INPUT FUNCTION   RESIDUE FUNCTION   TISSUE CONCENTRATION

Fig. 11. CBF, Tmax, and convolution. Each voxel has a "residue function" reflecting the proportion of an idealized, instantaneously injected unit-sized contrast bolus that remains in the voxel following its arrival. The tissue concentration function is the convolution of the arterial input function (which varies depending on complex variables such as contrast bolus injection rate, cardiac output, and patient anatomy), and a multiple of the residue function that has been scaled by the value of CBF. The amplitude of this scaled residue function is CBF, and the time at which it reaches its maximum is Tmax. The scaled residue function cannot be observed directly. If both the concentration function and an arterial input function are known, the scaled residue function can be calculated by deconvolution.

reflects arterial concentrations rather than tissue concentrations is technically complex.[81,82] The local AIF technique is not generally used in clinical practice.

Some postprocessing algorithms attempt to compensate for the arrival delay artifact by using a single global AIF, but shifting this AIF in time for each voxel, so that AIF arrival time matches the arrival of the bolus in the tissue.[83,84] Although this approach is used by some manufacturers of CT perfusion postprocessing software, in MR perfusion postprocessing, it has been largely supplanted by improved versions of the SVD algorithm that do not require curve shifting, because the techniques are insensitive to the delay artifact. One delay-insensitive SVD algorithm uses a block-circulant deconvolution matrix with oscillation index regularization.[85] This algorithm is sometimes known simply as "circular deconvolution"; however, using a block-circulant matrix for deconvolution without oscillation index regularization will likely underestimate normal to high flow rates, and precise description of the technique used is

important. There is increasing recognition of the potential importance of delay-compensated or delay-insensitive deconvolution in perfusion postprocessing.[27]

Mean Transit Time

MTT, like TTP, is frequently used in acute stroke imaging for putative identification of threatened brain tissue.[86–91] When MTT is used for this purpose, the region of DWI-MTT mismatch, like the region of DWI-TTP mismatch, is presumed to define tissue that is at risk. Like lesions in TTP maps, lesions in MTT maps are relatively easy to identify and delineate, because gray matter–white matter heterogeneity is minimized in MTT maps, and large vessels do not greatly impair lesion identification. MTT maps offer the advantage that they measure a parameter that is of more direct physiologic relevance, in that elevations in MTT reflect the autoregulatory response of the cerebral vasculature to a perceived drop in perfusion pressure. If a delay-insensitive deconvolution technique is used (see preceding discussion of CBF), MTT remains normal in regions where bolus arrival delay is delayed but perfusion is otherwise normal, and MTT is unlike TTP in this respect.

When MTT is used for identification of threatened tissue, it is sometimes stated that tissue with prolonged MTT is necessarily underperfused, which is a misconception. Although MTT prolongation occurs in regions of vasodilation with decreased CBF, MTT is also prolonged when vasodilation results in successful preservation of normal CBF. This situation can be appreciated by considering Table 1, and the relationship defined by the central volume theorem described earlier; if CBV is elevated but CBF is normal, then MTT, which is the quotient of CBV divided by CBF, is elevated. Tissue with elevated MTT but normal CBF may persist indefinitely in this state, without any threat to its survival, and this condition probably exists, for example, in many patients with chronic carotid stenosis. Nevertheless, although tissue metabolism remains normal if CBF is preserved, it is misleading to argue that tissue with elevated MTT but normal CBF should always be considered safe, for two reasons. First, if the vasodilation that leads to MTT elevation is caused by thromboembolic narrowing of a proximal artery, small emboli may break off of the main lesion and cause infarcts within the region of prolonged MTT. Second, preservation of normal CBF in regions of prolonged MTT often depends on collateral arterial supply, and collateral vessels may fail over time.

In light of these considerations, it is probably a reasonable approach to conclude that tissue with elevated MTT and reduced CBF is more severely and immediately threatened by ischemia, whereas tissue with elevated MTT but normal CBF experiences some smaller and perhaps less urgent degree of risk. Further complicating interpretation of MTT maps is the fact that MTT is sometimes prolonged in the setting of elevated CBF and elevated CBV, a condition that presumably does not pose any threat to tissue survival. In postischemic hyperperfusion, CBV and CBF are both elevated, and their quotient, MTT, may be either elevated or decreased, depending on which of CBV and CBF is the more elevated. Because tissue with elevated MTT may be at relatively high risk of infarction, low risk, or no risk, depending on the associated CBF value, it may be advisable to consult CBF maps when evaluating an MTT lesion.

In interpreting MTT maps, it is also worthwhile to consider how the algorithms that produce them may lead to artifacts. Postprocessing software usually generates an MTT value for each voxel by first computing CBV and CBF, using the methods described herein, and then dividing CBV by CBF. Most published studies in which MTT was evaluated as an indicator of tissue at risk have used delay-sensitive deconvolution to calculate CBF, which results in overestimation of MTT and overestimation of the size of the MTT lesion. Also, shorter perfusion scans, which lead to increasing flow-weighting and delay-weighting of CBV calculations, can lead to underestimation of MTT and underestimation of the size of MTT lesions (see Fig. 10). Other studies have measured MTT using parameters derived from the shape of the C(t) curve, and have then calculated CBF indirectly by dividing CBV by MTT.[92] Caution is therefore warranted when comparing results across studies.

Time of Maximum Value of the Residue Function

The third and final perfusion parameter that is derived from deconvolution is Tmax. Whereas CBF reflects the maximum value of the deconvolved residue function in each voxel, Tmax is the time at which this maximum value is reached. The value of Tmax therefore reflects bolus arrival time, with larger Tmax values reflecting later arrival of the injected contrast bolus in the voxel.

Tmax is a nonphysiological parameter, in that the viability of brain tissue presumably does not depend directly on how long it takes for blood to travel from the arm to the brain. Although high Tmax values have been correlated with lower likelihood of tissue survival,[93,94] Tmax may be prolonged in tissue with low, normal, or high CBF, and very large volumes of tissue may exhibit prolonged Tmax without proceeding to infarction.[95] Nevertheless, Tmax has been used as a predictor of tissue viability in various studies,[93,94,96,97] including two major trials testing the use of thrombolytic therapy outside of the usual 3-hour or 4.5-hour time windows.[98,99] Tmax has several advantages in this role. Like TTP and MTT maps, Tmax maps are relatively easy to interpret, with little gray matter–white matter heterogeneity, and relatively low conspicuity of large blood vessels that may complicate evaluation of brain parenchyma. Like TTP values, calculated Tmax values have discrete values that are equal to multiples of the TR that is used, and this often creates lesions that are easy to measure, because their boundaries are well defined. Tmax values are relatively unaffected by scan duration, provided the scan is long enough to detect the arrival of the contrast bolus in all parts of the brain (see Fig. 11). Some have speculated that Tmax is a reflection of extent of collateral perfusion.[100,101]

USING MR PERFUSION IMAGING IN PATIENT CARE

Diagnosis of Transient Ischemic Attack

DWI has become the gold standard for imaging detection of acute stroke, with sensitivity and specificity approaching 100%.[34,102–108] DWI's unique ability to confirm or exclude the diagnosis of stroke can be of critical importance, because the etiology of stroke-like symptoms is not always initially clear.[109] Establishing the diagnosis of cerebral ischemia can be especially difficult for transient ischemic attack (TIA) patients whose symptoms have resolved before the time of presentation, and therefore cannot be evaluated by physical examination. Correct diagnosis of TIA is critical because up to 17% of TIA patients suffer a stroke within 90 days of their TIA.[110–112] In approximately 44% of TIA patients, DWI shows an asymptomatic infarct that confirms the diagnosis.[113] Imaging of the major cervical arteries with ultrasonography, or with CT angiography or MR angiography, may also demonstrate stenosis that suggests a vascular origin. However, many TIAs, such as those due to cardiogenic emboli, can occur in patients without significant arterial pathology. In these patients, the presence of an abnormality on perfusion imaging may be the only objective indication of ischemic origin. In various studies, perfusion abnormalities have been found in between 3% and 25% of TIA patients who have no DWI abnormality.[114–116] It is likely that many of the patients in these studies would have been discharged home without a clear diagnosis if they had not undergone perfusion imaging, and therefore would have been deprived of a potentially life-saving admission for workup of their TIAs.

Selection of Patients for Thrombolysis

The most widely available treatment for acute stroke is recombinant tissue plasminogen activator (tPA), which can improve patients' outcomes by reperfusing and thereby rescuing ischemic tissue, but can also cause symptomatic intracranial hemorrhage (sICH). To maximize the potential for patients' benefit and minimize the risk of hemorrhage, tPA's use was initially restricted to patients who could be treated within three hours of the time when they were last known to be without symptoms. The particular choice of three hours as the time limit for tPA administration was based on the fact that the landmark 1995 National Institute of Neurological Disorders and Stroke (NINDS) trial[117] used a 3-hour limit and showed a benefit for tPA, whereas the European Cooperative Acute Stroke Study (ECASS)[118] used a 6-hour

limit and was not successful. The 3-hour cutoff was also supported by later thrombolysis trials that failed to show a benefit of thrombolysis when using 6-hour[119] or 5-hour[120] limits, as well as a 2007 retrospective study that confirmed that thrombolysis within three hours had been safe and effective in a large cohort.[121] A further refinement was provided in 2009, when the ECASS-III study[122] achieved success using a 4.5-hour window in a carefully selected stroke population, and this longer window consequently has been adopted by many centers.

The imposition of a strict time limit on thrombolytic therapy ignores the considerable variation that exists between individual stroke patients. In the aforementioned thrombolysis trials, the only imaging study that was required was a noncontrast CT scan, a study that is highly insensitive for acute stroke. It is likely that some patients who present only one hour after symptom onset have no remaining threatened tissue that could be rescued by thrombolysis, whereas some patients scanned eight hours after onset could still benefit from treatment. Furthermore, large numbers of patients are deemed ineligible for thrombolysis because the current time limit conservatively specifies that the patient must be treated within 3 or 4.5 hours of the time when he or she was last known to be without symptoms, not from the time when symptoms were discovered. Numerous patients are excluded from treatment because the exact stroke onset time cannot be ascertained with certainty, either because the patient's deterioration was not witnessed, or because the patient's symptoms were first noted when he or she awoke from sleep.[88,123] Only 1% to 7% of stroke patients receive thrombolytic therapy,[124–126] and the most common reason for ineligibility is inability to document the absence of symptoms within the required time window.[126,127]

MR perfusion imaging, when combined with DWI, offers the potential for customized patient-specific assessments of the potential risks and benefits of thrombolysis. This approach could allow for widening or even abandonment (see the article by Wu and colleagues elsewhere in this issue for further exploration of this topic) of the 3-hour or 4.5-hour time window, thereby making treatment available for vastly increased numbers of patients. Indeed, the search for a role for perfusion imaging in assessing eligibility for thrombolysis has formed one of the most active areas of research in MR perfusion imaging of acute stroke patients during recent years. Broadly speaking, this research has been guided by the following hypotheses. First, in an acute stroke MR imaging examination, the DWI lesion reflects the irreversibly injured infarct core. Second, the likelihood of infarct growth in the days following presentation can be predicted by perfusion imaging, because infarct expansion occurs into regions of moderately impaired perfusion that lie outside of the initial DWI lesion. Third, if the preceding hypotheses are correct, then the time window for thrombolytic therapy can be widened, provided that treatment is limited to those patients who have a significant mismatch between lesions in DWI and perfusion maps.

The first hypothesis is supported by observations that initially DWI-abnormal tissue usually proceeds to infarction in follow-up images, and that the volume of the early DWI lesion usually, though not always, is smaller than that of the ultimate infarct.[31,52,55–57,128,129] Some studies have contradicted this hypothesis by showing that reversal of DWI lesions can occur, usually in the setting of early vessel recanalization. In one such study,[96] six of seven patients demonstrated reversal of part of their DWI abnormalities following successful intra-arterial intervention with recanalization, although a subsequent increase in infarct volume was seen in three of those patients. In another study,[130] an ultimate reduction in the sizes of DWI lesions was seen in one of eleven patients whose infarcts did not recanalize, and in six of sixteen patients whose infarcts did recanalize. However, the median reduction in lesion size in this study was only 2.75 mL, and in some cases lesion size reduction may have been caused by encephalomalacic volume loss. A much larger study estimated the prevalence of DWI lesion reversal to be 0.2% to 0.4%.[131]

The second hypothesis, that perfusion imaging can be used to predict infarct growth, has received broad support from studies showing that infarct growth is more likely to occur in patients with a large mismatch between lesions seen in DWI images and those in perfusion maps, regardless of whether the perfusion parameter used is TTP,[31,33] CBF,[129] delay-sensitive MTT,[8,86,132] or, in one study, a nondeconvolution-based parameter that provided an estimate of MTT.[133] These results suggest that, even if thrombolytic therapy is not under consideration, perfusion imaging may help in prognostication by suggesting the possibility of impending clinical worsening.

The final hypothesis, that the therapeutic window can be safely widened if thrombolysis is offered only to patients with a mismatch between lesions seen in DWI and perfusion maps, has been addressed by a small number of clinical trials, all but one of which were successful. The first[39] was a non–placebo-controlled trial in which patients were made eligible for tPA between three and six hours after stroke onset if they demonstrated at

least a 50% DWI-TTP mismatch, as estimated by gross visual inspection at the scanner console at the time of imaging. The study's report did not specify whether DWI lesion size or TTP lesion size was used as the denominator in this calculation. Among the 43 patients who were treated in the extended time window, rates of recanalization, hemorrhagic transformation, and neurologic improvement were similar to those seen in 79 patients who were treated between zero and 3 hours after stroke onset, using standard selection criteria.

The Desmoteplase in Acute Ischemic Stroke (DIAS) trial[134] was a double-blind, dose-finding, placebo-controlled phase II study in which patients presenting between three and nine hours after stroke onset were treated either with the thrombolytic drug, desmoteplase, or with placebo, provided that they met certain imaging criteria. Among these criteria was a requirement that a perfusion map chosen by each site in accordance with local practices demonstrated a lesion that was at least 120% of the size of the DWI lesion, as estimated by visual inspection. Favorable outcomes were seen in 22.2% of placebo-treated patients and in 60.0% of patients treated with the highest of three desmoteplase doses. Similarly positive results were achieved by the Dose Escalation of Desmoteplase for Acute Ischemic Stroke (DEDAS) trial,[135] which used the 3- to 9-hour time window, the same thrombolytic drug, and the same imaging criteria.

In the Diffusion and Perfusion Imaging Evaluation for Understanding Stroke Evolution (DEFUSE) study,[98] patients were treated with tPA between three and six hours after stroke onset. Patients underwent DWI and MR perfusion imaging before treatment, but all patients in the study were treated, regardless of their MR imaging findings. Reperfusion was associated with improved clinical outcomes in patients who had a significant diffusion-perfusion mismatch. However, patients without mismatch did not appear to benefit from reperfusion. In this study, perfusion lesions were defined as regions in Tmax was at least 2 seconds. Significant mismatch was defined as the presence of a Tmax lesion whose size was at least 120% of the DWI lesion's size, and patients were included only if the Tmax lesion was at least 10 mL larger than the DWI lesion.

The Echoplanar Imaging Thrombolytic Evaluation Trial (EPITHET)[99] provided further evidence of the utility of perfusion imaging in expanding the therapeutic time window for thrombolysis. In EPITHET, as in DEFUSE, patients presenting between three and six hours of onset were randomized to receive either tPA or placebo. As in DEFUSE, patients underwent MR imaging before treatment, and MR imaging results were not used to select patients for treatment. Perfusion lesions were defined as in the DEFUSE trial. EPITHET's primary endpoint was assessing whether, in patients with significant DWI and perfusion lesion mismatch, tPA decreased infarct growth, compared to placebo. Although this mismatch-related and treatment-related effect reached statistical significance only if patients with DWI lesions smaller than 5 mL were excluded, the effect was significant across all patients when the data were reanalyzed using a definition of mismatch volume as the volume of tissue that was included in the Tmax lesion but not in the DWI lesion, as opposed to the prespecified definition, which was the difference between the Tmax and DWI lesions volumes.[136] Treatment was associated with a significantly greater likelihood of reperfusion, and reperfusion was associated with significantly less infarct growth and significantly better clinical outcomes.

DIAS-2[137] attempted to replicate the results of the phase II DIAS trial in a phase III study of 186 patients, by again demonstrating a clinical benefit from desmoteplase in imaging-selected patients who presented between three and nine hours after stroke onset. As in the earlier DIAS study, patients were included if they had at least a 20% mismatch between lesions presumed to represent infarct core and "penumbra." However, in DIAS-2, each site was free to follow local practice not only in choosing the method used to estimate the "penumbra," but also in choosing the method used to estimate the "core." In DIAS-2, unlike DIAS, some sites used CT rather than MR imaging, and therefore did not have access to DWI as an indicator of the infarct core. The DIAS-2 trial failed to show a benefit of treatment. This result was speculated to be due to milder stroke population enrolled in the DIAS-2 study, low prevalence of occlusion on MR angiography or CT angiography, and lower absolute mismatch volumes, compared with DIAS and DEDAS studies.

These six trials defined DWI-perfusion mismatch in different ways. The trials used different thresholds for mismatch, and measurements of different perfusion parameters, none of which was an indicator of underperfusion and none of which was mentioned in the studies' abstracts. Despite these differences, five of the six trials succeeded in showing a benefit of thrombolysis outside of the usual 3-hour or 4.5-hour time window. It is likely that further refinements in imaging-based selection of patients for thrombolysis, perhaps incorporating multiparametric tissue modeling for even more accurate assessment of tissue risk,[138,139] might allow for yet further expansion of the therapeutic window.

Preservation of Collateral Perfusion

In moderately underperfused tissue that is at risk of infarction, preservation of residual blood flow, and therefore of tissue viability, is dependent to a large degree on collateral vascular channels. In recent years, understanding of these collateral vessels has progressed, and there has been increased interest in therapeutic maneuvers that attempt to preserve or enhance the effectiveness of collateral perfusion. Techniques that may be used in the future for acute stroke treatment include external counterpulsation[140] and partial aortic occlusion,[141] which seek to augment collateral perfusion; and supplemental oxygen administration, which seeks to forestall irreversible injury by enhancing oxygen delivery when blood flow is compromised.[142] However, there is one technique for improving collateral circulation that is already in widespread use, namely, blood pressure management.

Most acute stroke patients have elevated blood pressure.[143,144] Although there are many possible causes for this it may be adaptive, in that it can increase blood flow via narrowed arteries and enhance the effectiveness of collateral vascular pathways, thereby preserving threatened brain tissue. For this reason, hypertension is often allowed to remain untreated in the setting of acute stroke,[145–148] and hypertension may even be induced or augmented by pressor medications.[149–151] However, elevated blood pressure in the setting of acute stroke may also contribute to malignant brain edema,[152] increase the likelihood of hemorrhagic transformation,[153,154] and cause serious nonneurologic complications.[155]

Blood pressure management is an important issue in the management of virtually every acute stroke patient, and one that has been extensively researched. Most studies have found a U-shaped relationship between blood pressure in acute stroke and disability, with outcomes worsening if blood pressure is allowed to vary higher or lower than an optimal range.[155–157] However, in general these studies have treated stroke patients as a somewhat homogeneous group, without distinguishing between those who do and do not have persistently hypoperfused brain tissue, a distinction that can be made by MR perfusion imaging. Presumably the former might benefit from hypertension whereas the latter would not, and might only suffer only the negative consequences of elevated blood pressure. One small study, incorporating fifteen patients, demonstrated the effectiveness of induced hypertension therapy in patients who demonstrated a large DWI-perfusion mismatch. However, the intuitively appealing possibility of using the existence or absence of hypoperfused tissue to guide blood pressure management has yet to be tested in a large-scale trial.

SUMMARY

In acute stroke, MR perfusion imaging can be used to measure a variety of different parameters, which provide differing and complementary information about regional brain perfusion. Interpretation of MR perfusion images requires a basic qualitative understanding of the various perfusion states that may coexist in the brain of an acute stroke patient, and should incorporate knowledge of several important artifacts that occur in perfusion imaging. MR perfusion imaging has been used successfully to establish the diagnosis of cerebral ischemia in the absence of other objective evidence, and shows promise for selecting patients for thrombolytic therapy. As MR perfusion techniques undergo continuing technical refinement and are incorporated into new clinical trials, their utility in these clinical roles is likely to increase. It is also likely that MR perfusion imaging may play a larger role in guiding therapies designed to maintain and enhance collateral brain perfusion.

REFERENCES

1. Rosen BR, Belliveau JW, Chien D. Perfusion imaging by nuclear magnetic resonance. Magn Reson Q 1989;5:263–81.
2. Powers WJ. Cerebral hemodynamics in ischemic cerebrovascular disease. Ann Neurol 1991;29:231–40.
3. Grubb RL Jr, Phelps ME, Ter-Pogossian MM. Regional cerebral blood volume in humans. X-ray fluorescence studies. Arch Neurol 1973;28:38–44.
4. Grubb RL Jr, Phelps ME, Raichle ME, et al. The effects of arterial blood pressure on the regional cerebral blood volume by x-ray fluorescence. Stroke 1973;4:390–9.
5. Stewart GN. Researches on the circulation time in organs and on the influences which affect it, parts I-III. J Physiol (London) 1894;15:1–89.
6. Kety SS, King BD, Horvath SM, et al. The effects of an acute reduction in blood pressure by means of differential spinal sympathetic block on the cerebral circulation of hypertensive patients. J Clin Invest 1950;29:402–7.
7. Hossmann KA. Cerebral ischemia: models, methods and outcomes. Neuropharmacology 2008;55:257–70.
8. Parsons MW, Yang Q, Barber PA, et al. Perfusion magnetic resonance imaging maps in hyperacute stroke: relative cerebral blood flow most accurately identifies tissue destined to infarct. Stroke 2001;32:1581–7.
9. Jones TH, Morawetz RB, Crowell RM, et al. Thresholds of focal cerebral ischemia in awake monkeys. J Neurosurg 1981;54:773–82.
10. Astrup J, Siesjo B, Symon L. Thresholds in cerebral ischemia: the ischemic penumbra. Stroke 1981;12:723–5.
11. Siesjö BK. Pathophysiology and treatment of focal cerebral ischemia. Part I: pathophysiology. J Neurosurg 1992;77:169–84.
12. Cordes M, Henkes H, Roll D, et al. Subacute and chronic cerebral infarctions: SPECT and gadolinium-DTPA enhanced MR imaging. J Comput Assist Tomogr 1989;13:567–71.
13. Sette G, Baron JC, Mazoyer B, et al. Local brain haemodynamics and oxygen metabolism in cerebrovascular disease. Positron emission tomography. Brain 1989;112:931–51.
14. Weiller C, Ringelstein EB, Reiche W, et al. Clinical and hemodynamic aspects of low-flow infarcts. Stroke 1991;22:1117–23.
15. Zaharchuk G, Mandeville JB, Bogdanov AA Jr, et al. Cerebrovascular dynamics of autoregulation and hypoperfusion. An MRI study of CBF and changes in total and microvascular cerebral blood volume during hemorrhagic hypotension. Stroke 1999;30:2197–204 [discussion: 2204–5].
16. Rubin G, Firlik AD, Levy EI, et al. Xenon-enhanced computed tomography cerebral blood flow measurements in acute cerebral ischemia: review of 56 cases. J Stroke Cerebrovas Dis 1999;8:404–11.
17. Hakim AM, Pokrupa RP, Villanueva J, et al. The effect of spontaneous reperfusion on metabolic function in early human cerebral infarcts. Ann Neurol 1987;21:279–89.
18. Jorgensen HS, Sperling B, Nakayama H, et al. Spontaneous reperfusion of cerebral infarcts in patients with acute stroke. Incidence, time course, and clinical outcome in the copenhagen stroke study. Arch Neurol 1994;51:865–73.
19. Bowler JV, Wade JP, Jones BE, et al. Natural history of the spontaneous reperfusion of human cerebral infarcts as assessed by 99mTc HMPAO SPECT. J Neurol Neurosurg Psychiatry 1998;64:90–7.
20. Marchal G, Young AR, Baron JC. Early postischemic hyperperfusion: pathophysiologic insights from positron emission tomography. J Cereb Blood Flow Metab 1999;19:467–82.
21. Marchal G, Furlan M, Beaudouin V, et al. Early spontaneous hyperperfusion after stroke. A marker of favourable tissue outcome? Brain 1996;119:409–19.
22. Kidwell CS, Saver JL, Mattiello J, et al. Diffusion-perfusion MRI characterization of post-recanalization

hyperperfusion in humans. Neurology 2001;57: 2015–21.

23. Lassen NA. The luxury-perfusion syndrome and its possible relation to acute metabolic acidosis localised within the brain. Lancet 1966;2:1113–5.

24. Williams DS, Detre JA, Leigh JS, et al. Magnetic resonance imaging of perfusion using spin inversion of arterial water. Proc Natl Acad Sci U S A 1992;89:212–6.

25. Rosen BR, Belliveau JW, Vevea JM, et al. Perfusion imaging with NMR contrast agents. Magn Reson Med 1990;14:249–65.

26. Leenders KL, Perani D, Lammertsma AA, et al. Cerebral blood flow, blood volume and oxygen utilization. Normal values and effect of age. Brain 1990;113:27–47.

27. Wintermark M, Albers GW, Alexandrov AV, et al. Acute stroke imaging research roadmap. Stroke 2008;39:1621–8.

28. Boxerman JL, Hamberg LM, Rosen BR, et al. MR contrast due to intravascular magnetic susceptibility perturbations. Magn Reson Med 1995;34:555–66.

29. Donahue KM, Krouwer HG, Rand SD, et al. Utility of simultaneously acquired gradient-echo and spin-echo cerebral blood volume and morphology maps in brain tumor patients. Magn Reson Med 2000;43:845–53.

30. Kane I, Carpenter T, Chappell F, et al. Comparison of 10 different magnetic resonance perfusion imaging processing methods in acute ischemic stroke: effect on lesion size, proportion of patients with diffusion/perfusion mismatch, clinical scores, and radiologic outcomes. Stroke 2007;38:3158–64.

31. Beaulieu C, de Crespigny A, Tong DC, et al. Longitudinal magnetic resonance imaging study of perfusion and diffusion in stroke: evolution of lesion volume and correlation with clinical outcome. Ann Neurol 1999;46:568–78.

32. Marks MP, Tong DC, Beaulieu C, et al. Evaluation of early reperfusion and i.v. tPA therapy using diffusion- and perfusion-weighted MRI. Neurology 1999;52:1792–8.

33. Neumann-Haefelin T, Wittsack HJ, Wenserski F, et al. Diffusion- and perfusion-weighted MRI. The DWI/PWI mismatch region in acute stroke. Stroke 1999;30:1591–7.

34. Perkins CJ, Kahya E, Roque CT, et al. Fluid-attenuated inversion recovery and diffusion- and perfusion-weighted MRI abnormalities in 117 consecutive patients with stroke symptoms. Stroke 2001;32:2774–81.

35. Grandin CB, Duprez TP, Smith AM, et al. Which MR-derived perfusion parameters are the best predictors of infarct growth in hyperacute stroke? Comparative study between relative and quantitative measurements. Radiology 2002;223:361–70.

36. Wittsack HJ, Ritzl A, Fink GR, et al. MR imaging in acute stroke: diffusion-weighted and perfusion imaging parameters for predicting infarct size. Radiology 2002;222:397–403.

37. Derex L, Nighoghossian N, Hermier M, et al. Influence of pretreatment MRI parameters on clinical outcome, recanalization and infarct size in 49 stroke patients treated by intravenous tissue plasminogen activator. J Neurol Sci 2004;225:3–9.

38. Yamada K, Wu O, Gonzalez RG, et al. Magnetic resonance perfusion-weighted imaging of acute cerebral infarction: effect of the calculation methods and underlying vasculopathy. Stroke 2002;33:87–94.

39. Ribo M, Molina CA, Rovira A, et al. Safety and efficacy of intravenous tissue plasminogen activator stroke treatment in the 3- to 6-hour window using multimodal transcranial Doppler/MRI selection protocol. Stroke 2005;36:602–6.

40. Cenic A, Nabavi DG, Craen RA, et al. Dynamic CT measurement of cerebral blood flow: a validation study. AJNR Am J Neuroradiol 1999;20:63–73.

41. Nabavi DG, Cenic A, Dool J, et al. Quantitative assessment of cerebral hemodynamics using CT: stability, accuracy, and precision studies in dogs. J Comput Assist Tomogr 1999;23:506–15.

42. Wintermark M, Thiran JP, Maeder P, et al. Simultaneous measurement of regional cerebral blood flow by perfusion CT and stable xenon CT: a validation study. AJNR Am J Neuroradiol 2001;22:905–14.

43. Gillard JH, Antoun NM, Burnet NG, et al. Reproducibility of quantitative CT perfusion imaging. Br J Radiol 2001;74:552–5.

44. Furukawa M, Kashiwagi S, Matsunaga N, et al. Evaluation of cerebral perfusion parameters measured by perfusion CT in chronic cerebral ischemia: comparison with xenon CT. J Comput Assist Tomogr 2002;26:272–8.

45. Rempp KA, Brix G, Wenz F, et al. Quantification of regional cerebral blood flow and volume with dynamic susceptibility contrast-enhanced MR imaging. Radiology 1994;193:637–41.

46. Østergaard L, Smith DF, Vestergaard-Poulsen P, et al. Absolute cerebral blood flow and blood volume measured by magnetic resonance imaging bolus tracking: comparison with positron emission tomography values. J Cereb Blood Flow Metab 1998;18:425–32.

47. Hagen T, Bartylla K, Piepgras U. Correlation of regional cerebral blood flow measured by stable xenon CT and perfusion MRI. J Comput Assist Tomogr 1999;23:257–64.

48. Sakoh M, Rohl L, Gyldensted C, et al. Cerebral blood flow and blood volume measured by magnetic resonance imaging bolus tracking after acute stroke in pigs: comparison with [(15)O]H(2)O positron emission tomography. Stroke 2000;31:1958–64.

49. Smith AM, Grandin CB, Duprez T, et al. Whole brain quantitative CBF, CBV, and MTT measurements using MRI bolus tracking: implementation and

application to data acquired from hyperacute stroke patients. J Magn Reson Imaging 2000;12:400–10.

50. Lin W, Celik A, Derdeyn C, et al. Quantitative measurements of cerebral blood flow in patients with unilateral carotid artery occlusion: a PET and MR study. J Magn Reson Imaging 2001;14:659–67.

51. Endo H, Inoue T, Ogasawara K, et al. Quantitative assessment of cerebral hemodynamics using perfusion-weighted MRI in patients with major cerebral artery occlusive disease: comparison with positron emission tomography. Stroke 2006;37:388–92.

52. Sorensen AG, Buonanno FS, Gonzalez RG, et al. Hyperacute stroke: evaluation with combined multisection diffusion-weighted and hemodynamically weighted echo-planar MR imaging. Radiology 1996;199:391–401.

53. Rordorf G, Koroshetz WJ, Copen WA, et al. Regional ischemia and ischemic injury in patients with acute middle cerebral artery stroke as defined by early diffusion-weighted and perfusion-weighted MRI. Stroke 1998;29:939–43.

54. Ueda T, Yuh WT, Maley JE, et al. Outcome of acute ischemic lesions evaluated by diffusion and perfusion MR imaging. AJNR Am J Neuroradiol 1999; 20:983–9.

55. Sorensen AG, Copen WA, Østergaard L, et al. Hyperacute stroke: simultaneous measurement of relative cerebral blood volume, relative cerebral blood flow, and mean tissue transit time. Radiology 1999;210:519–27.

56. Karonen JO, Liu Y, Vanninen RL, et al. Combined perfusion- and diffusion-weighted MR imaging in acute ischemic stroke during the 1st week: a longitudinal study. Radiology 2000;217:886–94.

57. Schaefer PW, Hunter GJ, He J, et al. Predicting cerebral ischemic infarct volume with diffusion and perfusion MR imaging. AJNR Am J Neuroradiol 2002;23:1785–94.

58. Wintermark M. Brain perfusion-CT in acute stroke patients. Eur Radiol 2005;15(Suppl 4):D28–31.

59. Nagar VA, McKinney AM, Karagulle AT, et al. Reperfusion phenomenon masking acute and subacute infarcts at dynamic perfusion CT: confirmation by fusion of CT and diffusion-weighted MR images. AJR Am J Roentgenol 2009;193:1629–38.

60. Benner T, Heiland S, Erb G, et al. Accuracy of gamma-variate fits to concentration-time curves from dynamic susceptibility-contrast enhanced MRI: Influence of time resolution, maximal signal drop and signal-to-noise. Magn Reson Imaging 1997;15:307–17.

61. Lin W, Celik A, Paczynski RP. Regional cerebral blood volume: a comparison of the dynamic imaging and the steady state methods. J Magn Reson Imaging 1999;9:44–52.

62. delpolyi AR, Wu O, Schaefer PW, et al. Cerebral blood volume measurements in acute ischemic stroke are technique-dependent and cannot substitute for DWI. American Society for Neuroradiology 48th Annual Meeting. Boston (MA), May 15–20, 2010.

63. Kwong KK, Reese TG, Nelissen K, et al. Early time points perfusion imaging. Neuroimage 2011;54: 1070–82.

64. King RB, Deussen A, Raymond GM, et al. A vascular transport operator. Am J Physiol 1993;265:H2196–208.

65. van Osch MJ, Vonken EJ, Wu O, et al. Model of the human vasculature for studying the influence of contrast injection speed on cerebral perfusion MRI. Magn Reson Med 2003;50:614–22.

66. Rausch M, Scheffler K, Rudin M, et al. Analysis of input functions from different arterial branches with gamma variate functions and cluster analysis for quantitative blood volume measurements. Magn Reson Imaging 2000;18:1235–43.

67. Carroll TJ, Rowley HA, Haughton VM. Automatic calculation of the arterial input function for cerebral perfusion imaging with MR imaging. Radiology 2003;227:593–600.

68. Mouridsen K, Christensen S, Gyldensted L, et al. Automatic selection of arterial input function using cluster analysis. Magn Reson Med 2006;55: 524–31.

69. Østergaard L, Weisskoff RM, Chesler DA, et al. High resolution measurement of cerebral blood flow using intravascular tracer bolus passages. Part I: mathematical approach and statistical analysis. Magn Reson Med 1996;36:715–25.

70. Østergaard L, Sorensen AG, Kwong KK, et al. High resolution measurement of cerebral blood flow using intravascular tracer bolus passages. Part II: experimental comparison and preliminary results. Magn Reson Med 1996;36:726–36.

71. Kudo K, Sasaki M, Yamada K, et al. Differences in CT perfusion maps generated by different commercial software: quantitative analysis by using identical source data of acute stroke patients. Radiology 2010;254:200–9.

72. Calamante F, Gadian DG, Connelly A. Delay and dispersion effects in dynamic susceptibility contrast MRI: simulations using singular value decomposition. Magn Reson Med 2000;44:466–73.

73. Calamante F, Gadian DG, Connelly A. Quantification of perfusion using bolus tracking magnetic resonance imaging in stroke: assumptions, limitations, and potential implications for clinical use. Stroke 2002;33:1146–51.

74. Wu O, Østergaard L, Koroshetz WJ, et al. Effects of tracer arrival time on flow estimates in MR perfusion-weighted imaging. Magn Reson Med 2003;50:856–64.

75. Lythgoe DJ, Ostergaard L, William SC, et al. Quantitative perfusion imaging in carotid artery stenosis using dynamic susceptibility contrast-enhanced

magnetic resonance imaging. Magn Reson Imaging 2000;18:1–11.

76. Calamante F, Morup M, Hansen LK. Defining a local arterial input function for perfusion MRI using independent component analysis. Magn Reson Med 2004;52:789–97.

77. Lorenz C, Benner T, Lopez CJ, et al. Effect of using local arterial input functions on cerebral blood flow estimation. J Magn Reson Imaging 2006;24:57–65.

78. Lorenz C, Benner T, Chen PJ, et al. Automated perfusion-weighted MRI using localized arterial input functions. J Magn Reson Imaging 2006;24: 1133–9.

79. Christensen S, Mouridsen K, Wu O, et al. Comparison of 10 perfusion MRI parameters in 97 sub-6-hour stroke patients using voxel-based receiver operating characteristics analysis. Stroke 2009; 40:2055–61.

80. Lee JJ, Bretthorst GL, Derdeyn CP, et al. Dynamic susceptibility contrast MRI with localized arterial input functions. Magn Reson Med 2010;63: 1305–14.

81. Duhamel G, Schlaug G, Alsop DC. Measurement of arterial input functions for dynamic susceptibility contrast magnetic resonance imaging using echoplanar images: comparison of physical simulations with in vivo results. Magn Reson Med 2006;55:514–23.

82. Bleeker EJ, van Buchem MA, van Osch MJ. Optimal location for arterial input function measurements near the middle cerebral artery in first-pass perfusion MRI. J Cereb Blood Flow Metab 2009;29:840–52.

83. Rose SE, Janke AL, Griffin M, et al. Improving the prediction of final infarct size in acute stroke with bolus delay-corrected perfusion MRI measures. J Magn Reson Imaging 2004;20:941–7.

84. Rose SE, Janke AL, Griffin M, et al. Improved prediction of final infarct volume using bolus delay-corrected perfusion-weighted MRI: implications for the ischemic penumbra. Stroke 2004;35:2466–71.

85. Wu O, Østergaard L, Weisskoff RM, et al. Tracer arrival timing-insensitive technique for estimating flow in MR perfusion-weighted imaging using singular value decomposition with a block-circulant deconvolution matrix. Magn Reson Med 2003;50:164–74.

86. Baird AE, Benfield A, Schlaug G, et al. Enlargement of human cerebral ischemic lesion volumes measured by diffusion-weighted magnetic resonance imaging. Ann Neurol 1997;41:581–9.

87. Grandin CB, Duprez TP, Smith AM, et al. Usefulness of magnetic resonance-derived quantitative measurements of cerebral blood flow and volume in prediction of infarct growth in hyperacute stroke. Stroke 2001;32:1147–53.

88. Fink JN, Kumar S, Horkan C, et al. The stroke patient who woke up: clinical and radiological features, including diffusion and perfusion MRI. Stroke 2002;33:988–93.

89. Coutts SB, Simon JE, Tomanek AI, et al. Reliability of assessing percentage of diffusion-perfusion mismatch. Stroke 2003;34:1681–3.

90. Ay H, Koroshetz WJ, Vangel M, et al. Conversion of ischemic brain tissue into infarction increases with age. Stroke 2005;36:2632–6.

91. Yoo AJ, Barak ER, Copen WA, et al. Combining acute diffusion-weighted imaging and mean transmit time lesion volumes with national institutes of health stroke scale score improves the prediction of acute stroke outcome. Stroke 2010;41:1728–35.

92. Rivers CS, Wardlaw JM, Armitage PA, et al. Do acute diffusion- and perfusion-weighted MRI lesions identify final infarct volume in ischemic stroke? Stroke 2006;37:98–104.

93. Shih LC, Saver JL, Alger JR, et al. Perfusion-weighted magnetic resonance imaging thresholds identifying core, irreversibly infarcted tissue. Stroke 2003;34:1425–30.

94. Olivot JM, Mlynash M, Thijs VN, et al. Optimal Tmax threshold for predicting penumbral tissue in acute stroke. Stroke 2009;40:469–75.

95. Bang OY, Lee KH, Kim SJ, et al. Benign oligemia despite a malignant MRI profile in acute ischemic stroke. J Clin Neurol 2010;6:41–5.

96. Kidwell CS, Saver JL, Mattiello J, et al. Thrombolytic reversal of acute human cerebral ischemic injury shown by diffusion/perfusion magnetic resonance imaging. Ann Neurol 2000;47:462–9.

97. Kakuda W, Lansberg MG, Thijs VN, et al. Optimal definition for PWI/DWI mismatch in acute ischemic stroke patients. J Cereb Blood Flow Metab 2008; 28:887–91.

98. Albers GW, Thijs VN, Wechsler L, et al. Magnetic resonance imaging profiles predict clinical response to early reperfusion: the diffusion and perfusion imaging evaluation for understanding stroke evolution (DEFUSE) study. Ann Neurol 2006;60:508–17.

99. Davis SM, Donnan GA, Parsons MW, et al. Effects of alteplase beyond 3 h after stroke in the echoplanar imaging thrombolytic evaluation trial (EPITHET): a placebo-controlled randomised trial. Lancet Neurol 2008;7:209–309.

100. Liebeskind DS. Collaterals in acute stroke: beyond the clot. Neuroimaging Clin N Am 2005;15:553–73, x.

101. Christensen S, Calamante F, Hjort N, et al. Inferring origin of vascular supply from tracer arrival timing patterns using bolus tracking MRI. J Magn Reson Imaging 2008;27:1371–81.

102. Lövblad KO, Laubach HJ, Baird AE, et al. Clinical experience with diffusion-weighted MR in patients with acute stroke. AJNR Am J Neuroradiol 1998; 19:1061–6.

103. Singer MB, Chong J, Lu D, et al. Diffusion-weighted MRI in acute subcortical infarction. Stroke 1998;29: 133–6.

104. van Everdingen KJ, van der Grond J, Kappelle LJ, et al. Diffusion-weighted magnetic resonance imaging in acute stroke. Stroke 1998;29:1783–90.

105. Gonzalez RG, Schaefer PW, Buonanno FS, et al. Diffusion-weighted MR imaging: diagnostic accuracy in patients imaged within 6 hours of stroke symptom onset. Radiology 1999;210:155–62.

106. Urbach H, Flacke S, Keller E, et al. Detectability and detection rate of acute cerebral hemisphere infarcts on CT and diffusion-weighted MRI. Neuroradiology 2000;42:722–7.

107. Fiebach JB, Schellinger PD, Jansen O, et al. CT and diffusion-weighted MR imaging in randomized order: diffusion-weighted imaging results in higher accuracy and lower interrater variability in the diagnosis of hyperacute ischemic stroke. Stroke 2002; 33:2206–10.

108. Mullins ME, Schaefer PW, Sorensen AG, et al. CT and conventional and diffusion-weighted MR imaging in acute stroke: study in 691 patients at presentation to the emergency department. Radiology 2002;224:353–60.

109. Hand PJ, Kwan J, Lindley RI, et al. Distinguishing between stroke and mimic at the bedside: the brain attack study. Stroke 2006;37:769–75.

110. Johnston SC, Gress DR, Browner WS, et al. Short-term prognosis after emergency department diagnosis of TIA. JAMA 2000;284:2901–6.

111. Furie KL, Kasner SE, Adams RJ, et al. Guidelines for the prevention of stroke in patients with stroke or transient ischemic attack. A guideline for healthcare professionals from the American Heart Association/American Stroke Association. Stroke 2011; 42(1):227–76.

112. Coutts SB, Sylaja PN, Choi YB, et al. The aspire approach for TIA risk stratification. Can J Neurol Sci 2011;38:78–81.

113. Ovbiagele B, Kidwell CS, Saver JL. Epidemiological impact in the United States of a tissue-based definition of transient ischemic attack. Stroke 2003;34:919–24.

114. Restrepo L, Jacobs MA, Barker PB, et al. Assessment of transient ischemic attack with diffusion- and perfusion-weighted imaging. AJNR Am J Neuroradiol 2004;25:1645–52.

115. Krol AL, Coutts SB, Simon JE, et al. Perfusion MRI abnormalities in speech or motor transient ischemic attack patients. Stroke 2005;36:2487–9.

116. Mlynash M, Olivot JM, Tong DC, et al. Yield of combined perfusion and diffusion MR imaging in hemispheric TIA. Neurology 2009;72:1127–33.

117. NINDS rt-PA Study Group. Tissue plasminogen activator for acute ischemic stroke. The National Institute of Neurological Disorders and Stroke rt-PA Stroke Study Group. N Engl J Med 1995;333:1581–7.

118. Hacke W, Kaste M, Fieschi C, et al. Intravenous thrombolysis with recombinant tissue plasminogen activator for acute hemispheric stroke. The European Cooperative Acute Stroke Study (ECASS). JAMA 1995;274:1017–25.

119. Hacke W, Kaste M, Fieschi C, et al. Randomised double-blind placebo-controlled trial of thrombolytic therapy with intravenous alteplase in acute ischaemic stroke (ECASS II). Second European-Australasian Acute Stroke Study investigators. Lancet 1998;352:1245–51.

120. Clark WM, Wissman S, Albers GW, et al. Recombinant tissue-type plasminogen activator (Alteplase) for ischemic stroke 3 to 5 hours after symptom onset. The Atlantis Study: a randomized controlled trial. Alteplase thrombolysis for acute noninterventional therapy in ischemic stroke. JAMA 1999;282:2019–26.

121. Wahlgren N, Ahmed N, Davalos A, et al, SITS-MOST investigators. Thrombolysis with alteplase for acute ischaemic stroke in the safe implementation of thrombolysis in stroke-monitoring study (SITS-MOST): an observational study. Lancet 2007;369:275–82.

122. Bluhmki E, Chamorro A, Davalos A, et al. Stroke treatment with alteplase given 3.0-4.5 h after onset of acute ischaemic stroke (ECASS III): additional outcomes and subgroup analysis of a randomised controlled trial. Lancet Neurol 2009;8:1095–102.

123. Boode B, Welzen V, Franke C, et al. Estimating the number of stroke patients eligible for thrombolytic treatment if delay could be avoided. Cerebrovasc Dis 2007;23:294–8.

124. Smith MA, Doliszny KM, Shahar E, et al. Delayed hospital arrival for acute stroke: the Minnesota stroke survey. Ann Intern Med 1998;129:190–6.

125. Katzan IL, Furlan AJ, Lloyd LE, et al. Use of tissue-type plasminogen activator for acute ischemic stroke: the Cleveland area experience. JAMA 2000;283:1151–8.

126. Barber PA, Zhang J, Demchuk AM, et al. Why are stroke patients excluded from TPA therapy? An analysis of patient eligibility. Neurology 2001;56: 1015–20.

127. O'Connor RE, McGraw P, Edelsohn L. Thrombolytic therapy for acute ischemic stroke: why the majority of patients remain ineligible for treatment. Ann Emerg Med 1999;33:9–14.

128. Tong DC, Yenari MA, Albers GW, et al. Correlation of perfusion- and diffusion-weighted MRI with NIHSS score in acute (<6.5 hour) ischemic stroke. Neurology 1998;50:864–70.

129. Karonen JO, Vanninen RL, Liu Y, et al. Combined diffusion and perfusion MRI with correlation to single-photon emission CT in acute ischemic stroke. Ischemic penumbra predicts infarct growth. Stroke 1999;30:1583–90.

130. Parsons MW, Barber PA, Chalk J, et al. Diffusion- and perfusion-weighted MRI response to thrombolysis in stroke. Ann Neurol 2002;51:28–37.

131. Grant PE, He J, Halpern EF, et al. Frequency and clinical context of decreased apparent diffusion coefficient reversal in the human brain. Radiology 2001;221:43–50.

132. Barber PA, Darby DG, Desmond PM, et al. Prediction of stroke outcome with echoplanar perfusion- and diffusion-weighted MRI. Neurology 1998;51: 418–26.

133. Schlaug G, Benfield A, Baird AE, et al. The ischemic penumbra: operationally defined by diffusion and perfusion MRI. Neurology 1999;53:1528–37.

134. Hacke W, Albers G, Al-Rawi Y, et al. The desmoteplase in acute ischemic stroke trial (DIAS): a phase II MRI-based 9-hour window acute stroke thrombolysis trial with intravenous desmoteplase. Stroke 2005;36:66–73.

135. Furlan AJ, Eyding D, Albers GW, et al. Dose escalation of desmoteplase for acute ischemic stroke (DEDAS): evidence of safety and efficacy 3 to 9 hours after stroke onset. Stroke 2006;37:1227–31.

136. Nagakane Y, Christensen S, Brekenfeld C, et al. EPITHET: positive result after reanalysis using baseline diffusion-weighted imaging/perfusion-weighted imaging co-registration. Stroke 2011;42:59–64.

137. Hacke W, Furlan AJ, Al-Rawi Y, et al. Intravenous desmoteplase in patients with acute ischaemic stroke selected by MRI perfusion-diffusion weighted imaging or perfusion CT (DIAS-2): a prospective, randomised, double-blind, placebo-controlled study. Lancet Neurol 2009;8:141–50.

138. Rose SE, Chalk JB, Griffin MP, et al. MRI based diffusion and perfusion predictive model to estimate stroke evolution. Magn Reson Imaging 2001;19:1043–53.

139. Wu O, Koroshetz WJ, Østergaard L, et al. Predicting tissue outcome in acute human cerebral ischemia using combined diffusion- and perfusion-weighted MR imaging. Stroke 2001;32: 933–42.

140. Han JH, Wong KS. Is counterpulsation a potential therapy for ischemic stroke? Cerebrovasc Dis 2008;26:97–105.

141. Uflacker R, Schonholz C, Papamitisakis N. Interim report of the SENTIS trial: Cerebral perfusion augmentation via partial aortic occlusion in acute ischemic stroke. J Cardiovasc Surg (Torino) 2008; 49:715–21.

142. Singhal AB, Benner T, Roccatagliata L, et al. A pilot study of normobaric oxygen therapy in acute ischemic stroke. Stroke 2005;36:797–802.

143. International Stroke Trial Collaborative Group. The international stroke trial (IST): a randomised trial of aspirin, subcutaneous heparin, both, or neither among 19435 patients with acute ischaemic stroke. International stroke trial collaborative group. Lancet 1997;349:1569–81.

144. CAST (Chinese Acute Stroke Trial) Collaborative Group. CAST: randomised placebo-controlled trial of early aspirin use in 20,000 patients with acute ischaemic stroke. CAST (Chinese Acute Stroke Trial) Collaborative Group. Lancet 1997;349:1641–9.

145. Barer DH, Cruickshank JM, Ebrahim SB, et al. Low dose beta blockade in acute stroke ("BEST" trial): an evaluation. Br Med J (Clin Res Ed) 1988;296: 737–41.

146. Ahmed N, Nasman P, Wahlgren NG. Effect of intravenous nimodipine on blood pressure and outcome after acute stroke. Stroke 2000;31:1250–5.

147. Horn J, Limburg M. Calcium antagonists for ischemic stroke: a systematic review. Stroke 2001;32:570–6.

148. Ahmed N, Wahlgren NG. Effects of blood pressure lowering in the acute phase of total anterior circulation infarcts and other stroke subtypes. Cerebrovasc Dis 2003;15:235–43.

149. Rordorf G, Cramer SC, Efird JT, et al. Pharmacological elevation of blood pressure in acute stroke. Clinical effects and safety. Stroke 1997;28:2133–8.

150. Hillis AE, Ulatowski JA, Barker PB, et al. A pilot randomized trial of induced blood pressure elevation: effects on function and focal perfusion in acute and subacute stroke. Cerebrovasc Dis 2003;16:236–46.

151. Mistri AK, Robinson TG, Potter JF. Pressor therapy in acute ischemic stroke: systematic review. Stroke 2006;37:1565–71.

152. Krieger DW, Demchuk AM, Kasner SE, et al. Early clinical and radiological predictors of fatal brain swelling in ischemic stroke. Stroke 1999;30:287–92.

153. Bowes MP, Zivin JA, Thomas GR, et al. Acute hypertension, but not thrombolysis, increases the incidence and severity of hemorrhagic transformation following experimental stroke in rabbits. Exp Neurol 1996;141:40–6.

154. Fagan SC, Bowes MP, Lyden PD, et al. Acute hypertension promotes hemorrhagic transformation in a rabbit embolic stroke model: effect of labetalol. Exp Neurol 1998;150:153–8.

155. Vemmos KN, Spengos K, Tsivgoulis G, et al. Factors influencing acute blood pressure values in stroke subtypes. J Hum Hypertens 2004;18: 253–9.

156. Okumura K, Ohya Y, Maehara A, et al. Effects of blood pressure levels on case fatality after acute stroke. J Hypertens 2005;23:1217–23.

157. Ahmed N, Wahlgren N, Brainin M, et al. Relationship of blood pressure, antihypertensive therapy, and outcome in ischemic stroke treated with intravenous thrombolysis: retrospective analysis from safe implementation of thrombolysis in stroke-international stroke thrombolysis register (SITS-ISTR). Stroke 2009;40:2442–9.

Arterial Spin Label Imaging of Acute Ischemic Stroke and Transient Ischemic Attack

Greg Zaharchuk, PhD, MD

KEYWORDS

- Arterial spin labeling • Perfusion
- Cerebral blood flow • Cerebrovascular disease
- Stroke • Transient ischemic attack

Arterial spin labeling (ASL) is a noncontrast perfusion imaging method that relies on the magnetic labeling of arterial water.[1,2] This labeling can be performed in a variety of ways; the two major classes of ASL are distinguished from each other based on whether or not the label is applied during a single short-duration pulse (pulsed ASL [PASL]) or during an extended period (continuous ASL [CASL]). Although CASL techniques typically have higher signal-to-noise ratio (SNR), they have been limited in clinical practice by high radiofrequency energy deposition and more demanding requirements from the scanner hardware.[3–5] Primarily for this reason, PASL techniques were the first to enter routine clinical practice.[6–10] More recently, however, a hybrid approach, known as pulsed continuous or pseudocontinuous ASL (pcASL), has become popular, in which many short-duration RF pulses can be used to effectively label arterial water over a longer duration.[11,12] This method combines the high labeling efficiency of CASL with the reduced hardware demands of PASL. Regardless of the labeling approach, images are then acquired with and without labeling after allowing time for the labeled blood to pass from the site of labeling into the tissue of interest.

The difference in signal intensity between the two sets of images is approximately proportional to the local cerebral blood flow (CBF) (**Fig. 1**).

ASL images are sensitive to the exact parameters used to acquire the image, several of which are within the user's control. Choosing the appropriate labeling time for CASL is often a tradeoff between time and SNR; although longer label times lead to a larger buildup of labeled spins in the voxel, the increased time may be better spent on acquiring additional pairs of label and control images for signal averaging.[13] Postlabel delay (PLD) time, a parameter shared by PASL and CASL, is critical. It defines the time duration for spins to travel from the labeling plane or volume to the imaged slices and is typically between 1500 and 2000 ms. Because ischemic stroke is defined by reduced flow via proximal routes, any remaining flow to the tissue is often supplied via collateral routes, which leads to increased delays between the labeling of the spins and the arrival of those spins in the imaged voxel. Alsop and colleagues[14] demonstrated that longer PLDs lead to improved CBF quantification, although at the price of a loss in SNR; the longer the delay between the labeling and the imaging, the more

The author would like to acknowledge the funding sources that supported this article, including a Scholar Award from the American Society of Neuroradiology's Neuroradiology Education Research Fund (NERF), NIH R01-NS066506–01, and the Richard S. Lucas Center for Imaging at Stanford University.
Stanford University Medical Center, Stanford University, 1201 Welch Road, Mailcode 5488, Stanford, CA 94305-5488, USA
E-mail address: gregz@stanford.edu

Neuroimag Clin N Am 21 (2011) 285–301
doi:10.1016/j.nic.2011.01.003
1052-5149/11/$ – see front matter © 2011 Elsevier Inc. All rights reserved.

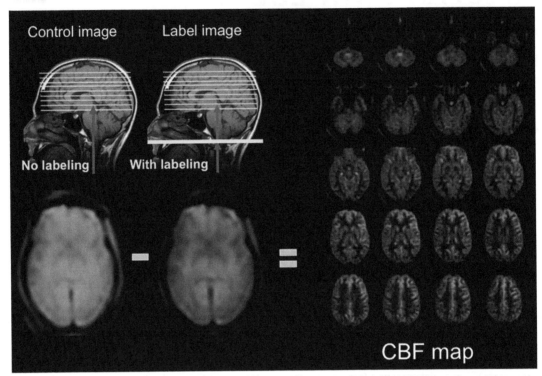

Fig. 1. ASL methodology. Images are acquired without (control) and with (label) application of arterial inversion at the site of the labeling plane. In this schematic, the inverted blood in the label image is shown in blue. Proton-density images are acquired after the labeling and the PLD time. The label image has slightly less signal intensity due to the infusion of inverted magnetization provided by the inflowing labeled blood. When subtracted from the control image, the ASL difference images are approximately proportional to CBF. At the right are CBF images of the central 20 slices of a 32-slice whole-brain 3D–FSE imaging set acquired at 3T requiring 4.5 minutes to acquire.

SNR penalty is paid due to T1-related decay of the labeled spins. Another approach is to obtain images at multiple PLDs, effectively mapping the inflow of label into the tissue[15,16]; such approaches offer the potential to quantify arrival times and then fit CBF to kinetic models,[17] although the approach is limited by reduced SNR in each of the individual images, challenges with nonlinear fitting of the inflow curves, and persistent inaccuracies in regions with severely delayed flow. An example of improved CBF quantitation with longer PLD times is shown as **Fig. 2** in a patient with bilateral moya-moya disease.

Often, on images in which the arterial arrival times are on the same scale or longer than the PLD, labeled spins are visualized in the arteries feeding

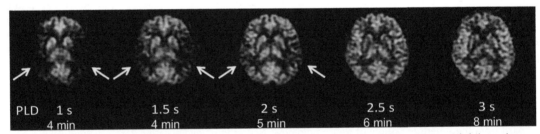

Fig. 2. CBF quantitation is improved on long PLD images using pcASL at 3T in this patient with bilateral moya-moya disease. On images with relatively short PLDs, there is less ASL signal in the bilateral MCA territories (*arrows*). As PLD increases, these regions with arterial arrival delay fill-in, indicating that CBF in these regions is normal. Longer PLD images have lower SNR, however, requiring longer acquisition time. In practice, a compromise must be made between these two competing effects, with most clinical ASL images having PLDs between 1.5 and 2 seconds.

the ischemic tissue, a finding termed, arterial transit artifact (ATA).[18] This is particularly evident if no vascular suppression is used; vascular suppression is a method whereby small diffusion gradients are applied to the ASL images so that spins moving above a certain velocity (presumably vascular) are not imaged.[19] ATA, although problematic in terms of quantification, can actually be a useful marker for pathology. ATA in the borderzone regions, often seen bilaterally, is more sensitive than bolus perfusion-weighted imaging (PWI) for identifying subtle perfusion alterations.[12] Also, the presence of ATA in patients with carotid disease is predictive of poor cerebrovascular reactivity after an acetazolamide challenge.[18] One prior stroke study suggested that patients with ATA had improved outcomes[20] and suggested that ATA may represent collateral flow.[5,21,22]

ASL differs from the more widely used bolus-based dynamic susceptibility contrast PWI method in several important ways (Table 1). Because of the lack of the use of contrast agents, ASL can be repeated frequently within the same imaging session and, therefore, can be used for challenge-type paradigms.[18,23] It can give some measure of perfusion in patients in whom gadolinium-based contrast agents are contraindicated due to poor renal function or allergy. As discussed previously, ASL is more susceptible to errors in patients with long arterial arrival times and may overestimate regions of decreased perfusion. Bolus PWI has higher contrast-to-noise per unit time and is an excellent method for measuring cerebral blood volume (CBV), assuming that the blood-brain barrier is intact, but measuring CBF with PWI remains challenging and highly model-dependent.[24,25] Recently, an approach combining ASL and PWI to more accurately measure CBF has been described that takes advantage of the superior relative perfusion properties of PWI and used ASL to provide a proper scaling factor.[26]

Although the basic method for measuring CBF with ASL was described more than 20 years ago, ASL has only recently entered the clinical arena. The reasons for this are multifactorial. The more widespread use of 3T neuroimaging has led to markedly improved ASL, due to the inherent higher SNR as well as the longer blood T1 at high field. Another important advance was the recognition of the importance of static background tissue signal suppression. To image the spatial distribution of the labeled blood, brain images acquired with and without the label (the control image) must be subtracted from one another. Typically the difference between the label and control images is approximately 1% of the signal intensity of either image. This means that even small amounts of motion between the label and control scans leads to large errors on subtraction images. By suppressing the static tissue signal using multiple inversion pulses, errors associated with patient motion can be significantly reduced; additionally, any biologic or gaussian noise in the individual label and control images is also reduced using this technique, leading to increased SNR of the final CBF images.

Another advance that has facilitated clinical ASL imaging is the ability to use more optimized readout strategies. Traditionally, single-shot echo-planar imaging (ssEPI) has been used to create the label and control images. This was largely because of the high SNR efficiency of this sequence, because the center of k-space is acquired during each acquisition. Many pairs of label and control ssEPI images are collected, and the subsequent difference images are combined using data averaging to improve SNR. This approach, in theory, also allows the elimination of image pairs with patient motion. Once SNR improved and the sequences became less sensitive to motion with the advent of robust background suppression (as described previously), however, it was possible to use other

Table 1
Comparison between ASL and bolus contrast PWI

ASL	Bolus PWI
Powerful technique to measure CBF	Powerful technique to measure CBV and Tmax
Cannot measure CBV	CBF challenging
Noncontrast	Requires gadolinium-containing agents
Spin-echo	High contrast-to-noise
Repeatable	Gradient-echo (primarily)
Microvascular measurement of perfusion	Clinical experience
Insensitive to blood-brain barrier damage	Errors due to blood-brain barrier damage
Errors in tissue with long arrival time	2 min scan time
3–5 min scan time	

readout approaches, such as steady-state free precession,[27] gradient- and spin-echo (GRASE),[28] and fast spin-echo (FSE).[11] Compared with ssEPI, these methods are more robust in regions with high magnetic susceptibility differences, allowing imaging of structures not typically amenable to ssEPI, such as the posterior fossa, midbrain, and inferior temporal and frontal lobes. FSE imaging also improves performance in patients with aneurysm clips, coils, and blood products. Finally, the use of 3D acquisition methods has entered clinical practice[11,29]; the advantages include the acquisition of isotropic voxels, allowing reformatting in different planes, as well as the fact that all slices can be obtained at the same PLD.

INDICATIONS FOR ASL PERFUSION IMAGING

Given that bolus PWI has gained some level of acceptance in the clinical arena during the past decade, the question arises as to why one would want to perform a perfusion study using an alternative method, particularly one with less SNR. The recent recognition of the relationship between gadolinium-containing contrast agents and nephrogenic systemic fibrosis has led to both absolute and relative contraindications to such agents at many institutions. In such patients, ASL is the only option for obtaining information about tissue perfusion. Also, intravenous access is challenging in certain patient groups, in particular children and intravenous drug users. Finally, ASL sequences can be easily repeated during a single clinical examination, which is useful for performing cerebrovascular reserve studies using either acetazolamide or breath-hold paradigms.

Specifically, in patients with cerebrovascular disease, ASL has several potential advantages. Although the acquisition time of the study is often a few minutes longer than that of bolus PWI, this is offset by the time-saver of not needing to place an intravenous line or hook up a power injector. Additionally, reconstruction times for ASL tend to be shorter than those for bolus PWI, especially because the background-suppressed ASL variants do not typically require motion correction, as do many bolus PWI studies. ASL excels at identifying bilateral disease, which can occur in this patient group, because it can be used in a quantitative rather than qualitative manner. Finally, the ability of ASL to detect perfusion alterations that are more subtle than those seen with bolus PWI make it an ideal methodology to study minor stroke and transient ischemic attack (TIA), where the ability to ascribe the event to a vascular etiology is of paramount importance,

because this may affect treatment triage and outcome.

PREVIOUS LITERATURE ON ASL FINDINGS IN TIA AND STROKE

Several early studies documented that ASL imaging could be used to image cerebrovascular disease, such as carotid stenosis and occlusion, as well as acute ischemic stroke. Chalela and colleagues[20] reported on 15 patients imaged within the first 24 hours after acute ischemic stroke. Using CASL, they found perfusion changes in the ipsilateral hemisphere consistent with the diffusion and clinical findings. They found that the quantitative CBF levels in the affected hemisphere correlated with National Institute of Health Stroke Scale (NIHSS) and Rankin Scale at 30-day follow-up. Also, they observed ATA in approximately half of their patients and suggested that this was a good prognostic sign, perhaps reflecting the presence of collateral flow. Detre and colleagues[18] examined the role of ASL imaging with acetazolamide challenge in patients with symptomatic intracranial internal carotid artery (ICA) or MCA stenosis. They showed that the presence of ATA correlated with poor cerebrovascular reactivity after acetazolamide challenge and suggested that ATA could possibly be used to avoid the risks associated with acetazolamide. ASL has also been applied to large vessel disease, as, for example, in a study by Hendrikse and colleagues[15] in patients with unilateral ICA occlusion. They used a PASL method with multiple PLD times, which were then fit to a model to determine CBF in the symptomatic hemispheres of 9 patients and 11 controls. The benefit of their approach was that the results were presumably independent of arrival time, because this is included in the model, although the maximum PLD used (1600 ms) is probably not long enough to ensure that late-arriving flow is appropriately counted. They found a 20% CBF decrease in the hemisphere ipsilateral to the carotid occlusion compared with the contralateral hemisphere or normal subjects.

More recently, Deibler and colleagues,[8,9] in a series of articles, demonstrated a clinically feasible ASL method and further examined various hypoperfusion patterns. They described the application of a PASL method, called quantitative imaging of perfusion using a single subtraction, second version,[7,30] which is relatively insensitive to errors associated with slow flow in 3000 clinical patients over a 12-month period. They show examples of the expected CBF changes in the core and penumbra of acute ischemic stroke. They also point out that ASL is not well suited to examine the white-matter perfusion in patients with suspected chronic microvascular ischemia, given the low absolute CBF and the prolonged transit times. Chen and colleagues[31] showed that ASL was useful clinically in 10 pediatric patients with acute ischemic stroke. They also noted that ATA was often present surrounding the ischemic core and tended to be associated with lack of progression to infarct and better clinical outcome.

Finally, relatively little has been reported on perfusion in general, and ASL in particular, in TIA patients. A recent study of lacunar syndromes in minor stroke and TIA patients suggested that the presence of a bolus PWI lesion could predict early deterioration (defined as ≥3 points on the NIHSS in

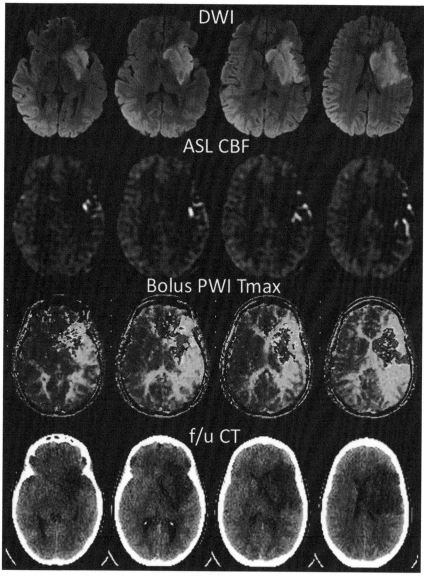

Fig. 3. A 25-year-old woman 6 hours after aortic coarctation repair and inability to speak or move her right side. MR angiogram (not shown) demonstrated no flow-related enhancement in the left MCA. DWI confirm acute ischemic stroke in the left MCA territory. ASL CBF images show hypoperfusion in the regions with high DWI signal, with ATA in the periphery. Bolus contrast normalized Tmax maps show a severe abnormality in the regions corresponding to the DWI lesion, with a milder abnormality in the region of ATA on ASL. The patient received no treatment due to her recent surgery. Coregistered slices from a follow-up noncontrast CT examination 3 days later reveal that there was no increase in the size of the lesion into the region with ATA on ASL. This is consistent with prior reports suggesting that ATA may reflect the beneficial effects of collateral flow and that such tissue has a good prognosis.

the first 72 hours).[32] In the only ASL study specifically focusing on this population, Macintosh and colleagues[33] describes ASL findings in 4 patients with TIA and 11 with minor stroke (NIHSS ≤6).

They used a 3D–GRASE-PASL method with multiple PLDs (500–2500 ms) to characterize the CBF and the arterial arrival time (AAT). This attempt to use ASL to measure arrival times quantitatively

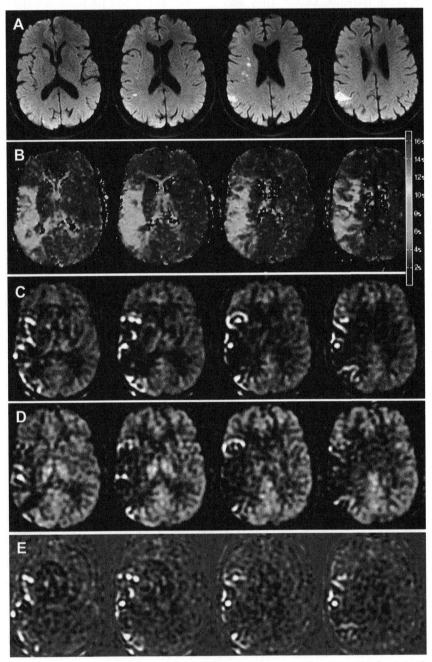

Fig. 4. A 74-year-old man with mild right facial droop. (*A*) DWI shows small, scattered infarcts in the right MCA territory. (*B*) Bolus PWI shows a mild Tmax lesion in a larger region. ASL images without (*C*) and with (*D*) vessel suppression demonstrate a similar region of abnormality. Serpiginous high ASL signal is seen throughout the affected territory, much of which is removed on the vessel-suppressed ASL images, confirming that the high signal is vascular. (*E*) Difference images between the two ASL images yield an image of the region of collateral flow. The patient was not treated due to his mild symptoms and had no worsening of his symptoms and no change in the pattern of infarcts on a 2-day follow-up MR imaging.

in stroke patients is significant, given that bolus arrival time markers, such as the normalized time-to-maximum contrast arrival (Tmax), seem to be useful in bolus PWI stroke studies.[34,35] They proposed an asymmetry index to detect the differences in AAT between hemispheres, and found that AAT was significantly increased in the affected hemisphere. Such an approach, however, is challenging in these patients, because often they have bilateral carotid disease and are abnormal on both sides to some degree. To evaluate this, Zaharchuk and colleagues[36,37] have begun to systematically examine ASL images in TIA patients with the goal of establishing a vascular etiology for the symptomatology. They have found that approximately 50% of such patients have

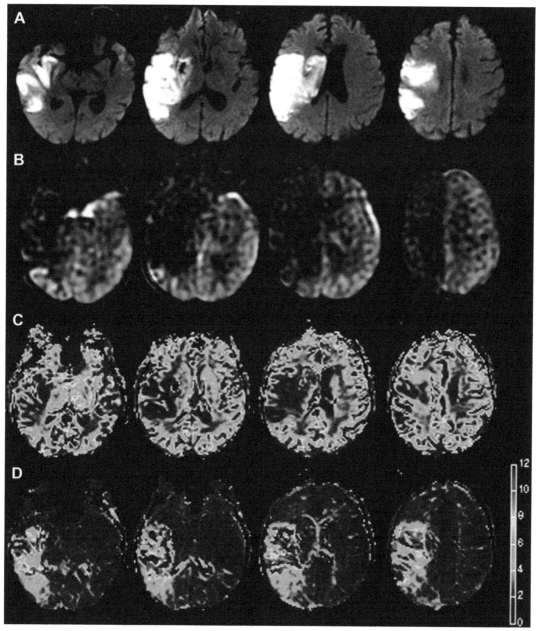

Fig. 5. A 79-year-old woman with dense left hemiparesis. (*A*) Large right MCA diffusion lesion is present. (*B*) ASL shows hypoperfusion in a region larger than the DWI lesion without significant ATA. Bolus contrast PWI (*C*) relative CBF and (*D*) Tmax in the same slices. The ASL lesion appears slightly larger than either of the bolus PWI maps. The absence of ATA suggests that this patient lacks significant collateral flow to the right MCA territory.

abnormalities, which exceeds the published yield of bolus PWI in this population (16%).[38] In particular, in the clinically interesting population of 28 TIA patients without diffusion abnormalities, they found that 46% of patients had ASL abnormalities, compared with 18% on PWI, and that all patients with PWI lesions also had ASL lesions. A common abnormality was a bilateral borderzone sign.[12] These findings suggest that ASL alone may be a feasible perfusion method in TIA patients.

TYPICAL FINDINGS ON ASL STUDIES: STROKE

This section highlights some of the experiences at the author's institution with a 3D–FSE pcASL method at 1.5 T in patients with acute ischemic stroke and TIA. In addition, whenever possible, images from bolus PWI are included so that readers may contrast the information gained from each modality.

Fig. 3 demonstrates an example of acute ischemic stroke in a 25-year-old woman 6 hours after repair of aortic coarctation. Hypoperfusion is noted within a large region of the left middle cerebral artery (MCA) territory on both ASL and bolus PWI Tmax map. Posterior to this core region, the ASL images show multiple serpiginous high-intensity structures compatible with ATA; this region on bolus PWI shows a milder Tmax abnormality than the core. The findings are compatible

with collateral flow, and in this patient, who did not receive therapy due to her recent surgery, these regions did not convert to infarction based on a 3-day follow-up noncontrast CT scan.

Confirmation that this serpiginous high ASL signal is intravascular is shown in Fig. 4. This 74-year-old man presented with right facial droop and received bolus PWI as well as two separate ASL scans, one with and one without vascular suppression using diffusion gradients.[19,39] The magnetic resonance (MR) angiogram showed distal occlusion of the M1 segment of the right MCA. Here, the diffusion-positive region is fairly small, consistent with the mild symptoms. Bolus PWI Tmax maps show a larger area of abnormality, suggesting tissue at risk of infarction. ASL without vessel suppression showed low parenchymal CBF with extensive regions of ATA throughout the affected territory, which was less evident on the vessel-suppressed ASL images. This suggests that the high serpiginous signal is related to slow flow in excellent collateral vessels; in this patient, fluid-attenuated inversion recovery (FLAIR) images also showed evidence of slow flow.[22] The patient was not treated due to the mild initial symptoms and did not show progression either clinically or on follow-up MR imaging.

Not all stroke patients show the same pattern of central hypoperfusion with surrounding ATA. Fig. 5 demonstrates a case of a right M1 MCA

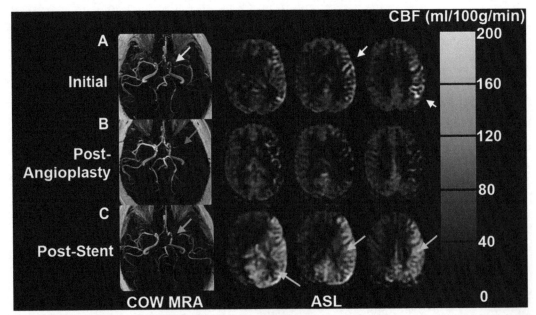

Fig. 6. Repeat ASL CBF imaging in a 58-year-old man with symptomatic left MCA stenosis. (A) Initial ASL images show ATA in the left MCA territory as expected due to the stenosis of the M1 segment of the left MCA (arrows). (B) Immediately after angioplasty, the patient had clinical deterioration and reduced CBF in the affected territory. This was determined to be related to rapid in-stent restenosis. (C) Imaging after emergent angioplasty and stenting show high CBF in the left MCA and bilateral PCA territories, presumably related to luxury perfusion (arrows).

occlusion in a 79-year-old woman with a dense left hemiparesis who received intra-arterial thrombectomy with removal of the main clot 8 hours after symptom onset. ASL images obtained 3 days later demonstrate a large right MCA infarct with associated region of hypoperfusion without significant ATA; the lack of ATA may reflect the loss of any collateral circulation at this time.

The value of repeated quantitative CBF imaging is suggested by the case of a 58-year-old man who underwent elective angioplasty for symptomatic MCA stenosis (**Fig. 6**). His initial ASL images

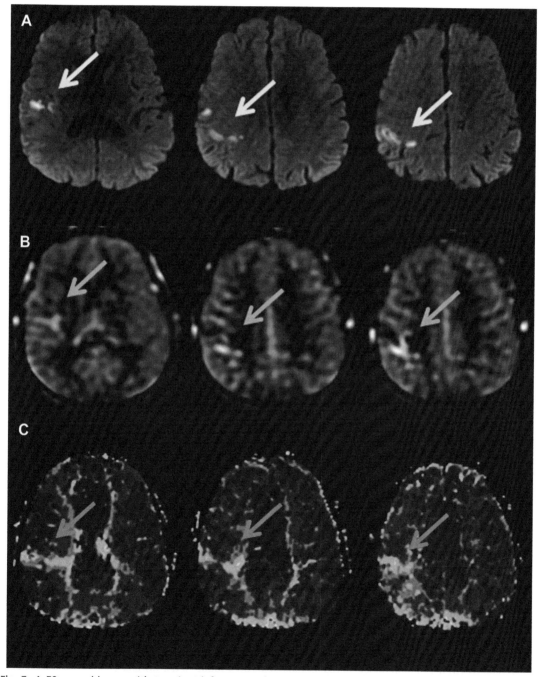

Fig. 7. A 59-year-old man with transient left arm weakness, ABCD2 score was 5. (*A*) DWI images show a small infarct in the right frontoparietal region (*arrows*). This is accompanied by a subtle region of ATA on (*B*) ASL CBF images and (*C*) mild Tmax prolongation on bolus PWI (*arrows*).

showed ATA in the left MCA territory, as expected from his severe stenosis. Immediately after the procedure, the patient clinically deteriorated, with aphasia and right hemiparesis. ASL images acquired at this time showed markedly reduced CBF and ATA in the left MCA territory, which was associated with rapid in-stent restenosis.

The patient underwent emergent repeat angioplasty with stenting with resolution of his symptoms. Follow-up imaging 3 days later demonstrated hyperperfusion to the left MCA territory as well as the bilateral posterior cerebral artery (PCA) territories. Subsequent ASL studies over the next several months showed a persistent

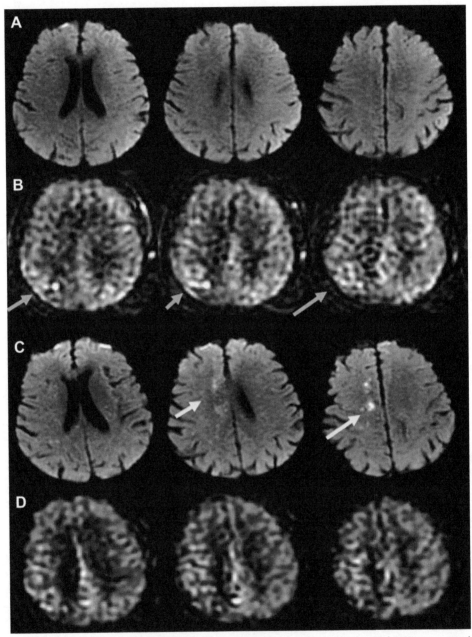

Fig. 8. A 79-year-old man with transient left leg weakness. ABCD2 score was 5. (*A*) Initial DWI was normal. (*B*) ASL shows mild ATA in the right paramedian region (*orange arrows*) suggesting a vascular etiology for the patient's symptoms. Two days later, the patient returned with new onset of left leg weakness and (*C*) the DWI study shows new small infarcts in the right paramedian region (*yellow arrows*) near the prior ATA abnormality from the initial ASL. (*D*) ASL shows slightly more pronounced ATA in the same territory.

but less pronounced region of increased CBF in the same distribution.

TYPICAL FINDINGS ON ASL STUDIES: TIA

Imaging plays an important role in the work-up of TIA, given that patients are asymptomatic at clinical presentation. Although clinical scales, such as the ABCD2 scale,[40] have gained acceptance as a way to predict the risk of recurrent stroke, many studies have shown that imaging can improve the predictive ability of these scales.[41,42] Because approximately 30% of TIA patients have diffusion changes, it is not unexpected that such patients also may demonstrate perfusion lesions, either with bolus contrast PWI[38] or ASL (Fig. 7). The author has also seen patients without diffusion-weighted image (DWI) changes who have perfusion abnormalities, which are most evident as ATA on ASL imaging. Fig. 8 shows an example in a 79-year-old man presenting with transient left leg weakness. Initial studies were DWI negative, but there was evidence of subtle ATA in the right paramedian frontal lobe, suggesting a vascular etiology for the patient's symptoms. He was discharged but returned 2 days later with a new DWI lesion in the right MCA-ACA borderzone region, associated with increased conspicuity of the previously noted ATA. This case highlights the high sensitivity of ASL to minor perfusion alterations, which can be particularly helpful in TIA patients.

Another finding that can be seen in the setting of TIA is the borderzone sign; this finding, that of ASL signal dropout in the MCA-ACA borderzone regions with associated ATA, is most commonly seen in a bilateral distribution.[12] Because of this, it is frequently occult on bolus PWI, because this is usually interpreted in a qualitative fashion in which the two hemispheres are compared with each other. Although the etiology of this finding is unclear, given that it is rarely associated with significant large vessel stenosis or occlusion, it may represent overall decreased cardiac output or microvascular disease. Fig. 9 shows an example of the bilateral borderzone sign in a 79-year-old man with transient expressive aphasia. In this case, a subtle DWI lesion is present in the left centrum semiovale, suggesting a vascular etiology. Although there is some suggestion of bilateral mild Tmax prolongation in the borderzone regions, the ASL images demonstrate a moderate borderzone sign. In the author's limited experience, the presence of a borderzone sign is a poor prognostic feature.

Finally, the author has begun to explore whether or not there is a role for cerebrovascular reserve (CVR) assessment in TIA patients. ASL can be used in this setting, because it can be repeated easily. Also, the relatively mild perfusion

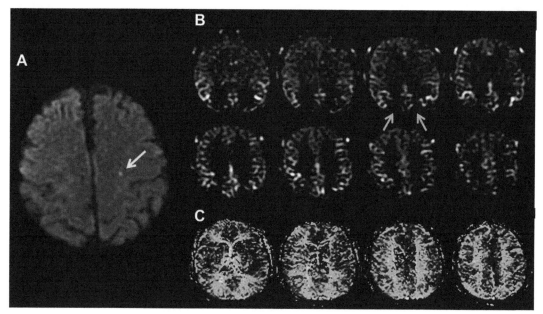

Fig. 9. A 79 year-old man with 10 minutes of transient expressive aphasia. (A) There is a small subtle DWI lesion in the left centrum semiovale (*yellow arrow*). (B) ASL imaging shows a moderate bilateral borderzone sign, evidenced by ASL signal dropout in the MCA-ACA and MCA-PCA borderzone regions (eg, *orange arrows*). (C) Bolus PWI Tmax maps show mild prolongation bilaterally but was read as normal. The presence of the borderzone sign suggests a vascular etiology for the patient's symptoms.

abnormalities in TIA lessen the impact of delayed flow in this population. An example of reduced CVR after acetazolamide challenge in the hemisphere thought to be responsible for clinical symptoms is shown as **Fig. 10**. This patient had several hours of transient left lower-extremity weakness and had reduced CVR in the right hemisphere, consistent with her symptoms. The author hypothesizes that such a finding points to a vascular cause of symptoms and may put her at higher risk for subsequent infarction in this territory.

PROBLEMS WITH ASL IMAGING IN STROKE AND TIA

Although it is likely that ASL will have an important role in the diagnosis or monitoring of stroke and TIA, it is important to recognize its limitations. The most important of these is the sensitivity of ASL to delayed transit times. As discussed previously, this is a double-edged sword; the sensitivity allows the recognition of subtle changes based on ATA. In severe cases and in the presence of large artery stenosis and occlusion, however, ASL may overestimate the region of CBF abnormality. This is frequently seen in patients with chronic occlusions, such as moyamoya disease (**Fig. 11**). Longer PLD sequences mitigate this problem, but it remains a problem for very long transit times. Also, although the borderzone sign is helpful to identifying a vascular etiology, in some cases it obscures the presence of a more focal lesion (**Fig. 12**).

Finally, other artifacts that can mimic stroke exist. One of particular concern is that of poor labeling of arterial spins due to magnetic susceptibility inhomogeneities, which can occur if there is a poor shim of the magnet or if a patient has metallic substances

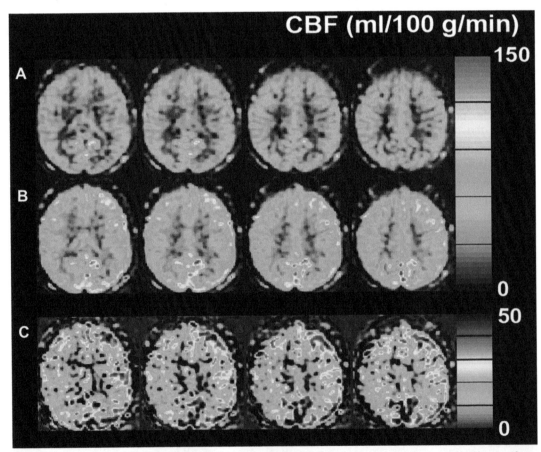

Fig. 10. CVR abnormality detected with MR imaging ASL CBF study in a 51-year-old woman with 3 hours of transient left leg weakness. ABCD2 score was 3. ASL CBF maps obtained (*A*) before and (*B*) 20 minutes after 1 g of intravenous acetazolamide. (*C*) The pre–post difference image demonstrates that both sides show CBF augmentation, with the left increasing by approximately 30–50 mL/100 g/min. The right hemisphere also increases but not as much as the left, with CBF augmentation of approximately 10–30 mL/100 g/min. The lower CVR localizes to the expected hemisphere of the patient's symptoms and may put her at higher risk of future infarct in this territory.

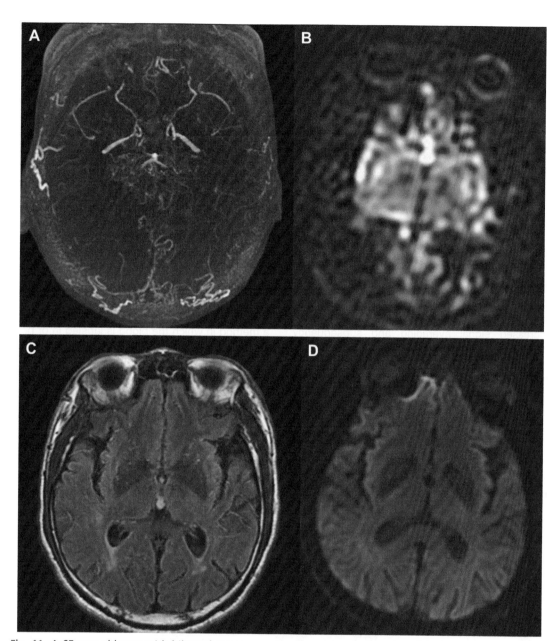

Fig. 11. A 65-year-old man with bilateral moyamoya disease, as demonstrated on (A) MR angiogram. (B) ASL images show normal signal in the deep gray matter but no ASL signal in the bilateral MCA cortices. The patient did not have any evidence of low flow in these regions based on xenon CT (not shown), (C) FLAIR, or (D) DWI. This demonstrates that severely delayed flow will be underestimated using ASL with a PLD used for routine clinical work (2 seconds).

in his or her body, such as dental hardware, stents, or surgical clips. In these situations, often the labeling from one artery is affected and can mimic a large artery occlusion. An example of this, in a patient who was scanned for acute ischemic stroke, is shown as Fig. 13. In this patient, there was partial reperfusion of the left basal ganglia region, but no ASL signal was seen in the right ICA territory. Given the lack of any clinical symptoms referable to the right

MCA territory, it was decided that this represented an artifact related to poor proximal labeling due to susceptibility related to dental hardware in the right neck.

Other issues with ASL include the advanced age of most patients with acute stroke and the corresponding reduced CBF levels associated with age. Also, it has been suggested that arterial arrival times are longer in elderly patients.[43] Both of these

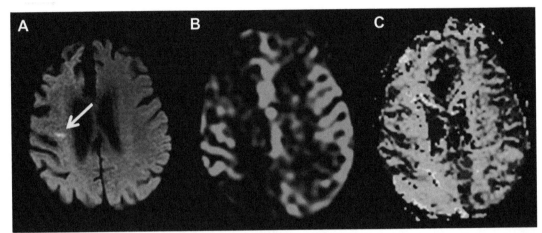

Fig. 12. A 93-year-old woman with recent cerebrovascular accident and new-onset confusion. A small infarct (*arrow*) is seen on the (*A*) DWI study. (*B*) ASL shows bilateral ATA with more prominent signal dropout in the right borderzone region. (*C*) Bolus PWI Tmax shows asymmetric prolongation in the same region.

lead to reduced SNR, suggesting the need for increased signal averaging and subsequently longer imaging scans. Because the efficacy of stroke treatment is known to decrease with time, increasing scan time is suboptimal. Longer scan times are more susceptible to artifacts related to patient motion, although motion correction methods can be applied to ASL.[44]

FUTURE OF ASL IN STROKE AND TIA

Two newer ASL methods may prove to be useful in the work-up of patients with cerebrovascular disease. Velocity-selective ASL (VS-ASL) is a method in which the blood is labeled in or near the voxel of interest rather than at a distant labeling plane, and this may mitigate the errors and artifacts associated with delayed transit.[45] Despite theoretic advantages, this technique has not yet been applied in a systematic fashion to patients with long delay times. Some initial evidence at the author's institution suggests, however, that VS-ASL images in moyamoya disease patients with high-grade stenoses and occlusions are less affected by ATA or ASL signal loss in regions known to have normal CBF on stable xenon CT

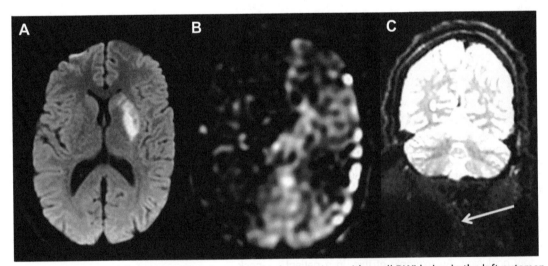

Fig. 13. Poor proximal labeling can mimic large vessel infarct. Patient with small DWI lesion in the left putamen (*A*). (*B*) ASL images show a small region in the left hemisphere with low CBF but a much larger region extending over the entire right ICA territory. Given the lack of symptoms referable to the right MCA territory, it was concluded that this represented a labeling artifact. (*C*) This is further suggested by the region of signal dropout (*arrow*) on coronal B0 maps obtained as part of the diffusion study, indicating magnetic susceptibility artifact in this region, possibly due to dental hardware.

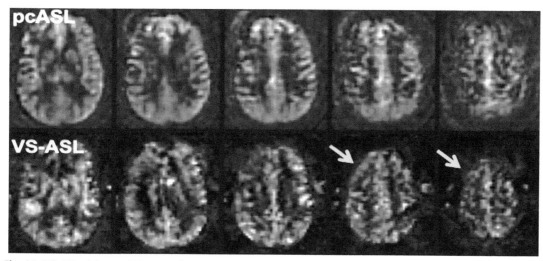

Fig. 14. VS-ASL mitigates CBF errors due to arterial arrival delays. Coregistered images from pcASL and VS-ASL are shown in a patient with moyamoya disease and bilateral MCA occlusion. The pcASL images were obtained using a PLD of 2 seconds, which is too short to image the CBF in the high right frontal lobe. There is preserved ASL signal on the VS-ASL images in this region (*arrows*), suggesting that the errors associated with conventional ASL are reduced with this technique. Note the lower SNR in the VS-ASL images, which is largely due to the fact that the label images can only saturate rather than invert flowing blood.

studies (Fig. 14). A current drawback to routine clinical use of VS-ASL is that currently feasible VS-RF pulses saturate rather than invert affected spins, resulting in 2-fold reduction in SNR. Also, it has yet to be integrated into a sequence with background-suppressed 3D imaging readout, limiting its clinical utility.

Perfusion territory imaging strives to provide separate CBF images that demonstrate how much flow is provided from individual cerebral arteries.[46–48] In theory, such information may be helpful to distinguish antegrade from collateral flow[21] and to assess the perfusion territories supplied by bypass grafts.[49] As such, it yields a more complete view of the cerebrovasculature and for this reason is likely to provide clinical value. It is not yet in widespread clinical use, because most implementations require additional time either for the imaging itself or for the planning of which arteries are to be interrogated.

Finally ASL has not yet been incorporated into a major imaging-based stroke or TIA trial. More clinical experience is necessary to better understand the role of ASL and whether it adds value in this population.

SUMMARY

ASL is a promising technique for evaluating patients with cerebrovascular disease. Recent improvements in pulse sequence design, the more widespread use of 3T neuroimaging, and the recognition of nephrogenic systemic fibrosis

have driven renewed clinical interest in this technique. Although prolonged transit times can lead to quantitative errors in ASL CBF maps, the increased sensitivity to minor perfusion alterations may be of clinical value in patients with TIA and minor stroke. Initial experience with ASL in this patient population is encouraging and suggests that the time may be ripe to consider including ASL in imaging-based stroke and TIA protocols to better understand its practical utility.

REFERENCES

1. Dixon WT, Du LN, Faul DD, et al. Projection angiograms of blood labelled by adiabatic fast passage. Magn Reson Med 1986;3:454–62.

2. Detre JA, Leigh JS, Williams DS, et al. Perfusion imaging. Magn Reson Med 1992;23:37–45.

3. Roberts DA, Detre JA, Bolinger L, et al. Quantitative magnetic resonance imaging of human brain perfusion at 1.5 T using steady-state inversion of arterial water. Proc Natl Acad Sci U S A 1994; 91:33–7.

4. Alsop DC, Detre JA. Multisection cerebral blood flow MR imaging with continuous arterial spin labeling. Radiology 1998;208:410–6.

5. Detre JA, Alsop DC. Perfusion magnetic resonance imaging with continuous arterial spin labeling: methods and clinical applications in the central nervous system. Eur J Radiol 1999;30:115–24.

6. Edelman RR, Siewert B, Darby DG, et al. Qualitative mapping of cerebral blood flow and functional localization with echo-planar MR imaging and signal

targeting with alternating radio frequency. Radiology 1994;192:513–20.

7. Wong EC, Buxton RB, Frank LR. Quantitative imaging of perfusion using a single subtraction (QUIPSS and QUIPSS II). Magn Reson Med 1998; 39:702–8.

8. Deibler AR, Pollock JM, Kraft RA, et al. Arterial spin-labeling in routine clinical practice, part 1: technique and artifacts. AJNR Am J Neuroradiol 2008;29: 1228–34.

9. Deibler AR, Pollock JM, Kraft RA, et al. Arterial spin-labeling in routine clinical practice, part 2: hypoperfusion patterns. AJNR Am J Neuroradiol 2008;29: 1235–41.

10. Deibler AR, Pollock JM, Kraft RA, et al. Arterial spin-labeling in routine clinical practice, part 3: hyperperfusion patterns. AJNR Am J Neuroradiol 2008;29(8): 1428–35.

11. Dai W, Garcia D, de Bazelaire C, et al. Continuous flow driven inversion for arterial spin labeling using pulsed radiofrequency and gradient fields. Magn Reson Med 2008;60:1488–97.

12. Zaharchuk G, Bammer R, Straka M, et al. Arterial spin-label imaging in patients with normal bolus perfusion-weighted MR imaging findings: pilot identification of the borderzone sign. Radiology 2009; 252:797–807.

13. Wong EC, Buxton RB, Frank LR. A theoretical and experimental comparison of continuous and pulsed arterial spin labeling techniques for quantitative perfusion imaging. Magn Reson Med 1998;40: 348–55.

14. Alsop DC, Detre JA. Reduced transit time sensitivity in noninvasive magnetic resonance imaging of human cerebral blood flow. J Cereb Blood Flow Metab 1996;16:1236–49.

15. Hendrikse J, van Osch MJ, Rutgers DR, et al. Internal carotid artery occlusion assessed at pulsed arterial spin-labeling perfusion MR imaging at multiple delay times. Radiology 2004;233:899–904.

16. Petersen ET, Lim T, Golay X. Model-free arterial spin labeling quantification approach for perfusion MRI. Magn Reson Med 2006;55:219–32.

17. Buxton RB, Frank LR, Wong EC, et al. A general kinetic model for quantitative perfusion imaging with arterial spin labeling. Magn Reson Med 1998;40: 383–96.

18. Detre JA, Samuels OB, Alsop DC, et al. Noninvasive magnetic resonance imaging evaluation of cerebral blood flow with acetazolamide challenge in patients with cerebrovascular stenosis. J Magn Reson Imaging 1999;10:870–5.

19. Wang J, Alsop DC, Song HK, et al. Arterial transit time imaging with flow encoding arterial spin tagging (FEAST). Magn Reson Med 2003;50:599–607.

20. Chalela JA, Alsop DC, Gonzalez-Atavales JB, et al. Magnetic resonance perfusion imaging in acute ischemic stroke using continuous arterial spin labeling. Stroke 2000;31:680–7.

21. Chng SM, Petersen ET, Zimine I, et al. Territorial arterial spin labeling in the assessment of collateral circulation: comparison with digital subtraction angiography. Stroke 2008;39:3248–54.

22. Liebeskind DS. Collateral circulation. Stroke 2003;34: 2279–84.

23. Yen Y-F, Field AS, Martin EM, et al. Test-retest reproducibility of quantitative CBF measurements using FAIR perfusion MRI and acetazolamide challenge. Magn Reson Med 2002;47:921–8.

24. Calamante F, Gadian DG, Connelly A. Quantification of perfusion using bolus tracking magnetic resonance imaging in stroke: assumptions, limitations, and potential implications for clinical use. Stroke 2002;33:1146–51.

25. Calamante F, Vonken EJ, van Osch MJ. Contrast agent concentration measurements affecting quantification of bolus-tracking perfusion MRI. Magn Reson Med 2007;58:544–53.

26. Zaharchuk G, Straka M, Marks MP, et al. Combined arterial spin label and dynamic susceptibility contrast measurement of cerebral blood flow. Magn Reson Med 2010;63:1548–56.

27. Koktzoglou I, Edelman RR. Fast projective carotid MR angiography using arterial spin-labeled balanced SSFP. J Magn Reson Imaging 2008;28: 778–82.

28. Guenther M, Oshio K, Feinberg D, editors. Very fast 3D perfusion measurement with high signal-to-noise ratio using single-shot 3D-GRASE: application to improve perfusion quantitation. Kyoto (Japan): ISMRM; 2004. p. 714.

29. Guenther M, Oshio K, Feinberg DA. Single-shot 3D imaging techniques improve arterial spin labeling perfusion measurements. Magn Reson Med 2005;54: 491–8.

30. Luh WM, Wong EC, Bandettini PA, et al. QUIPSS II with thin-slice TI1 periodic saturation: a method for improving accuracy of quantitative perfusion imaging using pulsed arterial spin labeling. Magn Reson Med 1999;41:1246–54.

31. Chen J, Licht DJ, Smith SE, et al. Arterial spin labeling perfusion MRI in pediatric arterial ischemic stroke: initial experiences. J Magn Reson Imaging 2009;29:282–90.

32. Poppe AY, Coutts SB, Demchuk AM. Transient ischemic attack etiologic subtype and early risk of stroke. Stroke 2008;39:e108 [author reply: e109–10].

33. Macintosh BJ, Lindsay AC, Kylintireas I, et al. Multiple inflow pulsed arterial spin-labeling reveals delays in the arterial arrival time in minor stroke and transient ischemic attack. AJNR Am J Neuroradiol 2010;31(10):1428–35.

34. Albers GW, Thijs VN, Wechsler L, et al. Magnetic resonance imaging profiles predict clinical

response to early reperfusion: the diffusion and perfusion imaging evaluation for understanding stroke evolution (DEFUSE) study. Ann Neurol 2006; 60:508–17.

35. Davis SM, Donnan GA, Parsons MW, et al. Effects of alteplase beyond 3 h after stroke in the Echoplanar Imaging Thrombolytic Evaluation Trial (EPITHET): a placebo-controlled randomised trial. Lancet Neurol 2008;7:299–309.

36. Zaharchuk G, Olivot JM, Bammer R, et al, editors. Arterial spin label imaging of transient ischemic attack. Stockholm (Sweden): Internat Soc Magn Reson Med (ISMRM); 2010. p. 4418.

37. Zaharchuk G, Olivot JM, Mlynash M, et al, editors. Yield of perfusion mr imaging in diffusion negative transient ischemic attack patients. Boston: Am Soc Neuroradiology; 2010. p. 27.

38. Mlynash M, Olivot JM, Tong DC, et al. Yield of combined perfusion and diffusion MR imaging in hemispheric TIA. Neurology 2009;72:1127–33.

39. Zaharchuk G, Shankaranarayanan A, Alsop DC, editors. Removing large vessel contamination from arterial spin label MR perfusion images using T2 preparation. In: Proceedings of RSNA. Chicago: RSNA; 2008. VN31-10.

40. Johnston SC, Rothwell PM, Nguyen-Huynh MN, et al. Validation and refinement of scores to predict very early stroke risk after transient ischaemic attack. Lancet 2007;369:283–92.

41. Ay H, Arsava EM, Johnston SC, et al. Clinical- and imaging-based prediction of stroke risk after transient ischemic attack: the CIP model. Stroke 2009; 40:181–6.

42. Coutts SB, Eliasziw M, Hill MD, et al. An improved scoring system for identifying patients at high early risk of stroke and functional impairment after an acute transient ischemic attack or minor stroke. Int J Stroke 2008;3:3–10.

43. Campbell AM, Beaulieu C. Pulsed arterial spin labeling parameter optimization for an elderly population. J Magn Reson Imaging 2006;23: 398–403.

44. Zhang J, Zaharchuk G, Moseley M, et al, editors. Pulsed continuous arterial spin labeling (pcASL) with prospective motion correction (PROMO). Stockholm (Sweden): Internat Soc Magn Reson Med (ISMRM); 2010. p. 5034.

45. Wong EC, Cronin M, Wu W-C, et al. Velocity-selective arterial spin labeling. Magn Reson Med 2006; 55:1334–41.

46. Hendrikse J, Hartkamp MJ, Hillen B, et al. Collateral ability of the circle of Willis in patients with unilateral internal carotid artery occlusion: border zone infarcts and clinical symptoms. Stroke 2001;32: 2768–73.

47. Wong EC. Vessel-encoded arterial spin-labeling using pseudocontinuous tagging. Magn Reson Med 2007;58:1086–91.

48. Zaharchuk G, Ledden P, Kwong K, et al. Multislice perfusion and perfusion territory imaging in humans with separate label and image coils. Magn Reson Med 1999;41:1093–8.

49. van Laar PJ, van der Grond J, Hendrikse J. Brain perfusion territory imaging: methods and clinical applications of selective arterial spin-labeling MR imaging. Radiology 2008;246:354–64.

Transient Ischemic Attack: Definition, Diagnosis, and Risk Stratification

A. Gregory Sorensen, MD[a], Hakan Ay, MD[b],*

KEYWORDS

- Transient ischemic attack • Definition
- Diffusion-weighted imaging • Imaging • Risk stratification
- Risk scores

Each year, approximately 200,000 to 500,000 patients are diagnosed by a physician as having experienced a transient ischemic attack (TIA) in the United States.[1,2] An additional 300,000 to 700,000 individuals experience neurologic symptoms suggestive of a TIA but never seek medical attention for their symptoms.[1,2] The clinical syndrome of TIA designates that the abnormality in the cardiovascular system leading to compromised blood flow to the brain is unstable and, if not properly treated, may also cause a debilitating ischemic stroke. The most remarkable characteristic of TIA is, perhaps, the temporal information it conveys that relates to the timing of an upcoming stroke. The excess risk after TIA can be imminent; the risk is highest within hours of a TIA and declines steadily within the ensuing days, weeks, and months[3]; nearly half of strokes occurring within the next 30 days occur within the first 24 hours after a TIA. It is estimated that 12% to 30% of patients report a history of TIA soon before their stroke and approximately a quarter of them occur during the hours before the stroke.[4,5] TIA constitutes a true medical emergency. Early initiation of preventive treatment of TIA (for instance within 24 hours instead of 20 days) can reduce the 90-day risk of stroke by approximately 80%.[6]

Although rapid and accurate diagnosis and urgent initiation of treatment are key to the management of TIA, given that nearly half of the population reports a brief episode of focal loss of brain function (either TIA or TIA mimics) at one point in their lifetime,[7] indiscriminate use of diagnostic and therapeutic resources may exhaust the health care system. It is critical to accurately identify patients who are most likely to benefit from further diagnostic investigations and rapid treatment. The purpose of this review is to provide an overview on the traditional TIA concept, introduce the new tissue-based definition, and discuss the potential utility of advanced diagnostic imaging and risk stratification in TIA.

CLINICAL DIAGNOSIS OF TIA

According to the World Health Organization criteria proposed in 1988, TIA is defined as rapidly developed clinical signs of focal or global disturbance of cerebral function, lasting less than 24 hours, with no apparent nonvascular cause.[8] The National Institute of Neurologic Disorders and Stroke Report published in 1990 defines TIA as brief episodes of focal loss of brain function for less than 24 hours, thought to be caused by

Disclosures: HA: NIH grant R01-NS059710 and AGS: NIH grant R01-NS038477. Full disclosures are listed in http://www.biomarkers.org/NewFiles/disclosures.html.
[a] Department of Radiology, A.A. Martinos Center for Biomedical Imaging, Massachusetts General Hospital, Harvard Medical School, 13th Street, CNY149-2301, Boston, MA 02129, USA
[b] Stroke Service, A.A. Martinos Center for Biomedical Imaging, Massachusetts General Hospital, Harvard Medical School, 13th Street, CNY149-2301, Boston, MA 02129, USA
* Corresponding author.
E-mail address: hay@partners.org

Neuroimag Clin N Am 21 (2011) 303–313
doi:10.1016/j.nic.2011.01.013
1052-5149/11/$ – see front matter © 2011 Elsevier Inc. All rights reserved.

neuroimaging.theclinics.com

ischemia, which can usually be localized to that portion of the brain supplied by one vascular system.[9] Both of these traditional definitions are based on the assumption that rapid resolution of symptoms in TIA indicates an ischemic insult that is transient at the tissue level. Traditional definitions also assume that clinical judgment as to whether the pattern of signs and symptoms fit into a specific arterial territory is an accurate means of attributing transient symptoms to ischemia. Recent advances in neuroimaging have substantially changed our understanding of TIA. At present, we know that none of these assumptions are quite correct. TIA is not necessarily transient at the tissue level; approximately one-third of traditionally defined TIAs are associated with permanent ischemic tissue injury.[10] Likewise, focal symptoms localizable to an arterial territory do not a priori indicate an ischemic mechanism; several nonischemic mechanisms, including seizures, subdural hemorrhage, intracerebral hemorrhage, brain tumors, multiple sclerosis, and migraine, can cause transient neurologic symptoms confined to a vascular territory.[11,12]

Transient events characterized by symptoms that are focal but not clearly attributable to a known cause are considered atypical or uncertain TIA.[9,13] Clinical features that are not considered to be typical of an ischemic attack include gradual buildup of symptoms (more than 5 minutes), spread of symptoms from one body part to another (without passing the midline), progression of symptoms from one type to another, isolated disturbance of vision in both eyes characterized by the occurrence of positive phenomena, isolated sensory symptoms with remarkably focal distribution, isolated brain stem symptoms, and the occurrence of identical spells over a period longer than 1 year.[9,14] Transient focal atypical spells are common, corresponding to approximately 1 of every 5 emergency room visits because of transient neurologic symptoms.[13] Approximately 10% of patients with atypical symptom characteristics reveal an acute brain lesion on diffusion-weighted magnetic resonance imaging (DWI), suggesting that atypical spells do not exclusively represent a nonischemic subset and may, therefore, not be as benign as previously considered [Hakan Ay, MD, unpublished Massachusetts General Hospital data, 2011].

The opportunity for objective assessment of clinical deficit in TIA is very limited. Approximately 60% of TIAs last for less than 1 hour, and two-thirds of those lasting for less than 1 hour last for less than 10 minutes.[15,16] Only less than 10% of patients can be examined by physicians when they are fully symptomatic.[17] The inevitable use of historical information contributes to the variability in TIA diagnosis; reported rates of disagreement in the diagnosis of TIA by history vary between 42% and 86% among neurologists.[18,19] This variability in TIA diagnosis obviously hampers the clinical and research utility of the term TIA. Recent advances in neuroimaging have revolutionized the evaluation of TIA and provided an opportunity to overcome many of the shortcomings of the clinical-based approach by introducing an objective component to its definition. The following section summarizes the current state of knowledge on the utility of neuroimaging in attributing a transient spell to brain ischemia.

BRAIN IMAGING FINDINGS IN TIA

The introduction of first computed tomography (CT) and later magnetic resonance imaging (MRI) to the evaluation of TIA have challenged the conventional view by demonstrating that clinically transient events are not necessarily transient at the tissue level. Approximately one-third of patients with the clinical syndrome of TIA develop a clinically relevant brain infarct.[10,20,21] The first report of imaging proof of brain infarct in patients with TIA dates back to 1979. Perrone and coworkers[22] reported small hypodense areas on CT consistent with infarction in 12 of the 35 patients with TIA. Four years later, in 1983, Waxman and Toole[23] coined the term "cerebral infarction with transient deficit" to describe transient episodes associated with CT evidence of brain infarction in a clinically relevant location. Since then several researchers have used CT to observe patients with TIA and reported variable rates of brain infarcts ranging from 4% to 34%.[22,24] Subsequent studies with MRI have revealed somewhat higher rates of infarcts changing between 21% and 67%.[25,26] Although infarct rates on CT and MRI are similar, the diagnostic yield of these two imaging methods in identifying the clinically relevant or clinically appropriate infarct is quite different. The ability to distinguish acute infarcts from chronic lesions is critical to be able to tie a brain infarct to the transient clinical event. CT has limited sensitivity in identifying clinically related infarcts because infarcts observed in TIA are often very small, lack edema and mass effect, and demonstrate no or very subtle contrast enhancement. In a study of 149 patients with TIA, only 16% of infarcts suspected to be acute based on CT assessment had lesion characteristics consistent with acute infarcts detected on DWI.[27] In another study of 57 patients with TIA, lesions designated as clinically appropriate and acute on conventional MRI

(Fluid-attenuated inversion recovery (FLAIR)- and T2-weighted images) overlapped with an acute lesion detected by DWI in only 48% of the patients, indicating that the so-called appropriate lesion on conventional MRI was not acute and therefore not related to the transient clinical event in more than half of the patients (Fig. 1).[28] DWI's ability to differentiate between acute and chronic infarcts is clearly a strength in conditions associated with small infarcts such as TIA. Another strength of DWI is its high signal to background contrast. Using DWI, acute small infarcts can be visualized that are not visible on CT or conventional MRI in approximately one-third of patients with TIA.[28] Current TIA guidelines recommend DWI as the preferred method of imaging in patients with TIA.[29] Nevertheless, MRI cannot be tolerated or is contraindicated in approximately 10% of patients, and this limits its widespread applicability.[17] In addition, availability, feasibility, and affordability of MRI for use in emergency management of TIA are limited in many practices. According to a survey based on emergency department visits in the United States between 1992 and 2001, MRI was the first line of imaging in only less than 5% of patients with TIA.[30] A more recent survey conducted in 2008 indicates that 15% of Canadian neurologists routinely use MRI in their practice for managing TIA.[31] Despite a trend toward more frequent use of MRI in recent years, most patients with TIA are currently underevaluated. Training of first-line physicians, formation of hospital systems that enable rapid access

to MRI, and development of newer imaging techniques with higher spatial resolution and lower cost are critical to enhance the diagnostic evaluation of TIA.

The most important characteristic of TIA-related infarcts on DWI is their strikingly small size (see Fig. 1; Figs. 2 and 3).[32] Infarcts as small as 0.07 mL can occur during a TIA. About 96% of all infarcts in TIA are smaller than 1 mL. The authors have previously coined the term "footprints of transient ischemia" to describe such punctate lesions on DWI that remain after complete resolution of TIA symptoms.[28] TIA-related infarcts can occur in any part of the brain including clinically important structures such as the brain stem, internal capsule, and motor cortex, as well as less important or silent brain regions. The probability of infarct on DWI increases as the symptom duration increases, yet this relationship is not consistent across all studies.[28,32,33] The authors have observed brain infarcts occurring in patients with symptoms lasting for as short as 30 seconds as well as normal DWI despite symptoms lasting for several hours. Such evidence suggests that the pathophysiology of TIA includes not only tissue damage but also a component of recovery; it suggests the possibility of interplay between several factors such as the size of the ischemic insult and the robustness of the affected neuronal circuitry, including perhaps the strength of the axonal connections as well as of the underlying neurovascular substrate. There are clearly several fruitful areas for further investigation into how the

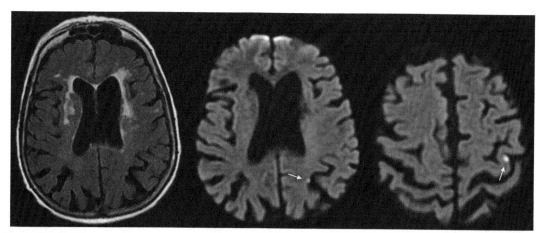

Fig. 1. The FLAIR image in an 86-year-old woman with incoherent speech and right facial droop for 5 minutes showing several scattered and confluent periventricular and subcortical white matter hyperintense foci (left image). The diffusion-weighted images (middle and right images) show 2 punctate foci of restricted diffusion representing acute infarcts involving the left precentral gyrus and posterior left parietal lobe (arrows). Notice that lesions observed on FLAIR images are not associated with restricted diffusion on diffusion-weighted images, indicating that they are not acute.

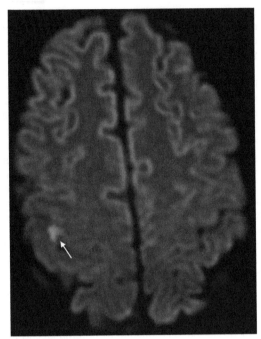

Fig. 2. The diffusion-weighted image in a 53-year-old man with a 2-minute episode of tingling and clumsiness of the left hand showing a 7-mm focus of restricted diffusion involving the right precentral gyrus (*arrow*). Notice the punctate nature of the lesion.

recovery from documentable tissue damage that is clearly present in patients with TIA might be able to be extended to larger stroke insults.

Although the presence of infarct on DWI indicates that the mechanism of transient clinical event is ischemic in origin, the opposite is not always true; DWI results can be negative when in fact transient symptoms are caused by ischemia. DWI has limited sensitivity for very small infarcts, particularly in the brain stem location.[34] In addition, a short lasting episode of ischemia that is not severe enough to cause permanent tissue injury may cause symptoms in the absence of lesions detected by DWI.[34,35] The combined use of DWI and perfusion-weighted MRI may improve the sensitivity for detection of tissue ischemia (**Fig. 4**). Based on observational case studies, perfusion-weighted MRI seems to provide evidence consistent with ischemia in an additional 3% to 16% of patients with TIA on top of DWI.[36–38] The diagnostic utility of perfusion-weighted MRI remains to be confirmed in unbiased large datasets. Limited spatial resolution of currently available perfusion-weighted MRI techniques is also of concern. Improvements in perfusion techniques in the future may overcome these concerns by enhancing the reliability of diagnoses for punctate regions of ischemia that typically occur in TIA.[39]

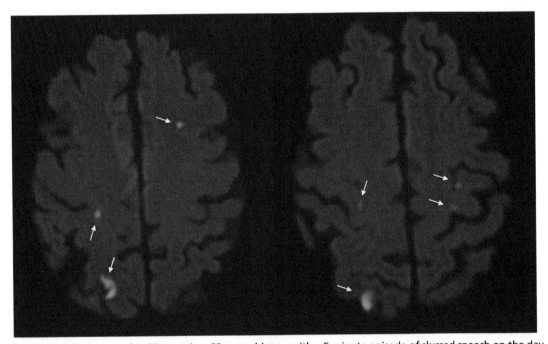

Fig. 3. The diffusion-weighted images in a 65-year-old man with a 5-minute episode of slurred speech on the day of admission showing multiple, mostly punctate foci of restricted diffusion (*arrows*) in both the right and left hemispheres, suggesting embolism from a proximal source.

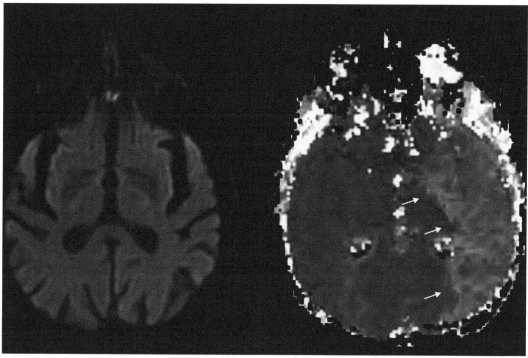

Fig. 4. The diffusion-weighted images in an 82-year-old man with 2 distinct episodes of aphasia, one lasting for 30 minutes and the other for 15 minutes, within a 2-hour period on the day of admission. There is no evidence of acute infarction on the diffusion-weighted image (*left image*). The time to peak map (*right image*), on the other hand, demonstrates signal changes consistent with hypoperfusion in the entire left middle cerebral artery territory (*arrows*), marking ischemia the cause of transient episodes.

TISSUE-BASED DEFINITION OF TIA

Advances in diagnostic imaging of TIA have led to the proposition of a new tissue-based definition.[29] This new definition classifies TIA as a transient episode of neurologic dysfunction caused by focal brain, spinal cord, or retinal ischemia, without evidence of acute infarction. All remaining neurologic events, regardless of whether symptoms are transient or permanent, are called ischemic stroke, as long as they are associated with brain infarction. The tissue-based definition provides a safe passage from subjectivity (arbitrary duration criterion) to objectivity (evidence of brain injury) in defining a TIA. This definition has gained widespread acceptance in a relatively short time and has been endorsed by the American Heart Association (AHA), the American Stroke Council, and the American Academy of Neurology.[29] One aspect of the tissue-based definition that may be perceived as a drawback is the dependency of categorizations on the sensitivity and availability of neuroimaging. The punctate nature of ischemic lesions in TIA particularly makes this problem more severe. Imaging techniques with lower sensitivity, such as CT or conventional MRI, would be expected to reveal a falsely higher prevalence of TIA than diffusion-based techniques that have higher contrast to noise for acute ischemic lesions and can distinguish between nonspecific chronic white matter lesions and acute ischemic lesions. The current pace of changes in diagnostic technology challenges the utility of the new definition in comparing studies from different periods or making uniform categorizations in longitudinal studies covering a long period. To ensure the comparability of studies, it is critical to explicitly acknowledge the method of imaging applied in research studies using the tissue-based definition. In addition, as the AHA/American Stroke Association recommendations also state, the term acute neurovascular syndrome may be used as an intermediate term to describe transient events when neuroimaging is not available or is insensitive to detect the brain infarct despite a strong clinical suspicion for ischemic stroke.

In contrast to the traditional concept that considers TIA as a medical emergency and a sign of an upcoming stroke, TIA, when using the new tissue-based definition, should be considered as an extremely low-risk condition. According to a recent pooled analysis of 4574 patients with TIA from 12 centers, the 7-day risk of stroke after a TIA with no infarction was 0.4%.[10] This risk is approximately 20 times smaller than the corresponding risk after imaging-positive TIA.[10,17,40–42] The early risk of stroke after imaging-positive TIA is not only higher than the risk after imaging-normal TIA but also substantially greater (5 to 10 times) than the corresponding risk for recurrent stroke after an ischemic stroke.[17,32,43,44] Thus, imaging-positive TIA represents an extremely unstable syndrome. These short-term prognostic estimates suggest that it may be operationally more accurate to stratify acute neurovascular syndromes into 3 prognostically different categories: TIA with normal imaging findings, transient symptoms with infarction (TSI), and ischemic stroke.[32,45] Acute cardiovascular syndromes are also classified into 3 major categories: stable angina pectoris, unstable angina pectoris or non–ST elevation myocardial infarction, and ST elevation myocardial infarction.[46] By analogy to the cardiac classification, ischemic stroke corresponds to ST elevation myocardial infarction (evidence of major ischemia and infarction by electrocardiography [ECG] and biochemical markers), TSI to unstable angina pectoris or non–ST elevation myocardial infarction (evidence of minor ischemia or infarction by ECG or biochemical markers), and TIA with no infarction to stable angina pectoris or the chest pain syndrome (no ECG or biomarker evidence of ischemia or infarction).[32,45] This syndromic classification not only takes into account the pathophysiology (the presence of tissue injury) but also incorporates prognostic estimates into definitions, providing the ability to serve as a means to guide treatment strategies. The syndromic classification, however, just like the conventional definition, is time based, necessitating the use of an arbitrary definition for transiency of symptoms.

PREDICTION OF STROKE RISK AFTER TIA

Although the stroke risk after TIA is high (approximately 10% in 7 days), most TIAs (approximately 90%) do not pose an imminent risk of stroke. Accurate differentiation of the 10% at risk from the remaining 90% is critical for optimal stroke prevention. Individualization of TIA management requires a risk-based approach, whereby high-risk and low-risk individuals follow different paths.[6,47] High-risk patients are expected to benefit from urgent referral to specialized stroke centers, timely identification of the underlying cause, and institution of specific preventive treatments, such

as antiplatelet agents, anticoagulants, and carotid endarterectomy. Admission of high-risk patients to specialized stroke centers may also provide the opportunity to administer immediate treatments in a timely manner in the event of a subsequent stroke. In contrast, elective evaluation offers benefit to low-risk patients by avoiding their exposure to the risks, discomforts, and costs of hospitalization. The high prevalence of TIA also makes identification of low-risk patients critical, particularly in settings in which resources are limited.

Several prognostic scores for the prediction of early stroke risk after TIA have been developed during the last decade (Table 1). There are briefly 2 types of prognostic scores: clinical scores and clinical-plus scores. The former is based on clinical predictors that are either baseline patient features or TIA characteristics and include the California score,[48] the ABCD score,[49] and the ABCD^2 score.[50] Clinical-plus scores provide risk estimates based on imaging and other diagnostic test findings in addition to clinical predictors and include the Clinical and Imaging-based Predictive (CIP) score,[17] the ABCD^2 plus imaging (ABCD^2-I) score,[10] the ABCD^2 plus dual TIA and imaging (ABCD^3-I) score,[21] and the Recurrence Risk Estimator (RRE) score.[51] Clinical and clinical-plus scores serve different purposes. Clinical scores are generally easy to apply because they require simple clinical information, such as patient age, history of vascular risk factors, and symptom characteristics that are available to physicians in most clinical settings. Clinical scores are particularly well suited for use in primary care and population-based settings to identify high-risk patients who may benefit from referral for assessment on an emergency basis. Clinical-plus scores, on the other hand, require burdensome laboratory testing for risk stratification. Nevertheless, the additional information provided by diagnostic evaluations helps to further segregate high-risk referrals based on clinical scores into different risk levels. Thus, the clinical-plus scores are more ideal for use in referral centers for individualizing immediate TIA management.

Table 1 summarizes important aspects of validated clinical and clinical-plus scores. The ABCD^2 score is one of the most widely used clinical scores. The ABCD^2 score is a unified clinical score generated from a combined dataset from 2 prior scores (the California score[48] and the ABCD score[49]). This score provides estimates for 2-day, 7-day, and 90-day risk of stroke across 8 possible scores changing from 0 to 7. Higher scores correlate with the presence of vascular risk factors, longer symptom duration, and certain clinical symptoms such as weakness and speech

Table 1
Prognostic scores for prediction of stroke risk after TIA

Score Characteristics	California	ABCD	ABCD²	CIPª	ABCD²-I	ABCD³-I	RREᶜ
Components (points assigned)							
Age >60 y	1	—	—	—	—	—	—
Age ≥60 y	1	1	1	1	1	1	—
Symptom duration >10 min	—	—	—	—	—	—	—
Symptom duration >10–59 min	—	1	1	1	1	1	—
Symptom duration ≥60 min	1	2	2	2	2	2	—
Focal weakness	1	2	2	2	2	2	—
Speech impairment	1	—	—	—	—	—	—
Speech impairment without weakness	—	1	1	1	1	1	—
Diabetes mellitus	—	—	1	1	1	1	—
SBP >140 mm Hg or DBP ≥90 mm Hgᵇ	—	1	—	—	—	—	—
SBP ≥140 mm Hg or DBP ≥90 mm Hg	—	—	1	1	1	1	—
DWI Evidence of acute infarction	—	—	—	1	3	2	1
TIA within the preceding 7 d	—	—	—	—	—	2	—
Ipsilateral carotid stenosis ≥50%	—	—	—	—	—	2	—
Etiologic TIA mechanism (CCS subtype)	—	—	—	—	—	—	1
Multiple infarcts of different ages on DWI	—	—	—	—	—	—	1
Simultaneous acute infarcts in different circulations	—	—	—	—	—	—	1
Multiple acute infarcts	—	—	—	—	—	—	1
Isolated cortical infarcts	—	—	—	—	—	—	1
TIA or stroke within the preceding 30 d	—	—	—	—	—	—	1
Total Possible Scores	5	6	7	—	10	13	7
Risk Prediction Interval (d)	90	7	2, 7, and 90	2 and 7	7 and 90	2, 7, 28, and 90	7, 14, and 90

Abbreviations: CCS, Causative Classification System; DBP, diastolic blood pressure; SBP, systolic blood pressure.
ª The CIP model provides risk estimates based on 4 possible combinations of DWI findings and dichotomized ABCD² score. No points are assigned in the CIP system.
ᵇ Systolic and diastolic blood pressures are based on measurements on first assessment after TIA.
ᶜ RRE score assigns 1 point to TIA etiology for CCS subtypes of large artery atherosclerosis and other uncommon causes.

abnormality. It has been suggested that the ABCD^2 score predicts stroke risk partly because of its ability to discriminate between a true TIA and a suspected TIA with eventual diagnosis of a nonvascular TIA mimic.[12,52,53] The major strength of the ABCD^2 score is its simplicity. The major weakness of this score is the limited discriminative ability. The area under the receiver operating characteristics curve (AUC) for the ABCD^2 score for prediction of 7-day stroke risk is 0.66 (95% confidence interval, 0.53–0.78).[10] Based on the most widely used cutoff score of 4, the ABCD^2 score identifies high- and low-risk patients with a sensitivity of 92% and a specificity of 33%. Nearly two-thirds of patients who do not develop a subsequent stroke are falsely classified as at high risk. This false classification obviously hampers the utility of the score in prioritization of resources in referral centers.

Clinical-plus scores have been developed to enhance the discriminative ability of clinical scores (see **Table 1**). The CIP model is a simple web-based system that combines DWI findings obtained within the first 24 hours of TIA and dichotomized ABCD^2 score (<4 vs $\geq$4) to predict the 7-day risk of subsequent stroke (available at http://cip.martinos.org).[17] Risk estimates are provided for each of the 4 possible combinations of imaging and dichotomous ABCD^2 score: 0% for normal DWI–low ABCD^2 score, 2% for normal DWI–high ABCD^2 score, 5% for positive DWI–low ABCD^2 score, and 15% for positive DWI–high ABCD^2 score. The CIP model provides superior predictive performance as compared with the ABCD^2 score (AUC, 0.80–0.66). It has been estimated that 25% of the patients graded as at low risk by the ABCD^2 score are classified as at high risk according to the CIP model. Likewise, 64% of the patients graded as at moderate or high risk per the ABCD^2 score are classified as at low risk by the CIP model. The CIP score does not assess the predictive value of DWI in simultaneous context with individual components of the ABCD^2 score. Therefore, strictly speaking, it is not a unified score. The ABCD^2-I score has been developed to integrate individual components of the ABCD^2 score and brain imaging in a pooled dataset of 4574 patients (3206 with DWI and 1368 with CT).[10] In this score, each component of the ABCD^2 score is weighted as originally described. The imaging component is weighted by 3 points. These components lead to an 11-point system in which the scores change from 0 to 10, with 10 indicating the highest-risk strata. Regardless of the type of imaging (DWI or CT) used, addition of imaging evidence of infarction to the ABCD^2 score significantly improves the discriminative ability of

predictions (AUC for 7-day risk predictions: 0.66 for ABCD^2, 0.78 for ABCD^2-I with CT, 0.78 for ABCD^2-I with DWI). Comparable performance of CT with DWI in the pooled analysis suggests that brain infarcts convey similar predictive value regardless of their age. Acute infarcts bear prognostic information by marking a spell truly ischemic. Chronic infarcts may also imply ischemia as the causative mechanism of transient symptoms by indicating a baseline ischemia-prone state. Caution, however, should be exercised before widespread application of CT for risk prediction in TIA. Only approximately a quarter of patients in the pooled dataset had CT as the initial line of imaging. The high variance in case mix, setting (population based, specialized neurovascular unit based, emergency based), timing of imaging, and the method of image assessment (blind assessment of one type of imaging to others) in published reports of CT-based datasets necessitates further studies in larger cohorts for conclusive evidence on the prognostic value of CT in TIA.

CIP and ABCD^2-I scores do not take into account the etiologic mechanism of TIA in risk predictions. The etiologic TIA mechanism is known to be an important predictor of stroke risk.[51] The ABCD^3-I score has been developed to partially fill this void.[21] The score adds 2 additional components to the ABCD^2-I score: history of another TIA within 7 days before the index TIA and ipsilateral carotid stenosis causing at least 50% narrowing. The score was generated in a pooled dataset consisting of 2654 patients from 8 studies and validated in a separate dataset of 1232 patients. The ABCD^3-I is a 14-point score system in which scores change between 0 and 13, 0 being the lowest and 13 being the highest risk category. The overall AUC for prediction of stroke risk in 7 days is 0.92 in the derivation and 0.71 in the validation datasets. The score also provides good discrimination for prediction of 28- and 90-day risks. Although incorporating the cause of TIA (carotid stenosis) into the risk prediction after TIA is a strength, the ABCD^3-I score does not take into account the whole spectrum of TIA causes (cardiac embolism, small artery occlusion, other uncommon causes, undetermined causes) that might provide additional prognostic information. The relatively poor performance of ABCD^3-I in the validation dataset is also of concern and suggests a need for further validation.

Since the early risk of stroke after a TIA with no infarction on DWI is negligibly low (0%–0.4%),[10,17] a clinically relevant question in the emergency setting is which patient with TIA with infarction is at imminent risk of developing a stroke. The RRE score has been developed to provide risk predictions in imaging-positive patients.[51] This score was originally generated to predict early risk of recurrent stroke in patients with ischemic stroke. The RRE is a web-based (http://www.nmr.mgh.harvard.edu/RRE/) 7-point score composed of 2 clinical and 4 imaging predictors each weighted by 1 point. Clinical predictors are prior ischemic event within the preceding month of TSI and etiologic stroke mechanism as classified by the Causative Classification System.[54] Imaging predictors include infarct characteristics such as age, location, distribution, and number of infarcts on DWI (see Table 1). The RRE provides risk estimates based on information available to the physician immediately after initial stroke evaluation in typical clinical practice. These include findings from clinical history, ECG, and baseline brain and vascular imaging. In a study of 257 patients with imaging-positive TIA, the RRE score applied within 24 hours of TIA provided an AUC of 0.85 for 7-day risk of stroke. The RRE score promises to further stratify high-risk patients at risk of developing stroke, but additional validation studies of this score in external settings need to be performed.

SUMMARY

Recent advances in neuroimaging have enhanced the understanding of TIA. Accumulated evidence indicates that clinically transient spells are not transient at the tissue level and leave infarct on the brain in nearly one-third of patients. TIA-related acute infarcts are typically extremely small and often are not detected by CT and conventional MRI. DWI is currently the preferred method of imaging in TIA. Recognition of acute infarcts in patients with TIA has challenged the long-standing conventional definition and led to the proposition of a new tissue-based definition. The tissue-based definition reserves the term TIA for transient episodes without evidence of acute infarction. TIA, as defined by the tissue-based definition, is not a medical emergency anymore; it is a very low-risk condition (early risk <0.4%). In contrast, TIA with infarction represents an extremely unstable condition with early risk of stroke that is as much as 20 times higher than the risk after TIA with normal imaging. The high prevalence of TIA necessitates accurate risk stratification to assure efficient use of resources. Several prognostic scores for prediction of early stroke risk after TIA with varying complexity and utility have been developed during the last 5 years. A staged approach to risk stratification in TIA based on availability of diagnostic resources should be advocated. Scores that are based on

baseline patient features and TIA characteristics, such as the California, the ABCD, and the $ABCD^2$ scores, are generally simple, can be widely applied, and are well suited for use in primary care and population-based settings for selection of patients for referral to specialized centers. Clinical-plus scores such as the CIP, the $ABCD^2$-I, the $ABCD^3$-I, and the RRE scores, on the other hand, require additional laboratory testing and are more difficult to apply but provide risk estimates with higher accuracy as compared with clinical scores. Clinical-plus scores could be used in specialized stroke centers to individualize TIA management and prioritize hospital resources. The RRE score could allow a more refined and targeted approach by further stratifying imaging-positive TIAs (the high-risk subset by other clinical-plus scores) into different risk levels. Future clinical studies must address the utility and cost benefit of individualized TIA management based on staged risk stratification.

REFERENCES

1. Johnston SC, Fayad PB, Gorelick PB, et al. Prevalence and knowledge of transient ischemic attack among US adults. Neurology 2003;60(9):1429–34.
2. Lloyd-Jones D, Adams RJ, Brown TM, et al. Heart disease and stroke statistics—2010 update: a report from the American Heart Association. Circulation 2010;121:e46–215.
3. Chandratheva A, Mehta Z, Geraghty OC, et al. Population-based study of risk and predictors of stroke in the first few hours after a TIA. Neurology 2009; 72:1941–7.
4. Rothwell PM, Warlow CP. Timing of TIAs preceding stroke: time window for prevention is very short. Neurology 2005;8(64):817–20.
5. Hackam DG, Kapral MK, Wang JT, et al. Most stroke patients do not get a warning: a population-based cohort study. Neurology 2009;73:1074–6.
6. Rothwell PM, Giles MF, Chandratheva A, et al. Effect of urgent treatment of transient ischaemic attack and minor stroke on early recurrent stroke (EXPRESS study): a prospective population-based sequential comparison. Lancet 2007;370:1432–42.
7. Toole JF, Lefkowitz DS, Chambless LE, et al. Self-reported transient ischemic attack and stroke symptoms: methods and baseline prevalence. The ARIC Study, 1987–1989. Am J Epidemiol 1996;144(9):849–56.
8. Who Monica. Project principal investigators. The World Health Organization MONICA Project (monitoring trends and determinants in cardiovascular disease): a major international collaboration. J Clin Epidemiol 1988;41(2):105–14.
9. National Institute of Neurological Disorders and Stroke. Special report from the National Institute of

Neurological Disorders and Stroke: classification of cerebrovascular diseases, III. Stroke 1990;21:637–76.

10. Giles MF, Albers GW, Amarenco P, et al. Addition of brain infarction to the ABCD2 Score (ABCD2I): a collaborative analysis of unpublished data on 4574 patients. Stroke 2010;41:1907–13.

11. Prabhakaran S, Silver AJ, Warrior L, et al. Misdiagnosis of transient ischemic attacks in the emergency room. Cerebrovasc Dis 2008;26:630–5.

12. Sheehan OC, Merwick A, Kelly LA, et al. Diagnostic usefulness of the ABCD2 score to distinguish transient ischemic attack and minor ischemic stroke from noncerebrovascular events: the North Dublin TIA Study. Stroke 2009;40:3449–54.

13. Koudstaal PJ, Algra A, Pop GA, et al. Risk of cardiac events in atypical transient ischaemic attack or minor stroke. The Dutch TIA Study Group. Lancet 1992;340:630–3.

14. Fisher CM. Late-life migraine accompaniments—further experience. Stroke 1986;17:1033–42.

15. Levy DE. How transient are transient ischemic attacks? Neurology 1988;38:674–7.

16. Shah SH, Saver JL, Kidwell CS, et al. A multicenter pooled patient-level data analysis of diffusion-weighted MRI in TIA patients. Stroke 2007;38:463a.

17. Ay H, Arsava EM, Johnston SC, et al. Clinical- and imaging-based prediction of stroke risk after transient ischemic attack: the CIP model. Stroke 2009; 40:181–6.

18. Tomasello F, Mariani F, Fieschi C, et al. Assessment of interobserver differences in the Italian Study on reversible cerebral ischemia. Stroke 1982;13:32–5.

19. Kraaijeveld CL, Van Gijn J, Schouten HJA, et al. Interobserver agreement for the diagnosis of transient ischemic attacks. Stroke 1984;15:723–5.

20. Ovbiagele B, Kidwell CS, Saver JL. Epidemiological impact in the United States of a tissue-based definition of transient ischemic attack. Stroke 2003;34: 919–24.

21. Merwick A, Albers GW, Amarenco P, et al. Addition of brain and carotid imaging to the ABCD^2 score to identify patients at early risk of stroke after transient ischaemic attack: a multicentre observational study. Lancet Neurol 2010;9(11):1060–9.

22. Perrone P, Candelise L, Scotti G. CT evaluation in patients with transient ischemic attack. Correlation between clinical and angiographic findings. Eur Neurol 1979;18:217–21.

23. Waxman SG, Toole JF. Temporal profile resembling TIA in the setting of cerebral infarction. Stroke 1983;14(3):433–7.

24. Douglas VC, Johnston CM, Elkins J, et al. Head computed tomography findings predict short-term stroke risk after transient ischemic attack. Stroke 2003;34:2894–8.

25. Crisostomo RA, Garcia MM, Tong DC. Detection of diffusion-weighted MRI abnormalities in patients with transient ischemic attack: correlation with clinical characteristics. Stroke 2003;34:932–7.

26. Rovira A, Rovira-Gols A, Pedraza S, et al. Diffusion-weighted MR imaging in the acute phase of transient ischemic attacks. AJNR Am J Neuroradiol 2002;23: 77–83.

27. Förster A, Gass A, Ay H, et al. Acute CT In TIA patients is unrevealing—a comparative CT/MRI Study. Stroke 2009;40:e195–6.

28. Ay H, Oliveira-Filho J, Buonanno FS, et al. "Footprints" of transient ischemic attacks: a diffusion-weighted MRI study. Cerebrovasc Dis 2002;14: 177–86.

29. Easton JD, Saver JL, Albers GW, et al. Definition and evaluation of transient ischemic attack: a scientific statement for healthcare professionals from the American Heart Association/American Stroke Association. Stroke 2009;40:2276–93.

30. Edlow JA, Kim S, Pelletier AJ, et al. National study on emergency department visits for transient ischemic attack, 1992–2001. Acad Emerg Med 2006;13:666–72.

31. Perry JJ, Mansour M, Sharma M, et al. National survey of Canadian neurologists' current practice for transient ischemic attack and the need for a clinical decision rule. Stroke 2010;41:987–91.

32. Ay H, Koroshetz WJ, Benner T, et al. Transient ischemic attack with infarction: a unique syndrome? Ann Neurol 2005;57:679–86.

33. Kidwell CS, Alger JR, Di Salle F, et al. Diffusion MRI in patients with transient ischemic attacks. Stroke 1999;30:1174–80.

34. Ay H, Buonanno FS, Rordorf G, et al. Normal diffusion-weighted MRI during stroke-like deficits. Neurology 1999;52:1784–92.

35. Minematsu K, Li L, Sotak C, et al. Reversible focal ischemic injury demonstrated by diffusion-weighted magnetic resonance imaging in rats. Stroke 1992; 23(9):1304–11.

36. Krol AL, Coutts SB, Simon JE, et al. Perfusion MRI abnormalities in speech or motor transient ischemic attack patients. Stroke 2005;36:2487–9.

37. Restrepo L, Jacobs MA, Barker PB, et al. Assessment of transient ischemic attack with diffusion- and perfusion-weighted imaging. AJNR Am J Neuroradiol 2004;25:1645–52.

38. Mlynash M, Olivot JM, Tong DC, et al. Yield of combined perfusion and diffusion MR imaging in hemispheric TIA. Neurology 2009;72:1127–33.

39. Ay H, Arsava EM, Vangel M, et al. Interexaminer difference in infarct volume measurements on MRI: a source of variance in stroke research. Stroke 2008;39:1171–6.

40. Prabhakaran S, Chong JY, Sacco RL. Impact of abnormal diffusion-weighted imaging results on short-term outcome following transient ischemic attack. Arch Neurol 2007;64:1105–9.

41. Calvet D, Touzé E, Oppenheim C, et al. DWI lesions and TIA etiology improve the prediction of stroke after TIA. Stroke 2009;40:187–92.

42. Asimos AW, Rosamond WD, Johnson AM, et al. Early diffusion weighted MRI as a negative predictor for disabling stroke after ABCD2 score risk categorization in transient ischemic attack patients. Stroke 2009;40:3252–7.

43. Lowett JK, Coull AJ, Rothwell PM. Early risk of recurrence by subtype of ischemic stroke in population-based incidence studies. Neurology 2004;62: 569–73.

44. Petty GW, Brown RD Jr, Whisnant JP, et al. Survival and recurrence after first cerebral infarction: a population-based study in Rochester, Minnesota, 1975 through 1989. Neurology 1998;50: 208–16.

45. Ay H, Koroshetz WJ. Transient ischemic attack: are there different types or classes? Risk of stroke and treatment options. Curr Treat Options Cardiovasc Med 2006;8(3):193–200.

46. Thygesen K, Alpert JS, White HD. Joint ESC/ACCF/AHA/WHF task force for the redefinition of myocardial, infarction. Universal definition of myocardial infarction. Eur Heart J 2007;28:2525.

47. Giles MF, Rothwell PM. Systematic review and pooled analysis of published and unpublished validations of the ABCD and ABCD2 transient ischemic attack risk scores. Stroke 2010;41:667–73.

48. Johnston SC, Gress DR, Browner WS, et al. Short-term prognosis after emergency department diagnosis of TIA. JAMA 2000;284:2901–6.

49. Rothwell PM, Giles MF, Flossmann E, et al. A simple score (ABCD) to identify individuals at high early risk of stroke after transient ischaemic attack. Lancet 2005;366:29–36.

50. Johnston SC, Rothwell PM, Nguyen-Huynh MN, et al. Validation and refinement of scores to predict very early stroke risk after transient ischaemic attack. Lancet 2007;369:283–92.

51. Ay H, Gungor L, Arsava EM, et al. A score to predict early risk of recurrence after ischemic stroke. Neurology 2010;74:128–35.

52. Josephson SA, Sidney S, Pham TN, et al. Higher ABCD2 score predicts patients most likely to have true transient ischemic attack. Stroke 2008;39:3096–8.

53. Quinn TJ, Cameron AC, Dawson J, et al. ABCD2 scores and prediction of noncerebrovascular diagnoses in an outpatient population: a case-control study. Stroke 2009;40:749–53.

54. Ay H, Benner T, Arsava EM, et al. A computerized algorithm for etiologic classification of ischemic stroke: the causative classification of stroke system. Stroke 2007;38:2979–84.

Measuring Permeability in Acute Ischemic Stroke

Andrea Kassner, PhD[a],*, Daniel M. Mandell, MD, FRCPC[b],
David J. Mikulis, MD, FRCPC[b]

KEYWORDS

- MRI • CT • Stroke • Dynamic contrast-enhanced imaging
- Hemorrhagic transformation • Permeability

Thrombolytic therapy with recombinant tissue plasminogen activators (rtPA) is the main treatment available for acute ischemic stroke, yet use of rtPA is currently limited to patients presenting within 4.5 hours of symptom onset, because of the increased risk of hemorrhagic transformation (HT) if it is administered later.[1,2] There is strong evidence that the HT process begins at the microvascular level.[3] There are also a growing number of reports implicating rtPA as either a primary cause or as an aggravating factor in BBB breakdown.[4–8] Following intravenous injection of contrast material, extravasation of contrast (through a damaged BBB) is an accurate predictor of subsequent HT. Imaging assessment of BBB integrity may predict the likelihood of hemorrhagic transformation on a patient-by-patient basis, rather than using the same simple 4.5-hour time limit for all patients. This could potentially extend the therapeutic time window in patients with evidence of BBB stability, and potentially exclude some patients from receiving rtPA if they have a high risk of hemorrhage despite falling within the 4.5-hour time window. In this article, we discuss the application of permeability imaging in acute ischemic stroke using MRI and CT.

MRI METHODS FOR THE ASSESSMENT OF BBB INTEGRITY

In the 1980s, the introduction of paramagnetic intravascular contrast agents, such as gadolinium chelate gadopentetate dimeglumine (Gd-DTPA), made possible the investigation of BBB integrity using MRI. Gd-DTPA is the most widely used MR contrast agent. It is a freely diffusible, extracellular tracer with a molecular size of 550 Da. The chelator moiety, DTPA, governs the kinetics of the entire compound and clearance occurs primarily via glomerular filtration. The contrast enhancement is produced by the paramagnetic Gd^{3+} core of the agent, which is known to reduce T1 in a concentration-dependent manner.[9]

For assessment of permeability, Gd-DTPA is administered intravenously, usually as a bolus (manual or power) injection. As the contrast agent passes through the microvasculature of the brain, it is almost entirely confined to the intravascular space. In regions of BBB breakdown, however, the contrast-agent can extravasate and accumulate in the interstitium. Once in the extravascular space, voxels with higher concentrations of contrast agent will appear bright on T1-weighted MR images. We will now discuss the use of

This work was supported by the Canada Research Chair Program and the Canadian Institutes of Health Research.

[a] Department of Medical Imaging, University of Toronto, 150 College Street, Room 125, Toronto, ON M5S 3E2, Canada

[b] Department of Medical Imaging, Toronto Western Hospital, University of Toronto, 399 Bathurst Street, Toronto, ON M5T 2S8, Canada

* Corresponding author.

E-mail address: andrea.kassner@utoronto.ca

Neuroimag Clin N Am 21 (2011) 315–325

doi:10.1016/j.nic.2011.01.004

standard (static) postcontrast T1-weighted MR imaging and dynamic contrast-enhanced MR imaging for the detection of BBB breakdown.

Postcontrast T1-Weighted MRI to Predict HT in Acute Ischemic Stroke

The detection of contrast leakage into brain parenchyma can be attempted with static T1-weighted MR imaging. As with brain tumors, the rationale for static contrast-enhanced MRI is that any tissue supplied by vessels with compromised BBB should eventually become conspicuous as a region of signal enhancement on T1-weighted images. Enhancement on T1-weighted images in hyperacute infarcts is indeed associated with subsequent HT.[10–12] High-resolution T1-weighted images are generally acquired at least several minutes after the intravenous (IV) bolus injection of contrast agent (usually 0.1 mmol/kg Gd-DTPA) to allow for sufficient tracer accumulation in the parenchyma at sites of BBB disruption. Although qualitative visual evidence of parenchymal enhancement (that is, contrast extravasation) on postcontrast T1-weighted MRI is a highly specific (specificity ∼85%) predictor of HT, it is infrequent during the crucial hours after symptom onset,[11,13–16] and insensitive (sensitivity ∼35%), which may make the test unsuitable for therapeutic decision making.[10–12] Because it provides only a "snapshot" of a dynamic process (ie, contrast extravasation via breaches in BBB integrity), postcontrast T1-weighted MRI could be problematic during the hyperacute or acute phase of injury in acute ischemic stroke. Postcontrast T1-weighted images of 2 HT cases imaged fewer than 6 hours after symptom onset at our institution are provided in **Fig. 1** to illustrate this problem. At present, it remains to be demonstrated that these images can be acquired at just the right moment to capture the onset of BBB breakdown and offer adequate sensitivity within the current 4.5-hour treatment window.

In part, the low sensitivity of postcontrast T1-weighted MRI for secondary hemorrhage may be a consequence of persistent ischemia or microvascular obstruction in the acute phase[17] such that contrast fails to accumulate sufficiently within the infarct despite local BBB disruption. A 1999 report demonstrated that the addition of a continuous low-dose infusion of contrast to the initial bolus dose could improve the sensitivity of postcontrast T1-weighted MRI.[13] Although a lengthy infusion is clearly unsuitable for the purpose of acute ischemic stroke treatment decision making, the development of convenient measures that increase the signal-to-noise ratio (SNR) may

enable us to detect BBB disruption, where it exists.

Dynamic Contrast-Enhanced MRI

Rationale and acquisition strategy

Dynamic contrast-enhanced MRI (DCE-MRI) typically involves intravenous bolus injection of a gadolinium contrast agent followed by T1-weighted gradient-recalled echo (GRE) imaging of the brain repeated dozens of times over the course of several minutes. Then, assuming a linear relationship between image MR signal intensity as a function of time ($SI[t]$) and contrast-agent concentration as a function of time ($C[t]$), one can generate a set of concentration versus time curves for each voxel or region of the brain. One also typically generates at least one curve consisting exclusively of blood plasma data ($C[p]$) (**Fig. 2**A). As with postcontrast T1-weighted imaging, evidence of enhancement indicates that contrast material has escaped the confines of the intravascular compartment via breaches in the BBB. The advantage of the dynamic T1-weighted imaging technique is that one can quantify contrast accumulation as a function of time, apply an appropriate pharmacokinetic model to the time-varying $C(t)$ and $C(p)$ data-sets, and estimate BBB permeability in standard units of mL/100 g/min.

The most common MRI sequence used in brain DCE-studies, including those performed at our institution, is a 3-dimensional (3D) GRE sequence with a short repetition-time (TR), short echo-time (TE), and a flip angle of approximately 20° at 1.5 T.[18] Three-dimensional volume acquisitions are favored over 2D equivalents in DCE-MRI of the brain, as they permit the simultaneous sampling of the signal intensity in tissue and in blood and are more likely to encompass a large vessel from which one can generate an arterial input function (a considerable challenge in brain DCE[19]). In addition to coverage, a 3D DCE acquisition offers the advantage of maximizing the saturation of inflowing blood while minimizing precontrast inflow enhancement.[20] Furthermore, the 3D GRE sequence is less sensitive to geometric distortions or magnetic susceptibility than equivalent echo-planar sequences.

The temporal resolution of the DCE sequence must be sufficient to capture the blood-brain flow of contrast anticipated for the pathology of interest. By definition, the temporal resolution of the acquisition will improve with shorter TRs (ie, more images can be collected per unit time); TE should also be short, but this choice is related more directly to mitigating susceptibility-related signal loss caused by the transit of the

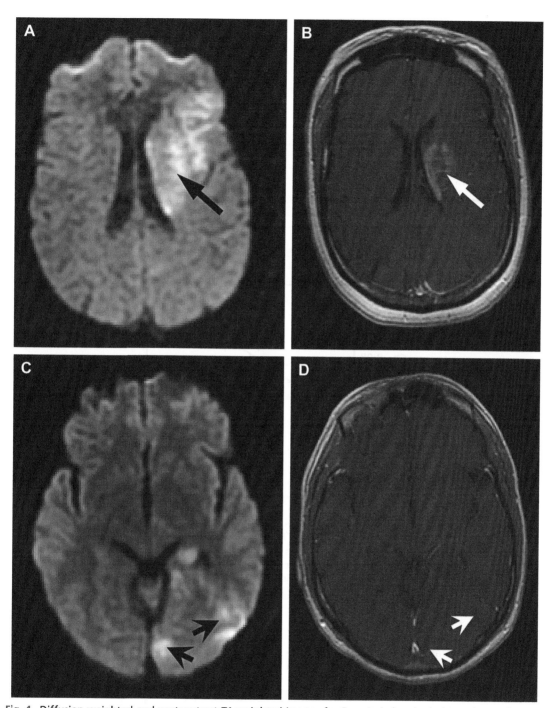

Fig. 1. Diffusion-weighted and postcontrast T1-weighted images for 2 acute ischemic stroke patients who proceeded to hemorrhage. Top: An 81-year-old female patient with acute ischemic stroke, visible as hyperintensity (*arrow*) on the diffusion-weighted image acquired at 3 hours after symptom onset (*A*). The acute ischemic stroke lesion in *A* (*arrow*) corresponds to an area of visible enhancement on the equivalent postcontrast T1-weighted image (*B, arrow*). Bottom: A 69-year-old male patient with acute ischemic stroke, visible as hyperintensity (*arrowhead*) on the diffusion-weighted image acquired at 5 hours 40 minutes after stroke (*C*). Unlike the previous case, the area of ischemia depicted by the diffusion-weighted image did not appear to correspond to any visible gadolinium enhancement in the equivalent T1-weighted image for this patient (*D, arrowhead*).

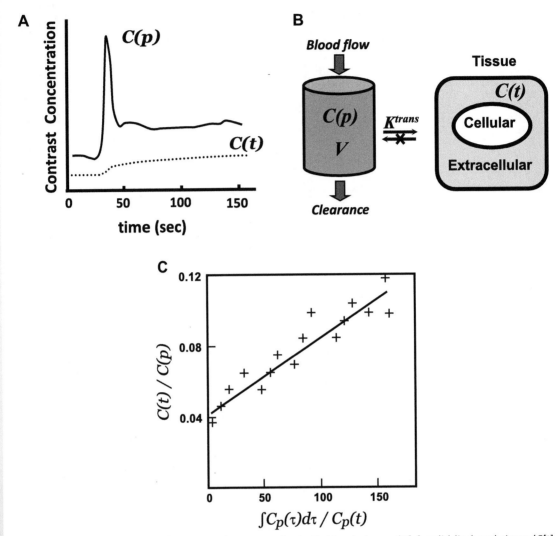

Fig. 2. The contrast concentration versus time curves for both blood plasma (*C[p]*, *solid line*) and tissue (*C[t]*, *dotted line*) are depicted in (*A*). Permeability can be estimated using a unidirectional 2-compartment tracer-kinetic model (*B*), such as the Patlak model.[27] Plotting the ratio *C(t)/C(p)* versus $\int C_p(\tau)d\tau/C_p(t)$ yields a linear relationship, where permeability (*KPS*) is the slope of best fit (*C*).

paramagnetic contrast-agent through the micro-vasculature.[21] The TR prescribed for brain DCE-MRI studies is typically less than 10 ms. Although a 3D volume acquisition necessarily increases TR relative to single-slice approaches, this is becoming less of an issue as more centers gain access to parallel imaging techniques (eg, sensitivity encoding using multiple receiver coils[22]).

Pharmacokinetic modeling The initial step in pharmacokinetic analysis is the conversion of MR signal intensity to contrast-agent concentration. The difference in SI between pre- and postcontrast

images using a T1-weighted GRE sequence can be expressed as:

$$\triangle SI = k\left(\frac{1}{T_{1post}} - \frac{1}{T_{1pre}}\right)$$

$$= k\triangle\left(\frac{1}{T_1}\right) = k\triangle R_1 \qquad (1)$$

where *k* is a proportionality constant, and R_1 is the longitudinal relaxation rate expressed as 1/T1. One has transitioned from $\triangle SI$ to $\triangle R_1$, and after that, one needs to determine the relationship between $\triangle R_1$ and *C(t)*. It is assumed that $\triangle R_1$ is related to *C(t)* by a linear scaling factor, r_1 (ie, T_1

relaxivity, in s^{-1} mM^{-1}). Given that local tissue environments can modulate tracer relaxivity, this simplification may introduce errors in the final parameter estimates.[23]

The next step is to model the relationship of the tissue contrast agent concentration $C(t)$ to the concentration time curve of the contrast agent in blood $C(p)$ to gain insight into the physiological process of exchange of the agent between the intravascular and the extracellular space. To achieve this, concentration time curves from both tissue of interest and reference vascular structures are mathematically fitted using a pharmacokinetic model, which enables the derivation of quantitative modeling parameters.

In many cases, the pharmacokinetic models that are applied to DCE-MRI data were originally developed for nuclear medicine tracers.[24–28] Most of these are compartmental models, which define the tissue space as a volume with both intravascular and extravascular compartments. The generalized 2-compartment analysis proposed by Tofts and colleagues[29] defines 2 tracer parameters of physiological interest: the transfer constant, K^{trans} $[s^{-1}]$ and the distribution volume, v_e (ie, the fraction of the extravascular-extracellular space occupied by tracer in mL/g):

$$\frac{dC_t(t)}{dx} = K^{trans}\left[C_p(t) - \left(\frac{C_t(t)}{v_e}\right)\right] \quad (2)$$

When the concentration of contrast in the tissue before injection is 0, that is $C(t)_0 = 0$, we can find a solution to Equation (2) and therefore determine the $C(t)$ for each time point postinjection:

$$C_t(t) = K^{trans}\int_0^t C_p(\tau)e^{-\frac{K^{trans}}{v_e}\cdot(t-\tau)} \quad (3)$$

$$d\tau = K^{trans}C_p(t) \otimes e^{-\frac{K^{trans}}{v_e}\cdot t} \quad (4)$$

where $C_t(t)$ is the tissue concentration $C(t)$, $C_p(t)$ is the plasma concentration $C(p)$ over time, and the $\otimes$ symbol indicates the convolution operator.

The physiological interpretation of K^{trans} will be specific to the tissue or pathology of interest. Furthermore, K^{trans} will depend on whether the intercompartmental movement of tracer is restricted primarily by capillary permeability or, rather, movement is limited by regional blood flow (F, in mL/min/g), ie, $K^{trans} = EF\rho$ $(1 - rHct)$, where E represents the fraction of contrast agent that extravasates during the first circuit through the vasculature (extraction fraction), ρ indicates the density of the tissue in g/mL, and Hct is the hematocrit (the fraction of blood-volume occupied by cells). In addition to flow, E is also related

to the permeability surface-area product (PS in mL/min/g), $E = 1 - exp(-PS/F)$. Taken together, we can see that K^{trans} will predominantly reflect regional blood flow when PS/F is high ($K^{trans} \sim F\rho$ $[1 - Hct]$). Conversely, if PS/F <1, as is typically the case for clinical MRI contrast media in normal brain parenchyma (and intact BBB), then K^{trans} will be equivalent to $PS\rho$.[18] (Note: K^{trans} is sometimes referred to as KPS under these conditions.)

If we consider the permeability-limited scenario and we further assume that there is no efflux of contrast, ie, the tracer becomes effectively "trapped" in the extravascular compartment, at least for the time-scale involved in the tracer-kinetic study, then we can simplify the pharmacokinetic model in the manner proposed by Patlak and colleagues[27] and depicted in **Fig. 2B**. The Patlak model is a graphical approach for estimating KPS that models the relationship between $C_t(t)$ and $C_p(t)$ (the input function) using linear regression:

$$\frac{C_t(t)}{C_p(t)} = KPS\cdot\int_0^t\frac{C_p(\tau)d\tau}{C_p(t)} + V \quad (5)$$

where V represents the fractional blood volume in each voxel. Plotting the ratio $C_t(t)/C_p(t)$ versus $\int C_p(\tau)d\tau/C_p$ yields a linear relationship, where KPS is the slope of best fit and V is the y-intercept (see **Fig. 2C**). This approach obviates the need for deconvolution (and its sensitivity to noise). The Patlak model has been adapted and successfully applied to DCE-MRI data obtained in both brain tumors[30] and acute ischemic stroke[20,31] for the estimation of KPS.

DCE-MRI for the prediction of HT in acute ischemic stroke

DCE-MRI may aid in selecting acute ischemic stroke patients for treatment based on imaging evidence of BBB integrity (that is, lack of BBB disruption). Using DCE-MRI in an ischemic stroke rat model, Knight and colleagues[32] found that progressive parenchymal enhancement was highly correlated with the presence of HT after reperfusion. After observing elevations in BBB permeability with DCE-MRI, even in the absence of visible postcontrast T1-weighted enhancement in patients who have subsequently hemorrhaged (**Fig. 3**), we added a DCE-MRI component to our acute ischemic stroke MRI protocol. A pilot study of 10 patients with acute ischemic stroke assessed within 24 hours of symptom onset (and not treated with rtPA) showed that it was feasible to measure KPS in a clinical acute ischemic stroke setting.[20] Follow-up imaging indicated that 3 of these patients converted to hemorrhage within 48 hours,

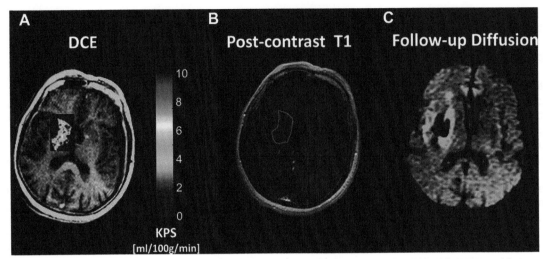

Fig. 3. *KPS* map superimposed on the equivalent DCE image obtained from a 73-year-old patient with acute ischemic stroke who subsequently hemorrhaged (*A*). There was no visible evidence of gadolinium enhancement on the equivalent static postcontrast T1-weighted image (*B*). Both (*A*) and (*B*) were acquired approximately 3 hours following stroke onset. Diffusion-weighted MR imaging performed 48 hours later (*C*) revealed a region of very low signal intensity within a region of hyperintensity, characteristic of hemorrhagic transformation.

and a retrospective analysis found significantly elevated *KPS* in infarcts that progressed to hemorrhage, compared with those in the non-HT group (*KPS* = 3.10 ± 0.44 mL/100 g/min in the HT group vs *KPS* = 0.12 ± 0.10 mL/100 g/min in the non-HT group; *P*<.02).[20] Intrigued by these results, we decided to perform a larger examination of DCE-MRI in acute ischemic stroke, comparing patients who received rtPA with untreated patients who presented to the emergency department within 4 hours of symptom onset.[33] Nine of the 33 patients with acute ischemic stroke who were studied showed progressive enhancement associated with increased permeability in the acute phase (5 received rtPA, 4 were untreated), all of whom proceeded to HT at 48 hours after symptom onset. The mean *KPS* in the HT infarcts was significantly elevated relative to the contralateral hemisphere (within-subjects), and significantly greater than in non-HT infarcts (between-subjects). This was observed in all HT cases, regardless of whether or not the subject received rtPA. With enough data, we may be able to derive a "permeability threshold," or *KPS* value capable of delineating between "low" and "high" risk of HT. The patients with acute ischemic stroke who would benefit the most from this type of stratification would be those who are otherwise excluded from thrombolytic therapy because they present beyond the current 4.5-hour time window for thrombolysis.

Establishing a single receiver operating characteristic (ROC) threshold for the prediction of HT, however, may be a challenge. Ding and colleagues[34] observed that BBB permeability appears to evolve over the course of the acute phase in their rat model of embolic stroke. The investigators found that at 3 hours after symptom onset, *KPS* measured in infarcts that later hemorrhaged was 44% greater than in those that did not, but this discrepancy rose to 167% by 24 hours. As with static postcontrast T1-weighted enhancement, DCE-MR imaging of BBB permeability may be attempting to image a "moving target." Curiously, and on a smaller time scale, a trend toward *decreasing KPS* estimates within the same scan has been observed in patients with acute ischemic stroke, with the *KPS* of HT infarcts exceeding 12 mL/100 g/min when the first 2.5 minutes of DCE-MRI data were used to calculate the estimate, and diminishing to approximately 3.5 mL/100 g/min when the full 4.8 minutes of data were used to approximate permeability in the same infarcts.[35] A similar phenomenon has been reported in the CT permeability imaging literature, whereby permeability values derived from first-pass data increased (3 minutes postcontrast) estimates by approximately fivefold in patients with acute ischemic stroke (7.6 vs 1.3 mL/100 g/min in infarcts).[36] We do not believe, however, that the decline in *KPS* reflects a true decrease in microvascular permeability during the course of DCE-MRI acquisition. Rather, accurate approximations of true microvascular permeability are more likely when the transfer of contrast between the blood and tissue compartments is "close" to equilibrium. To respect the assumptions inherent in the Patlak model, the tracer concentration versus time data must be acquired after blood-tissue equilibrium has been attained, that is, when the transfer of contrast between compartments is no longer dominated by the rapid changes associated with contrast wash-in.[27] Deviation from this assumption results in nonlinearity of the Patlak plot, perhaps manifesting in a steep rise followed by a rapid recession in C_t/C_p. Although it is still possible to perform linear regression, it is unlikely that the slope of best-fit would reflect true *KPS* in this scenario.

CT METHODS FOR THE ASSESSMENT OF BBB INTEGRITY

CT offers an alternative to MRI for mapping permeability in patients with acute ischemic stroke. Whereas DCE-MRI involves intravenous injection of a paramagnetic contrast agent and voxel-wise measurement of MR signal intensity as a function of time, dynamic contrast-enhanced CT involves intravenous injection of an iodinated contrast agent and voxel-wise measurement of attenuation coefficient (Hounsfield units) as a function of time. The subsequent pharmacokinetic modeling is similar for DCE-CT and DCE-MRI, as discussed previously. **Fig. 4** is an example of a CT permeability map obtained in an acute stroke patient. The image shows a region of increased permeability, with subsequent corresponding hemorrhagic transformation.

Advantages of the CT technique over MRI mainly pertain to availability, accessibility, and speed of CT in the acute stroke setting. These advantages are particularly realized at institutes already performing nonenhanced CT followed by CT angiography (CTA) and/or CT perfusion (CTP) for acute stroke. A major limitation of CTP has been limited craniocaudal spatial coverage, but this will not be an issue with the next generation of multidetector CT scanners.

In 2007, Lin and colleagues[37] reported the use of standard CTP data to map permeability. This group retrospectively reanalyzed first-pass dynamic CTP data (60-second cine acquisition) from 50 patients imaged within 3 hours of onset of acute ischemic stroke, and used the Patlak model to generate maps of permeability. In total, 6 of 50 patients had hemorrhagic transformation. Permeability surface area product (PS) ranged from 5.2 to 13.0 (mean: 9.8 ± 2.9) in infarcts with hemorrhage transformation, versus 0 to 5.9 (mean: 2.7 ± 2.0; *P*<.0001) in infarcts without hemorrhagic transformation. A PS threshold of 5.16 mL/100 mL/min yielded a sensitivity and specificity of 100% and 88.7% for prediction of hemorrhagic transformation, and the mean area under the ROC curve was 0.981. A limitation of this study was that the Patlak model was applied to first-pass data, but this model was intended for use only after a steady-state phase of contrast

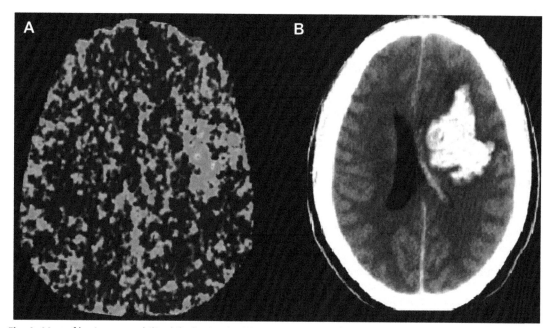

Fig. 4. Map of brain permeability (*A*) obtained using DCE-CT, in a patient with a left MCA territory acute ischemic stroke, demonstrates a large region of increased permeability (*green*) in the left MCA territory. A nonenhanced CT study performed 10 hours later shows hemorrhagic conversion (*B*) in the corresponding region. (Images courtesy of Dr Max Wintermark, Division of Neuroradiology, University of Virginia.)

transfer between the intravascular and extravascular compartments.

Dankbaar and colleagues[36] demonstrated empirically that, indeed, use of first-pass CTP data results in incorrect permeability values, and generates delayed perfusion information rather than permeability. Specifically, Dankbaar and colleagues found that first-pass CTP data yield an overestimation of permeability. Subsequently, Hom and colleagues[38] performed a study to determine how long a delay in acquisition is needed to achieve steady state, and generate accurate permeability values. They found that the CTP acquisition should extend for at least 210 seconds. A longer delay must be balanced against the increased likelihood of head motion with a longer acquisition, and potentially increased radiation dose as well.

Recognizing the need for a longer CTP acquisition, Aviv and colleagues[39] performed a prospective study using a 2-phase CTP acquisition to determine whether PS values distinguish patients with acute stroke who are likely to develop hemorrhagic transformation from those who are not. They reported on 41 patients with acute ischemic stroke who underwent imaging within 3 hours of symptom onset. A CTA was performed from the aortic arch through the vertex, followed by a second bolus of contrast injection, a 45-second continuous CTP acquisition, and then a 90-second CTP acquisition with an image acquired every 15 seconds. In this study, 23 of 41 patients developed hemorrhagic transformation. A PS threshold of 0.23 mL/100 mL/min yielded a sensitivity and specificity of 77% and 94% for prediction of hemorrhagic transformation, and the mean area under the ROC curve was 0.918. One question arising from this study was whether residual contrast material from the CTA affects the accuracy of the subsequent permeability measurement. Does saturation of the parenchymal compartment from the first bolus decrease the amount of contrast extravasation following the second bolus?[36] This theoretical possibility might require further investigation.

SUMMARY AND FUTURE DIRECTIONS FOR IMAGING ASSESSMENT OF BBB INTEGRITY

The term "permeability imaging" is currently used for MR and CT techniques to map disruption of the BBB. In the context of MRI, it involves either a qualitative (static postcontrast T1-weighted imaging) or quantitative (typically, DCE) technique. In the context of CT, it involves either standard or extended CTP acquisitions. Qualitative evidence of parenchymal contrast enhancement on T1-weighted static MRI is a specific, but not sensitive indicator of BBB disruption. Furthermore, visual assessment of gadolinium enhancement is unsuitable for the longitudinal study of permeability desired for clinical trials. There is a recognized need to identify incremental changes in microvascular permeability to evaluate the effectiveness of rtPA for acute ischemic stroke. In contradistinction, DCE-MRI may indeed provide a robust tool for assessing the effects of such therapies on HT, but more guidance is required regarding the appropriate selection of MR end points. Although we have endeavored to emphasize the relative strengths and weaknesses of both CT and MRI approaches, the choice of technique will also depend on institutional expertise. This is particularly true of the dynamic techniques, as they require familiarity with pharmacokinetic modeling or at least the interpretation of the parameter estimates provided by the software.

Several investigators have proposed MRI alternatives to T1-based DCE MRI, aimed to extract permeability-related information from routine clinical perfusion-weighted images.[40–42] Perfusion imaging with dynamic susceptibility contrast (DSC) MRI is a mainstay of most acute ischemic stroke evaluation protocols and can be acquired in less than 2 minutes. Like DCE, DSC imaging involves tracking the passage of an intravenously administered bolus of gadolinium contrast agent with a series of MR images. The high magnetic moment of gadolinium will alter the local magnetic field of blood (ie, change the susceptibility or T2*) relative to surrounding brain parenchyma. In principle, as long as the BBB remains intact, this change in susceptibility will be visualized as signal loss on T2*-weighted images. In the context of BBB disruption, however, the initial signal drop associated with gadolinium passing through the blood vessels within the voxel is followed by an increase in signal intensity as contrast begins to extravasate (ie, a competing T1 effect). Evidence of this secondary signal intensity increase, and/or its extent, forms the basis for exploring DSC-measures as potential surrogate markers of BBB disruption.

One such approach is to measure the relative recirculation of contrast (rR).[40] This DSC measure involves separating the intravascular (T2*) and extravascular/recirculation phases (T1) by fitting a theoretical first-pass curve to the ΔR_2^* versus time curve ($\Delta R_2^* = \Delta(1/T2^*)$) and measuring the difference in the areas encompassed by the measured and the fitted curves (**Fig. 5**). Given that contrast extravasation is also associated with BBB disruption in acute ischemic stroke, investigators have begun to evaluate DSC-based surrogates as predictors of hemorrhagic

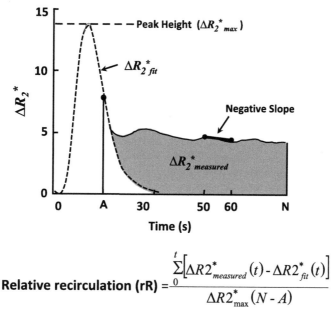

$$\text{Relative recirculation (rR)} = \frac{\sum\limits_{0}^{t}\left[\Delta R2^{*}_{measured}(t) - \Delta R2^{*}_{fit}(t)\right]}{\Delta R2^{*}_{max}(N-A)}$$

Fig. 5. A $\Delta R_2{}^*$ versus time curve ($\Delta R_2{}^*_{measured}$), as well as its gamma-variate fit ($\Delta R_2{}^*_{fit}$), depicting 3 DSC surrogate measures of BBB permeability: rR, Peak Height, and Slope = slope of $\Delta R_2{}^*_{measured}$ (t) between 50 and 60 seconds after injection.

complications. Bang and coworkers[42] hypothesized that the change in T2* relaxation rate ($\Delta R_2{}^*$) associated with the last 10 seconds of a 60-second bolus tracking study (negative slope) can predict HT in recanalized acute ischemic stroke patients. In fact, this simple DSC marker appeared to predict future HT with a sensitivity of 83%. More recently, we estimated rR in patients with acute ischemic stroke and compared this DSC metric with DCE-MRI estimates of BBB permeability (KPS).[43] Preliminary results indicated a strong and significant correlation between rR and KPS, as well as significant increases in both measures in stroke lesions that proceeded to hemorrhage (compared with those that did not). Taken together, these early findings provide support for our hypothesis that rR is related to the extent of BBB leakage and that rR may provide a reasonable surrogate for KPS.

Although encouraging, it is not presently known whether rR is strictly reflective of BBB permeability or rather just microvascular "abnormalities." A more prudent interpretation of these results is that rR reflects a superposition of microvascular features, including blood volume, vessel tortuosity and, perhaps, permeability.[40,44] As such, rR may be less suitable than KPS for the investigation of new therapies and their effects on BBB integrity (eg, where absolute quantification is desirable). Whether or not rR will ultimately prove valuable in treatment decision making in acute ischemic stroke remains to be demonstrated.

The next advancement in CT mapping of permeability is likely to be more widespread availability of CT scanners capable of whole-brain CTP coverage. Intrasubject comparison of permeability values obtained with CT versus MRI techniques may help clarify the relative merits of each of these approaches, but serial imaging with closely spaced CT and MRI will be challenging in an acute stroke setting. Perhaps animal model comparison will be useful.

With either CT or MRI, the ability to quickly and accurately predict the likelihood of hemorrhagic transformation may enable a transition from using a fixed therapeutic time window for rtPA administration to treatment decisions based on individual patient risk. This move to individualized risk assessment is certainly a promising area of imaging research in the broadest sense, and permeability imaging may be an early success.

REFERENCES

1. The National Institute of Neurological Disorders and Stroke rt-PA Stroke Study Group. Tissue plasminogen activator for acute ischemic stroke. N Engl J Med 1995;333:1581–7.

2. Hacke W, Kaste M, Bluhmki E, et al. Thrombolysis with alteplase 3 to 4.5 hours after acute ischemic stroke. N Engl J Med 2008;359:1317–29.

3. Hamann GF, Okada Y, del Zoppo GJ. Hemorrhagic transformation and microvascular integrity during

focal cerebral ischemia/reperfusion. J Cereb Blood Flow Metab 1996;16:1373–8.

4. Dijkhuizen RM, Asahi M, Wu O, et al. Rapid breakdown of microvascular barriers and subsequent hemorrhagic transformation after delayed recombinant tissue plasminogen activator treatment in a rat embolic stroke model. Stroke 2002;33:2100–4.

5. Busch E, Kruger K, Fritze K, et al. Blood-brain barrier disturbances after rt-PA treatment of thromboembolic stroke in the rat. Acta Neurochir 1997; 70:206–8.

6. Kelly MA, Shuaib A, Todd KG. Matrix metalloproteinase activation and blood-brain barrier breakdown following thrombolysis. Exp Neurol 2006;200:38–49.

7. Montaner J, Molina CA, Monasterio J, et al. Matrix metalloproteinase-9 pretreatment level predicts intracranial hemorrhagic complications after thrombolysis in human stroke. Circulation 2003;107: 598–603.

8. Yepes M, Sandkvist M, Moore EG, et al. Tissue-type plasminogen activator induces opening of the blood-brain barrier via the LDL receptor-related protein. J Clin Invest 2003;112:1533–40.

9. Weinmann HJ, Laniado M, Mutzel W. Pharmacokinetics of Gd-DTPA/dimeglumine after intravenous injection into healthy volunteers. Physiol Chem Phys Med NMR 1984;16:167–72.

10. Vo KD, Santiago F, Lin W, et al. MR imaging enhancement patterns as predictors of hemorrhagic transformation in acute ischemic stroke. AJNR Am J Neuroradiol 2003;24:674–9.

11. Kim EY, Na DG, Kim SS, et al. Prediction of hemorrhagic transformation in acute ischemic stroke: role of diffusion-weighted imaging and early parenchymal enhancement. AJNR Am J Neuroradiol 2005;26: 1050–5.

12. Kastrup A, Groschel K, Ringer TM, et al. Early disruption of the blood-brain barrier after thrombolytic therapy predicts hemorrhage in patients with acute stroke. Stroke 2008;39:2385–7.

13. Merten CL, Knitelius HO, Assheuer J, et al. MRI of acute cerebral infarcts, increased contrast enhancement with continuous infusion of gadolinium. Neuroradiology 1999;41:242–8.

14. Virapongse C, Mancuso A, Quisling R. Human brain infarcts: Gd-DTPA-enhanced MR imaging. Radiology 1986;161:785–94.

15. Mikulis DJ, Guo G, Wu R, et al. Gadolinium Enhancement Predicts Hemorrhagic Transformation in Acute Ischemic Stroke [abstract: 43]. In: 44th Annual Meeting of the American Society for Neuroradiology. San Diego (CA), May 2006.

16. Latour LL, Kang DW, Ezzeddine MA, et al. Early blood-brain barrier disruption in human focal brain ischemia. Ann Neurol 2004;56:468–77.

17. Wang X, Tsuji K, Lee SR, et al. Mechanisms of hemorrhagic transformation after tissue plasminogen activator reperfusion therapy for ischemic stroke. Stroke 2004;35:2726–30.

18. Kassner A, Roberts TP. Beyond perfusion: cerebral vascular reactivity and assessment of microvascular permeability. Top Magn Reson Imaging 2004;15: 58–65.

19. Cheng HL. Investigation and optimization of parameter accuracy in dynamic contrast-enhanced MRI. J Magn Reson Imaging 2008;28:736–43.

20. Kassner A, Roberts T, Taylor K, et al. Prediction of hemorrhage in acute ischemic stroke using permeability MR imaging. AJNR Am J Neuroradiol 2005; 26:2213–7.

21. Roberts TP. Physiologic measurements by contrast-enhanced MR imaging: expectations and limitations. J Magn Reson Imaging 1997;7:82–90.

22. Pruessmann KP, Weiger M, Scheidegger MB, et al. SENSE: sensitivity encoding for fast MRI. Magn Reson Med 1999;42:952–62.

23. Donahue KM, Weisskoff RM, Burstein D. Water diffusion and exchange as they influence contrast enhancement. J Magn Reson Imaging 1997;7: 102–10.

24. Larsson HB, Stubgaard M, Frederiksen JL, et al. Quantitation of blood-brain barrier defect by magnetic resonance imaging and gadolinium-DTPA in patients with multiple sclerosis and brain tumors. Magn Reson Med 1990;16:117–31.

25. Brix G, Semmler W, Port R, et al. Pharmacokinetic parameters in CNS Gd-DTPA enhanced MR imaging. J Comput Assist Tomogr 1991;15:621–8.

26. Tofts PS, Kermode AG. Measurement of the blood-brain barrier permeability and leakage space using dynamic MR imaging: 1. Fundamental concepts. Magn Reson Med 1991;17:357–67.

27. Patlak CS, Blasberg RG, Fenstermacher JD. Graphical evaluation of blood-to-brain transfer constants from multiple-time uptake data. J Cereb Blood Flow Metab 1983;3:1–7.

28. Patlak CS, Blasberg RG. Graphical evaluation of blood-to-brain transfer constants from multiple-time uptake data. Generalizations. J Cereb Blood Flow Metab 1985;5:584–90.

29. Tofts PS, Brix G, Buckley DL, et al. Estimating kinetic parameters from dynamic contrast-enhanced T(1)-weighted MRI of a diffusable tracer: standardized quantities and symbols. J Magn Reson Imaging 1999;10:223–32.

30. Roberts HC, Roberts TP, Brasch RC, et al. Quantitative measurement of microvascular permeability in human brain tumors achieved using dynamic contrast-enhanced MR imaging: correlation with histologic grade. AJNR Am J Neuroradiol 2000;21: 891–9.

31. Ewing JR, Knight RA, Nagaraja TN, et al. Patlak plots of Gd-DTPA MRI data yield blood-brain transfer constants concordant with those of 14C-sucrose

in areas of blood-brain opening. Magn Reson Med 2003;50:283–92.

32. Knight RA, Barker PB, Fagan SC, et al. Prediction of impending hemorrhagic transformation in ischemic stroke using magnetic resonance imaging in rats. Stroke 1998;29:144–51.

33. Kassner A, Liu F, Matta S, et al. Quantitative dynamic contrast-enhanced MRI: a potential tool for guiding treatment decisions in acute ischemic stroke. In: Joint Annual Meeting ISMRM-ESMRMB. Berlin (Germany), May 2007. p. 499.

34. Ding G, Jiang Q, Li L, et al. Detection of BBB disruption and hemorrhage by Gd-DTPA enhanced MRI after embolic stroke in rat. Brain Res 2006;1114: 195–203.

35. Vidarsson L, Thornhill RE, Liu F, et al. Quantitative permeability MRI in acute ischemic stroke: how long do we need to scan? Magn Reson Imaging 2009;27(9):1216–22.

36. Dankbaar JW, Hom J, Schneider T, et al. Dynamic perfusion CT assessment of the blood-brain barrier permeability: first pass versus delayed acquisition. AJNR Am J Neuroradiol 2008;29:1671–6.

37. Lin K, Kazmi KS, Law M, et al. Measuring elevated microvascular permeability and predicting hemorrhagic transformation in acute ischemic stroke using first-pass dynamic perfusion CT imaging. AJNR Am J Neuroradiol 2007;28:1292–8.

38. Hom J, Dankbaar JW, Schneider T, et al. Optimal duration of acquisition for dynamic perfusion CT assessment of blood-brain barrier permeability

using the Patlak model. AJNR Am J Neuroradiol 2009;30:1366–70.

39. Aviv RI, d'Esterre CD, Murphy BD, et al. Hemorrhagic transformation of ischemic stroke: prediction with CT perfusion. Radiology 2009;250:867–77.

40. Kassner A, Annesley DJ, Zhu XP, et al. Abnormalities of the contrast re-circulation phase in cerebral tumors demonstrated using dynamic susceptibility contrast-enhanced imaging: a possible marker of vascular tortuosity. J Magn Reson Imaging 2000; 11:103–13.

41. Lupo JM, Cha S, Chang SM, et al. Dynamic susceptibility-weighted perfusion imaging of high-grade gliomas: characterization of spatial heterogeneity. AJNR Am J Neuroradiol 2005;26: 1446–54.

42. Bang OY, Buck BH, Saver JL, et al. Prediction of hemorrhagic transformation after recanalization therapy using T2*-permeability magnetic resonance imaging. Ann Neurol 2007;62:170–6.

43. Wu SP, Vidarsson L, Winter J, et al. Estimates of relative contrast recirculation obtained from perfusion MRI: a potential tool for guiding treatment decision in acute ischemic stroke. In: 16th Scientific Meeting and Exhibition of the ISMRM. Toronto (ON), May 2008. p. 307.

44. Jackson A, Kassner A, Annesley-Williams D, et al. Abnormalities in the recirculation phase of contrast agent bolus passage in cerebral gliomas: comparison with relative blood volume and tumor grade. AJNR Am J Neuroradiol 2002;23:7–14.

Imaging Stroke Patients with Unclear Onset Times

Ona Wu, PhD[a],*, Lee H. Schwamm, MD[b],
A. Gregory Sorensen, MD[a]

KEYWORDS

- Stroke • Brain ischemia • Thrombolytic therapy
- Diffusion magnetic resonance imaging
- Perfusion magnetic resonance imaging • Time

Stroke is the fourth leading cause of death,[1] and the leading cause of serious long-term disability in the United States. Each year, approximately 795,000 people experience new or recurrent strokes; of these, 87% are ischemic.[2] The economic cost of this devastating disease for 2009 was estimated to be $68.9 billion.[2] The only current approved therapy for the treatment of acute ischemic stroke is intravenous (IV) alteplase or recombinant tissue plasminogen activator (rt-PA) administered within 3 hours from when the patient was last known to be well. More than a decade has passed since the US Food and Drug Administration (FDA) approved the use of IV rt-PA for the treatment of acute ischemic stroke. Yet, rt-PA is still underused worldwide and estimated to be given to less than 5% of patients.[3,4] The main reasons for this low rate are attributed to the delay in patient arrival, and the conservative definition of time of stroke onset in cases of unwitnessed onset, which is the time the patient was last known to be well. In 2008, the results from the third study of the European Cooperative Acute Stroke Study (ECASS 3), a randomized, double-blind, placebo-controlled, clinical trial, showed that in a carefully selected population, rt-PA could be safely given to patients treated within 4.5 hours from symptom onset.[5] Although this is a promising step toward expanding the use of rt-PA, according to the Paul Coverdell National Acute Stroke Registry Surveillance Report from 4 states (Georgia, Illinois, Massachusetts, and North Carolina), from 2005 to 2007, 57% of acute stroke patients arrived at the hospital with unknown time of symptom onset.[4] Because thrombolytic therapy is based on the patient's last known well time, these patients would be considered outside the treatment window. The key to offering thrombolytic therapy to patients with unwitnessed strokes is to clearly differentiate between the time when the patient was last known well and the time when the patient was discovered with symptoms. For witnessed strokes, these are one and the same. For strokes with unwitnessed onsets, the difference in times is unknown (by definition) and could be the difference between being eligible or ineligible for therapeutic intervention. Special cases of strokes with unknown onset are wake-up strokes, when there is no definite evidence that proves the strokes started before the patient woke up, and the stroke may have caused the patient to awaken. These patients are found in bed as opposed to on the floor or in the bathroom or kitchen. There are presumably no delays in bringing these patients directly to the hospital, whereas the patients with unknown onset

This work was supported by grants R01 NS059775, R01 NS038477, and P50NS051343 from the National Institutes of Health.
[a] Department of Radiology, MGH/MIT/HMS Athinoula A. Martinos Center for Biomedical Imaging, MGH, 149 Thirteenth Street Suite 2301, Charlestown, MA 02129, USA
[b] Neurology Service and TeleStroke & Acute Stroke Services, Department of Neurology, MGH, ACC 720, 55 Fruit Street, Boston, MA 02114, USA
* Corresponding author.
E-mail address: ona@nmr.mgh.harvard.edu

time may have been left unattended at home for minutes to hours. If a technique existed that could reliably substitute for the human witness and provide evidence that the duration of the stroke was within the therapeutic time window (eg, <4.5 hours), then these patients could be considered for IV rt-PA therapy. Several stroke researchers have suggested that imaging, in particular specific magnetic resonance (MR) imaging findings, could provide such information, and therefore could help bracket the time of onset based on tissue changes. **Fig. 1** shows an example of how imaging could potentially be used for triaging these patients for thrombolytic therapy. This article discusses the data supporting the use of imaging for selecting patients for thrombolytic therapy when precise stroke onset times are unavailable. First, background information on this population of stroke patients with unwitnessed onsets is presented, which includes a discussion of previous studies that investigated the feasibility of extending thrombolytic therapy. Imaging options that can potentially make giving rt-PA to this group safer are then investigated. One option is to use imaging as a surrogate for stroke duration and find techniques that can determine whether the patient is within the therapeutic time window or not. An alternative option is to use imaging as a surrogate for tissue viability. The idea of an MR imaging-based estimate of time of stroke onset is a separate, but closely linked concept of using imaging or other biomarkers to establish a "tissue clock" instead of a "wall clock" to identify candidates for intervention. The two distinct approaches are therefore discussed separately. Some of the proposed and ongoing clinical trials involving these patients are also briefly described.

PATIENTS WITH UNCLEAR STROKE ONSETS: BACKGROUND

The precise time from onset of symptoms to hospital arrival is not recorded or known for most patients with stroke.[4] Further, an estimated 16% to 28% of patients with stroke awaken with symptoms.[6–10] It was suggested early on by Marshall[11] that for most of these patients, the strokes may have occurred between 12:00 AM and 6:00 AM, making many of these patients outside the therapeutic time window if hospital arrival is delayed until discovery in the morning. Marshall posited that nighttime decreases in blood pressure in patients with dysfunctional autoregulation may result in reduced cerebral blood flow (CBF). His suppositions were based on findings from 554 patients with nonembolic ischemic stroke. However, other studies performed across all stroke subtypes found that most strokes occur in the early morning, between 6:01 AM and 12:00 PM.[7–10,12] A retrospective study[8] of 1272 patient datasets collected for the Trial of Org 10172 in Acute Stroke Treatment (TOAST),[13] in which patients who awakened with symptoms (N = 323, 25% of the datasets) were analyzed separately, found only 7% of the 1272 patient dataset (N = 87) had onsets between 12:01 AM and 6:00 AM. A meta-analysis of 31 publications, involving 11,816 patients, reported similar results, with a 49% increased risk of stroke between 6:00 AM and noon, and 35% decreased risk between midnight and 6:00 AM compared with the other 18 hours.[14] These observations have led many to conclude that there exists a circadian pattern in the frequency of stroke similar to that reported for myocardial infarction. This pattern may be partially explained by the circadian rhythm of blood pressure, cortisol secretion, blood viscosity, hematocrit, activated partial thromboplastin time, prothrombin time, and platelet aggregation.[10,12] Implications of these findings are that many patients with wake-up stroke, whose last known well time is the night before, may with high likelihood have had their onsets around awakening and could therefore be treated safely with rt-PA, assuming they meet all clinical and imaging criteria for the on-label use of IV rt-PA.

Several studies have investigated radiological differences between patients with wake-up stroke and patients with nonwake-up stroke to determine whether MR imaging could play a role in triaging these patients. Fink and colleagues[15] investigated apparent diffusion coefficient (ADC) differences between patients with well-known onset times and those who woke up with symptoms. In Fink and colleagues' study, 364 patients were retrospectively examined from a prospective dataset consisting of 100 patients with wake-up stroke. There was no statistical difference between times seen from symptom discovery for the two groups (6.0 vs 5.9 hours, $P = .83$), but fewer patients with wake-up stroke were imaged within 3 hours of symptom discovery (29% vs 45%, $P = .006$). The rates of mismatch on diffusion-weighted MR imaging (DWI) and perfusion-weighted MR imaging (PWI) in both groups (82% vs 73%, $P = .4$) were similar. Clinical features (eg, National Institutes of Health Stroke Scale [NIHSS] score, age, gender) were not significantly different between the two groups ($P>.05$). Using linear regression analysis, ADC values were found to be negatively associated with stroke onset time ($\beta = -0.184$, $P = .10$). ADC was lower in the wake-up stroke group compared with the nonwake-up group seen within 3 hours of onset (566 vs 665 $\mu m^2/s$, $P<.01$).

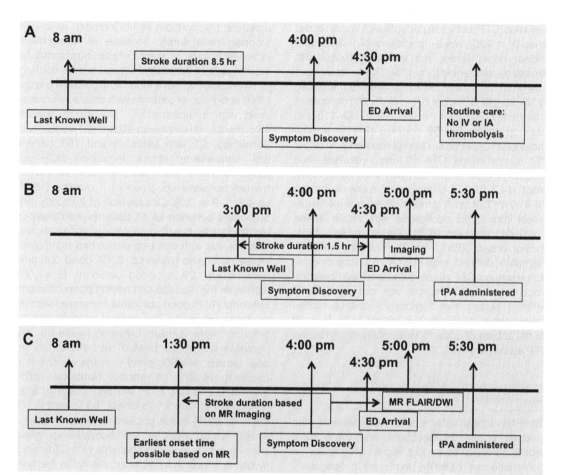

Fig. 1. Three different scenarios for assessing rt-PA eligibility based on time of stroke onset. Case example: a 68-year-old right-handed man, patient X, who was last seen well by his daughter at 8:00 AM was later discovered by her at 4:00 PM to be aphasic with a right hemiparesis, and rushed to the emergency department (ED) by 4:30 PM. He has no contraindications to IV rt-PA except for time of stroke onset. The following scenarios review the current guideline-based care (*A, B*) and the rationale for image-based "witnesses" (*C*). *Scenario A: Guideline-based care: not eligible for rt-PA treatment.* Under AHA guidelines and FDA indications, patient X's stroke onset is defined as 8:00 AM (ie, last known well time was 8:00 AM) and stroke duration is 8.5 hours. He is considered ineligible for guideline-based thrombolysis. *Scenario B: Guideline-based care: eligible for rt-PA treatment.* At 4:40 PM, the son (who is a reliable human witness) of patient X and who lives at home with him is called by the ED physician and states that he was with his father at 3:00 PM and that his father was normal at that time (ie, last known well time is 3:00 PM); therefore the stroke onset time is then defined as 3:00 PM, and stroke duration is calculated to be 1.5 hours. He is eligible for thrombolysis and receives IV rt-PA at 5:30 PM, which is 60 minutes after ED arrival. *Scenario C: Image-based witness: eligible for rt-PA treatment.* No human witness besides the daughter has seen patient X since 8:00 AM. However, clinically obtained MR imaging performed at 5:00 PM produces an MR imaging pattern that suggests the patient's stroke occurred less than 3.5 hours ago. Because he has no other contraindications to rt-PA, he is now eligible for off-label thrombolytic therapy. His daughter provides written informed consent and he receives study drug (IV rt-PA) at 5:30 PM. Based on the imaging hypothesis, he received rt-PA sometime between 1.5 and 4.0 hours since true stroke onset.

There have also been several studies investigating the possible role of computed tomography (CT) in triaging patients with unknown onset times. Todo and colleagues[16] researched differences on CT between patients with cardioembolic stroke imaged within 3 hours of symptom discovery. Patients were divided into 3 groups: patients with known times of onset (N = 46), patients with wake-up stroke (N = 17), and patients with unclear onset times who were not found on awakening (N = 18). The patients in the unclear onset time group presented with hypodense regions on CT more often than the wake-up stroke (56% vs 11%, *P* = .012) and known onset (56% vs 0%, *P*<.001) groups. Silva and colleagues[17] examined group differences in CT angiography (CTA) and CT perfusion (CTP) between patients with known onset times (N = 420), wake-up strokes (N = 131), and unclear onset times, not including those with strokes on awakening (N = 125). The unclear onset time group had more severe strokes as measured by NIHSS (NIHSS score 8 [3–16], $P<.01$) compared with the known onset (NIHSS score 5 [2–11]) and wake-up stroke (NIHSS score 5 [2–11]) groups. The unclear onset group also presented with larger CTA source image (CTA-SI) lesion volumes (46.6 [0–220.8] cm^3, $P = .04$) compared with the known onset (14.3 [0–137.4] cm^3) and wake-up stroke (14.4 [0–217.3] cm^3) groups. Presence of large-vessel intracranial occlusions was similar in the 3 groups (wake-up: 35%, known onset: 46%, unclear onset: 39%; $P = .2$). Frequency of CTP mismatch, defined as at least a 25% larger perfusion lesion on CBF maps compared with cerebral blood volume (CBV) maps, was not significantly different across the 3 groups (wake-up: 37%, known onset: 41%, unclear onset: 37%; $P = .9$) for the subset of patients who received admission CTP scans (N = 393).

Treating Patients with Wake-up and Unclear Onset Stroke

There have been attempts to treat patients with wake-up stroke prospectively, and these have shown some encouraging signs of efficacy in highly selected patients. Iosif and colleagues[18] presented case reports in two patients with wake-up stroke. Both patients exhibited mismatches in lesion volumes between DWI and CBF maps and little or no signal intensity changes on fluid-attenuated inversion recovery (FLAIR) images, which are believed to be indicative of early-stage stroke. Based on these findings, both patients were given a combination of intra-arterial (IA) mechanical and IV chemical thrombolytic therapy (rt-PA) and both had a good outcome as measured by modified Rankin Scale (mRS score<2). Hellier and colleagues[19] used CTP for deciding to treat two patients with unclear times of stroke onset with thrombolytic therapy. In this study, decision to treat with mechanical thrombectomy or IV rt-PA was based on subtle noncontrast CT (NCCT) hypodensity, and mismatch between CBV and time-to-peak (TTP) maps. For both patients, the TTP map indicated the entire ipsilateral middle cerebral artery (MCA) territory was at risk. As in the previous case study, both patients had good outcomes.

In addition to case studies, prospective studies involving larger patient cohorts have also been performed, and these have been less encouraging. A phase III trial of abciximab (AbESTT-II), a platelet glycoprotein IIb/IIIa inhibitor, which was stopped prematurely because of a significant increase in rate of symptomatic intracranial hemorrhage (sICH) and fatal intracranial hemorrhage (ICH) detected within 3 months, included a prespecified subgroup of patients with stroke who awakened with symptoms.[20,21] The study involved 43 patients with wake-up stroke (22 treated with abciximab, 21 with placebo) and 758 patients with nonwake-up stroke. Increased sICH was found in the treated wake-up arm versus the treated nonwake-up group at 3 months (18.2% vs 4.8%, $P = .03$). Comparison of 3-month mRS outcomes between all 43 patients with wake-up and 758 patients with nonwake-up stroke showed that patients with wake-up stroke had significantly worse outcomes (wake-up, 9.3% good outcome; nonwake-up, 29.2% good outcome; $P = .005$) with even the placebo arm having poorer 3-month outcome (14% good outcome) compared with the nonwake-up group. The general baseline characteristics were similar between wake-up and nonwake-up groups treated with abciximab (eg, age, gender, NIHSS score) with the exception of previous history of stroke (wake-up: 36%, nonwake-up 14%; $P = .04$) and imaging. More abnormalities were observed on baseline CT (86% vs 59%) in the abciximab-treated wake-up stroke group than in the nonwake-up group despite criteria excluding patients with CT findings involving more than 50% of the MCA territory. Potentially, more restrictive imaging criteria may have improved patient selection in terms of safety and likely-to-benefit profiles.

A retrospective single-center study by Barreto and colleagues[6] of patients with wake-up stroke who were treated with rt-PA on a compassionate basis suggest that rt-PA may be safely administered to a select population of patients with wake-up stroke. Patients were excluded if they presented with a hypodensity larger than one-third of the MCA territory on baseline noncontrast cranial CT scan, an imaging criterion more restrictive than that of AbESTT-II. Barreto and colleagues examined 46 rt-PA-treated and 34 non-rt-PA-treated patients with wake-up stroke as well as 174 on-label rt-PA-treated patients (treated within 3 hours from last known well). Of the 46 patients with wake-up stroke, 28 received IV rt-PA alone, 14 IA therapy alone and 4 combined full-dose IV rt-PA and IA treatment. The investigators found that the patients with wake-up stroke treated with thrombolytic therapy had a significantly higher rate of favorable outcome (discharge mRS score 0–2: 28% vs 13%, $P = .006$), but significantly higher mortality (15% vs 0%, $P = .02$) than nontreated patients with wake-up stroke. There was a 4.3% rate of sICH in the rt-PA-treated patients with wake-up stroke, compared with 0% in the non-rt-PA-treated group and 2.9% rate in the on-label-treated group. These differences were not statistically significant, likely because of the low incidence of sICH and small sample sizes involved. There was a higher rate of early changes on baseline CT (28% vs 12%; *P* = .009) and higher baseline NIHSS score (16 vs 11; *P* = .001) in the rt-PA-treated wake-up stroke group compared with the on-label-treated group. There were also more cases of cardioembolic strokes (44% vs 27%) in the treated wake-up stroke group, with fewer small-vessel (2% vs 14%) and unknown-cause (11% vs 23%) stroke subtypes compared with the on-label rt-PA-treated group. Imbalances in stroke subtypes and stroke severity may explain the slightly higher, but not statistically significant increased rates of sICH (4.3% vs 2.9%, *P* = .64) and mortality (15% vs 10%, *P* = .29) in the treated wake-up stroke group compared with the on-label-treated group. Rates of favorable outcome were statistically comparable (28% vs 48%, *P* = .64) between the two groups. The difference between mortality in the treated and nontreated wake-up stroke groups was attributed to greater stroke severity in the treated wake-up stroke group, because the more critically ill patients were more likely to receive rt-PA on a compassionate basis because of their expected poorer outcome without intervention. Since treatment was not randomized it is difficult to make definitive conclusions of safety and efficacy of rt-PA in patients with wake-up-stroke from this study.

A retrospective study of patients with unclear onset time by Cho and colleagues[22] involved 3 medical centers in Korea. Cho and colleagues examined the outcome in patients who arrived more than 3 hours from last known well time, and therefore were ineligible for on-label rt-PA therapy, but who showed favorable characteristics on MR imaging and were therefore treated with either IV rt-PA if the patient arrived within 3 hours of symptom discovery or IA urokinase if the arrival time was within 6 hours of symptom discovery. An MR-favorable profile was defined as patients showing a mismatch in DWI and PWI lesion volumes and absence of pronounced FLAIR hyperintensities in tissue spatially coincident with the acute DWI lesions. Based on this definition, 32 patients with unclear onset times (including wake-up strokes) and 223 with known onset times were examined. No significant differences were found in rates of recanalization, early neurologic improvement (4-point or greater improvement in

NIHSS score on Day 1 or Day 7), 24-hour to 48-hour sICH (6.3% vs 5.8%), and rates of 3-month favorable outcome (mRS score 0–1: 37.5% vs 35%; mRS score 0–2: 50% vs 49.3%) between the two groups, suggesting that thrombolysis can be safely administered to patients showing favorable MR imaging profiles. Furthermore, these MR imaging-selected patients with unclear onset time showed rates of favorable outcome comparable with patients with known onset time who received on-label IV rt-PA.

These preliminary results involving rt-PA administered to patients with unknown onset times are promising and suggest rt-PA can potentially be safely administered if careful selection of patients using neuroimaging criteria is performed.

IMAGING-BASED TRIAGE FOR THERAPEUTIC INTERVENTION

The next steps for extending thrombolytic therapy to patients with unclear onset times are large-scale clinical trials in which treatment is decided based on admission neuroimaging profiles. In the studies discussed earlier, a variety of inclusion and exclusion criteria have been used (from simple NCCT to multiparametric CT and MR imaging- favorable profiles) with varying degrees of success and failure. Therefore, which imaging criteria are used is critical for safely treating patients with unclear onset or wake-up stroke. Two approaches can be used in deciding these criteria: one is to determine which imaging parameter or combination of parameters best correlate with stroke onset time, and hence serve as a surrogate for time from stroke onset, and the other is to establish which parameters best correlate with severity of tissue injury. There are arguments supporting either approach, although both approaches likely produce similar results because time from symptom discovery is a surrogate for ischemic injury. Instead of identifying a surrogate (ie, stroke duration) for tissue pathophysiology, one may argue that one should instead concentrate on measuring tissue viability, regardless of time of imaging from stroke onset. Although this argument has merits, thrombolysis is approved only for treatment based on a time window of 3 hours,[23] and for a selected population 4.5 hours from last known well.[24] This time restriction supports research efforts for investigating imaging surrogates of stroke duration. Both approaches are discussed here, first describing attempts at correlating imaging findings with onset time, and then efforts toward identifying salvageable tissue. The focus is on MR imaging patterns of early imaging changes. Correlative studies involving CT patterns in the hyperacute stage is beyond the scope of this article.

Image-based Markers of Stroke Duration

Experimental studies correlating imaging and stroke duration

In one of the first studies reporting DWI sensitivity to early stroke changes, Moseley and colleagues[25] showed in an MCA stroke model in cats (N = 8) that the signal intensity ratio (SIR) of tissue in the ipsilateral MCA territory significantly increased on DWI within 1 hour after MCA occlusion (MCAO), whereas it stayed relatively unchanged on T2-weighted MR imaging (T2-WI) until 6 to 8 hours after MCAO. The hyperintense regions on DWI and T2-WI corresponded with regions of infarction identified by postmortem histology. In a transient MCAO model in rats (N = 18), Mintorovitch and colleagues[26] showed that DWI became abnormal within 15 minutes, whereas T2-WI became abnormal at approximately 2 hours after occlusion. No significant change in T2-WI was observed until immediately after reperfusion. The observed T2-WI changes were likely because of vasogenic edema from reperfusion injury. With reperfusion, DWI and T2-WI hyperintensities resolved by 4 hours after reperfusion. Jiang and colleagues[27] compared temporal ADC changes with histology after transient MCAO in rats (N = 14) using a neuronal grading score. Measuring MR imaging changes 0 to 2 hours during ischemia and 0 to 4 hours after restoration of perfusion, Jiang and colleagues showed that although ADC correlated well with neuronal grading score at 2 hours after MCAO before reperfusion, it correlated poorly at early time points and chronic time points (24, 48, 72, 96, and 168 hours) after reperfusion. Knight and colleagues[28] examined temporal changes on DWI, proton spin density (PD), T1-weighted (T1-WI) and T2-WI with regional neuronal grading, neuronal counts and hemispheric neutrophil counts in an MCA stroke model in rats (N = 34) at 2, 4, 6, 8, 24, 48, 96, and 168 hours after MCAO. The investigators found that DWI was the only parameter to correctly identify tissue injured by ischemia within 4 hours, whereas T1-WI and T2-WI abnormalities were not visually apparent until after 8 hours after MCAO because of poor contrast-to-noise. ADC values were observed to first sharply decrease within 2 hours after MCAO in the most severely injured regions of the brain before pseudonormalizing at approximately 24 to 48 hours, whereas T1-WI and T2-WI signal intensity steadily decreased and increased, respectively, peaking at 24 hours, and PD signal intensity steadily increased, peaking at 48 hours.

Diffusion-positive, FLAIR-negative mismatch

Findings from animal experiments support the hypothesis that mismatches between changes observed in DWI and T2-WI can be used to stage extent of ischemic injury. Based on previous experiments, it is reasonable to expect that tissue presenting with abnormal ADC and normal FLAIR or T2-WI represents tissue at an early stage of ischemia, likely within 3 to 4 hours of onset, and therefore has a high likelihood of recovering with restoration of blood flow. An example of such a DWI-positive FLAIR-negative mismatch is shown in **Fig. 2A**, from a patient imaged within 1.5 hours of symptom onset along with a patient considered DWI-positive and FLAIR-positive imaged at 6.2 hours from when he was last known to be well. Recent studies have shown that patients seen within 3 to 4.5 hours from stroke onset present with minimal abnormalities on FLAIR imaging.[29–32] **Tables 1** and **2** summarize the results from these studies for identifying patients imaged within 3 hours and 4.5 hours, respectively. Thomalla and colleagues[29] showed that in a consecutive series of patients with territorial infarction seen within 6 hours of stroke onset, negative FLAIR and positive DWI were 93% specific and 48% sensitive for classifying which patients were imaged within 3 hours of symptom onset. These investigators also found that patients who were FLAIR-positive (N = 65) were imaged significantly later (180 [120–240] minutes vs 120 [100–150] minutes; P<.001) and had more severe DWI Alberta Stroke Program Early CT Score (ASPECTS)[33] (6 [5–7] vs 8 [6–9]; P<.001) compared with FLAIR-negative patients (N = 39). The frequency of FLAIR-positive scans increased from 50% in patients imaged within 3 hours to 93.3% for patients imaged at 3 to 6 hours. Ebinger and colleagues[30] reported that for patients with DWI-positive lesions greater than 0.5 cm^3, FLAIR-negative scans were 80% specific and 51% sensitive for patients imaged within 3 hours. Aoki and colleagues[31] showed in MR imaging studies acquired within 24 hours from stroke onset that DWI-positive and FLAIR-negative scans were 83% sensitive and 71% specific for identifying stroke onsets within 3 hours. Petkova and colleagues[32] showed that for patients imaged within 12 hours of stroke onset, FLAIR-negative scans were 82% sensitive and 97% specific for identifying patients imaged within 3 hours of stroke onset (N = 63). When taking into consideration large DWI abnormalities with subtle FLAIR abnormalities limited to the cortex (for example see **Fig. 2C**) and classifying those to be FLAIR negative, results improved to 94% sensitivity with the same 97% specificity. The reduced specificity in

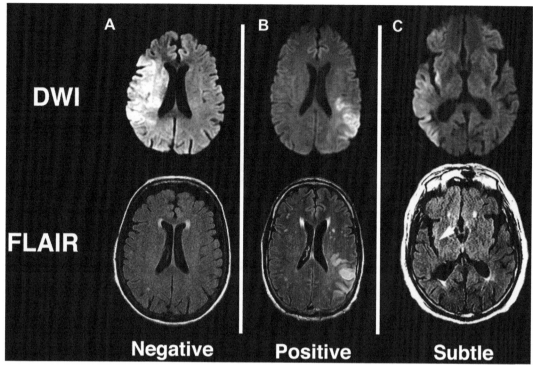

Fig. 2. Examples of (*A*) DWI-positive and FLAIR-negative image for an 80-year-old woman imaged 1.5 hours from last known well with admission NIHSS score of 20, (*B*) DWI-positive, FLAIR-positive image for a 48-year-old man imaged 6.2 hours of last known well with admission NIHSS score of 3 and (*C*) DWI-positive, subtle FLAIR lesion abnormality (*arrowhead*) for an 85-year-old man imaged 2.5 hours from last known well and admission NIHSS score of 6 who would be classified as FLAIR-negative using the algorithm described by Petkova and colleagues.[32]

Ebinger and colleagues' study compared with the other 3 studies may be because of the milder strokes investigated, involving small lesion volumes (1.47 [0.49–4.33] cm³), although some differences could be because of the use of a 3-T magnet[32] for Ebinger and colleagues' study, whereas the others used 1.5-T systems. All 4 studies are limited by being retrospective single-center studies; hence, the generalizability of the results have been questioned, despite consistency with another. This situation stems in part from poor interrater agreement ($\kappa = 0.29$) reported by Thomalla and colleagues compared with good ($\kappa = 0.65$) to excellent agreement ($\kappa = 0.97$) reported by Aoki and colleagues and Petkova and colleagues, respectively. The differences in these studies may be because of the use of 4 raters in Thomalla and colleagues' study (for which 2 of the raters were neurologists and 2 were neuroradiologists) and only 2 raters with similar training in Aoki and colleagues' (neurologists) and Petkova and colleagues' (neuroradiologists) studies. There may also have been differences in the level of training and instruction provided to the readers

before evaluation of images. The observational PRE-FLAIR study[34] tests the generalizability of the preliminary results of Thomalla and colleagues[29] by investigating on a multicenter basis the performance of combining FLAIR with DWI as a surrogate marker for lesion age. The results of this study should address concerns of reproducibility of these findings across different scanners using diverse imaging protocols.

Whether a FLAIR lesion is considered negative or positive, and hence an early-stage or late-stage stroke, likely depends on the degree of contrast that is used to display the image (**Fig. 3**) and may explain the varying degrees of consensus reported across studies. This observation has led to the investigation of relative signal intensities (rSI) or SIRs of FLAIR voxels coincident with abnormal DWI with respect to normal contralateral voxels as a predictor of stroke age. Using a FLAIR SIR of tissue in abnormal DWI to mirrored normal tissue in the contralateral hemisphere, Petkova and colleagues[32] found that classifying patients with less than or equal to 7% increase in SIR as "early" resulted in 90% sensitivity and 92%

Table 1
Summary of DWI-positive and FLAIR-negative studies identifying patients within 3 hours of stroke onset

Author Year	Admission NIHSS Score (Interquartile Range)	Time Range (h)	MR Imaging Scans	Studies Within 3 h (%)	Sensitivity (%)	Specificity (%)	κ (Readers)	Field Strength (T) (Manufacturer)
Thomalla et al 2009[29]	14 (8–17)[a]	0–6	101	71 (70)	48	93	0.29 (4)	1.5 (Siemens)
Ebinger et al 2010[30b]	4 (1–7)[a]	0–12	71	41 (58)	51	80	NA	3 (Siemens)
Aoki et al 2010[31]	5 (2–11)	0–24	361	140 (39)	83	71	0.65[a] (2)	1.5 (General Electric)
Petkova et al 2010[32]	11[c]	0–12	130	63 (48)	82	97	0.97 (2)	1.5 (General Electric)

[a] All patients including DWI-negative studies.
[b] Patients with DWI lesions >0.5 cm³.
[c] Mean NIHSS score calculated from Table 1 in Petkova and colleagues.[32]

Table 2
Summary of DWI-positive and FLAIR-negative studies identifying patients within 4.5 hours of stroke onset

Author Year	MR Imaging Scans	Studies Within 4.5 h (%)	Sensitivity (%)	Specificity (%)
Thomalla et al 2009[29]	101	92 (91)	38	89
Ebinger et al 2010[30,a]	71	51 (72)	49	90
Aoki et al 2010[31]	361	212 (59)	74	85

[a] Patients with DWI lesions >0.5 cm³.

specificity in identifying patients imaged within 3 hours from symptom onset. Ebinger and colleagues[30] found that FLAIR SIR poorly correlated with time from stroke onset with a Spearman correlation coefficient of −0.152 ($P = .128$). In contrast, Petkova and colleagues found a significant correlation between FLAIR SIR and time from stroke onset with a Pearson's coefficient $R = 0.63$ ($P<.001$). The discrepancies in the results of the 2 studies may be partly explained by differences in the methodology. Ebinger and colleagues correlated rSI based only on FLAIR lesions, whereas Petkova and colleagues measured SIR based on back-projected DWI lesions, which resulted in the inclusion of tissue that was FLAIR negative, leading to lower SIR measured in early-stage stroke, and significant correlation of SIR with respect to onset time. The differences in results may also be because of the more severe strokes involved in Petkova and colleagues' cohort (which excluded patients with NIHSS score ≤3) compared with Ebinger's cohort (median NIHSS score 4 [interquartile range 1–7]).

Advanced neuroimaging markers

In addition to DWI-positive and FLAIR-negative imaging, investigators have proposed using advanced imaging sequences that may provide better prediction of stroke duration. A study by Siemonsen and colleagues[35] proposed using quantitative T2 (qT2) mapping for predicting time of stroke onset in place of the qualitative assessment currently available with FLAIR imaging and T2-WI. Much of the experimental literature supporting T2 as an accurate marker for stroke duration is based on quantitative T2 imaging. Using a triple-echo T2 sequence in 36 patients imaged within 6 hours of stroke onset, the investigators found that the predictive accuracy of qT2 for identifying patients imaged within 3 hours of onset was 0.794 compared with 0.676 using FLAIR. This finding suggests that qT2 may provide a more objective metric for identifying early lesions than afforded by visual assessment of FLAIR lesions.

Sodium MR imaging has been shown to increase linearly with stroke onset time 2 to 7 hours after MCAO in rats[36] and 0 to 6 hours after MCAO in

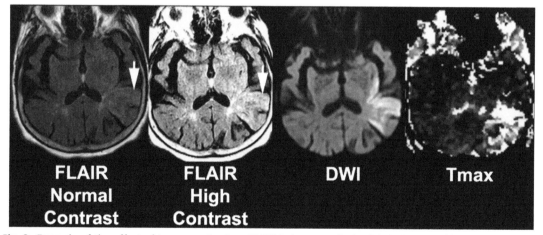

FLAIR Normal Contrast   **FLAIR High Contrast**   **DWI**   **Tmax**

Fig. 3. Example of the effect of image contrast on FLAIR lesion conspicuity for an 89-year-old woman imaged 6 hours from witnessed onset. Using default contrast, the FLAIR appears normal and would be classified FLAIR negative. However, by changing the contrast, the lesion becomes more evident (*arrow*), changing the classification to FLAIR-positive.

nonhuman primate models.[37] For human studies, sodium MR imaging performed more than 24 hours from stroke onset (N = 31) showed mean tissue sodium concentrations greater than 70 mmol/L, suspected to be a threshold for identifying infarcted tissue.[37] Another study in patients imaged between 4 and 104 hours (N = 21) also found that sodium imaging SI nonlinearly increased with stroke duration.[38] Within 7 hours of stroke onset, the increase was noted to be 10% or less, whereas beyond 9 hours from symptom onset the rate more than doubled to 23%, saturating at approximately 48 hours. Analysis of sodium changes in the area of DWI and PWI mismatch in 9 patients imaged 4 to 32 hours after onset showed no changes.[39] However, in the DWI lesion for these patients, sodium MRI SI was found to increase with stroke duration after 17 hours but showed no significant difference for studies within 7 hours. These results have led some to speculate that patients who present with minimal abnormality on sodium imaging could be safely treated with reperfusion therapy.

$T_{1\rho}$ has also been shown to correlate with time of symptom onset in experimental rat models of stroke imaged up to 7 hours after onset.[40] $T_{1\rho}$ has been found to correlate with regions of irreversible ischemia in models of transient stroke, increasing within minutes after occlusion.[41,42] Because $T_{1\rho}$ is less affected by blood-oxygenation-level–dependent effect than T2, $T_{1\rho}$ increases earlier than T2. In comparison, T2 images acquired simultaneously with the $T_{1\rho}$ were shown to first decrease within minutes after stroke,[40] consistent with reports in human patients with stroke,[43] before increasing. This very early decrease in T2 may contribute to the specificity of FLAIR-negative scans for identifying early-stage stroke.

Image-based Markers of Tissue Salvageability

Beyond serving as a surrogate for stroke duration, many investigators postulate that imaging can be used a marker of tissue salvageability. A few studies have explored this hypothesis. Studies have shown that MR imaging-based thrombolysis selection improved safety profiles irrespective of time window.[44,45] ECASS 3 reported that in a carefully selected population, rt-PA could be safely administered to patients treated between 3 and 4.5 hours since last known well.[5] Even with this expanded time window, by defining onset of stroke symptoms in the most conservative manner, namely using the time the patient was last known well, many patients whose onsets are unwitnessed are ineligible for IV rt-PA therapy even if their true time of onset (if it could be established) would qualify them for treatment. This situation has led some to propose the use of a "tissue clock," in place of a "wall clock," for determining treatment options for patients because time is essentially a surrogate for tissue injury. Welch and colleagues[46] speculated that histopathophysiologic changes in human stroke can be noninvasively tracked by monitoring changes in MR imaging profiles. These investigators' hypothesis was based on imaging findings from experimental animal models of stroke for which times of stroke onset were well defined and histopathology samples were available.[25,28] Based on animal experiments described earlier,[28,47] Welch and colleagues[46] formulated a tissue signature model combining MR imaging changes to predict histopathology after stroke.[48] The investigators describe six MR imaging signatures that can be used to characterize degree of tissue injury and chance of recovery (Table 3). As can be noted from the table, the DWI-positive and FLAIR-

Table 3
MR tissue signatures

Signature	ADC	T2-WI	Interpretation	Prediction
A	Normal	Normal	Normal	Normal
B	Low	Normal	Compromised tissue	May or may not recover
C	Low	High	Transition to cellular necrosis	Less likelihood of recovery
D	Normal	High	Transition to pannecrosis	Not likely
E	Normal	High	Necrosis	Unlikely
F	High	Normal	Necrosis	Unlikely

Adapted from Welch KM, Windham J, Knight RA, et al. A model to predict the histopathology of human stroke using diffusion and T2-weighted magnetic resonance imaging. Stroke 1995;26(11):1983–9; and Jiang Q, Chopp M, Zhang ZG, et al. The temporal evolution of MRI tissue signatures after transient middle cerebral artery occlusion in rat. J Neurol Sci 1997;145(1):15–23.

negative pattern proposed as a surrogate for early stroke onset is consistent with Signature B, which is representative of not only early-stage stroke but tissue with the greatest likelihood of recovery with reperfusion. **Fig. 4** shows an example of these temporal changes on DWI, ADC, and FLAIR images from a 54-year-old patient imaged within 2.9 hours since last known well. FLAIR is a T2-WI with signal from cerebrospinal fluid suppressed, which improves lesion conspicuity.[49] Also shown is the admission NCCT for comparison. For the acute scans, DWI and ADC are clearly abnormal, whereas NCCT appears negative and the FLAIR shows a subtle lesion. Over time, the lesion becomes more conspicuous on FLAIR, whereas it pseudonormalizes on ADC. ADC values for human stroke have been observed to

pseudonormalize approximately 1 to 2 weeks after onset for patients not given reperfusion therapy,[50] with maximal T2-WI lesion volumes observed at approximately 1 week, before stabilizing at approximately 30 days.[51] The observed differences in ADC and T2-WI lesion evolutions between stroke in humans and experimental animal stroke models are likely because animal models are imprecise replicas of human stroke,[52] in which ADC and T2-WI changes depend on often unmodeled clinical factors such as age, gender, and stroke subtype.[53] Furthermore, because both ADC and T2-WI temporal changes have been shown to differ with severity of ischemic insult, variations in collateral blood flow can contribute to these discrepancies.[28] In our example (see **Fig. 4**) ADC appears pseudonormal

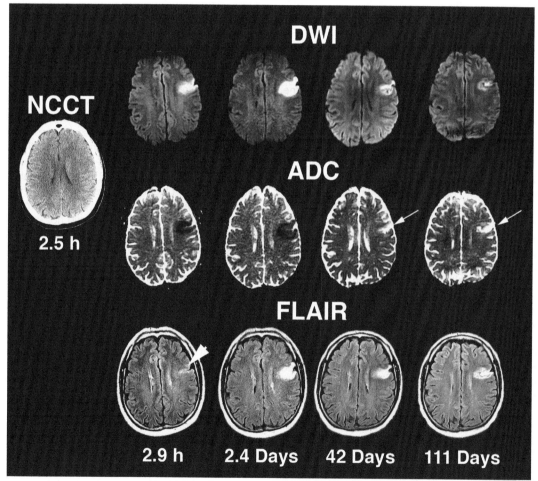

Fig. 4. Example of temporal changes in DWI, ADC, FLAIR images along with admission NCCT for a 54-year-old male patient imaged serially with MR imaging at 2.9 hours, 2.4 days, 42 days, and 111 days after onset. Admission NIHSS score was 1, 3-month mRS score was 2. Both DWI and ADC are readily abnormal by admission, whereas FLAIR shows subtle signs of abnormality (*arrowhead*). NCCT appears normal. Regions of ADC appear pseudonormal on the subacute scan, increasing by 1 month (*arrows*). DWI appears hyperintense across all time points. FLAIR lesion volume appears largest at day 2 as a result of edema, before stabilizing its infarct size at 42 days.

by day 2 in some regions (although T2 is abnormal, as seen on FLAIR images).

ADC values

Studies have investigated imaging parameters other than DWI-positive and FLAIR-negative mismatch to provide insight into severity of ischemic injury. Some have reported that patients with known onset times were safely treated with rt-PA despite presenting with FLAIR-positive patterns, with similar clinical and radiological outcomes as the FLAIR-negative group.[54] Thus, excluding those patients with wake-up stroke or unclear onset stroke who are FLAIR positive, may be overly restrictive, and other more sensitive, but just as specific, criteria should perhaps be used, such as degree of ADC reduction. Although Petkova and colleagues[32] showed a significant positive association in relative ADC values with respect to stroke onset time ($R = 0.47$, $P<.001$), these results may be confounded by the biphasic nature of ADC. ADC values dramatically decrease within the first minutes to hours after stroke onset, followed by pseudonormalization, eventually increasing in chronic stages of stroke.[46,50] Some have speculated that the rates of these transitions across patients depend on stroke etiology, severity of ischemic insult, and extent of collateral flow. As a result, some have focused on identifying thresholds for predicting when tissue has become irreversibly injured and no longer suited for reperfusion therapy. Some studies suggest that there may be a threshold of severe ADC reduction for which thrombolytic therapy may be unsuitable,[55,56] although other reports have suggested that this may not be the case,[57,58] and the discrepancies may potentially be caused by the heterogeneity of values found in the ADC lesion.[59] An ADC threshold (0.65×10^{-3} mm^2/s) was found to be an excellent predictor of tissue infarction measured on histology.[60] Consistent with the hypothesis that the amount of salvageable tissue after ischemia is a function of degree and duration of flow deficit,[61] the correlation between the ADC threshold and CBF values varied with stroke duration. At 30 minutes, this ADC threshold corresponded with severe flow deficit (15 mL/100 g/min) whereas at 60 minutes, the threshold reflected moderate deficits (40 mL/100 g/min).[60] Tissue showing severe initial ADC reductions was also found likely to infarct even with reperfusion in human stroke. The threshold for defining irreversible injury also varied by mechanism for reperfusion intervention, being 50% for IV rt-PA therapy[62] and 0.55×10^{-3} mm^2/s for IA therapy.[63] Tissue with ADC values less than 0.55×10^{-3} mm^2/s was also found more frequently in regions that eventually experienced hemorrhagic transformation secondary to infarction.[55] The use of a threshold for predicting infarction assumes that tissue with ADC values higher than this cutoff, albeit reduced, can potentially be saved. Although tissue showing increased ADC restriction has been shown to reverse after restoration of CBF, histologic evidence from experimental stroke studies has shown persistent neuronal injury despite normal-appearing ADC.[64] In addition, for both experimental and human studies, secondary injury has been noted in tissue in which the ADC apparently recovered, only to be discovered infarcted by later imaging[65,66] or histologic studies.[64,67–70]

DWI and PWI mismatches

Although DWI is extremely sensitive to ischemic injury, detecting changes as early as 3 minutes after onset,[71] by definition, PWI, by either bolus tracking[72] or arterial spin labeling,[73] is the most sensitive technique for detecting ischemia-induced alterations, reflecting areas that are at risk of infarction without reperfusion. PWI is discussed in detail by Copen and colleagues in this issue. DWI and PWI have been shown to be highly sensitive and specific in diagnosing acute human cerebral ischemia.[74–77] Examples of mismatch patterns are shown in **Fig. 5**. The patient without a mismatch (see **Fig. 5**A) is the same case shown in **Fig. 4**, with admission MR imaging obtained within 3 hours of last known well. There are signs of spontaneous reperfusion (hypointense mean transit time [MTT]) and the lesion did not expand. The patient with mismatch (see **Fig. 5**B) woke up with symptoms and was last known well before he went to bed. He was found by his wife with symptoms in the morning. MR imaging was performed 14.4 hours from last known well and 4.6 hours from symptom discovery; subtle signs of FLAIR hyperintensity can be noted that match the DWI lesion. However, there is a larger perfusion deficit noted on CBF, MTT, and T$_{max}$ (the time point for which the deconvolved residue function reaches maximum value[78]) maps, into which the infarct expanded by 5 days. Extensive tissue loss and cavitation are noted at 115 days. Patients presenting with patterns similar to those shown in our examples have led to the proposed use of DWI and PWI mismatches for triaging patients for thrombolytic therapy, even those whose onset time is known to be beyond the therapeutic time window of 3 to 4.5 hours, such as **Fig. 5**B. The Diffusion and Perfusion Imaging Evaluation for Understanding Stroke Evolution (DEFUSE; N = 74) trial[79] and Echoplanar Imaging Thrombolytic Evaluation Trial (EPITHET; N = 101)

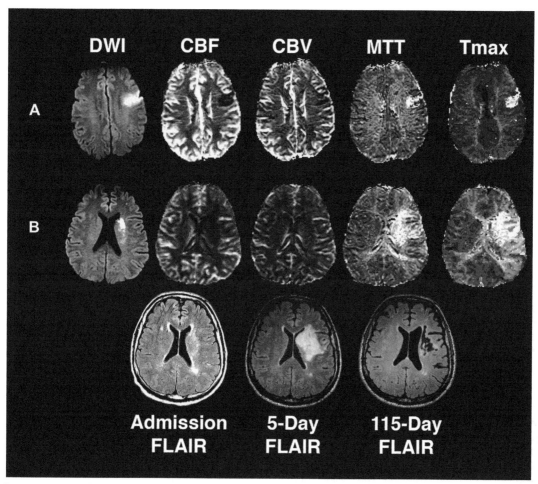

Fig. 5. Examples of (*A*) DWI and PWI without mismatch for the same patient imaged serially in Fig. 4 and (*B*) DWI and PWI lesion mismatch for a 59-year-old man with unknown onset who awakened with symptoms. Admission MR imaging was performed 14.4 hours from last known well with an NIHSS score of 9. For the case with mismatch (*B*), the patient's lesion expanded into the perfusion deficit, whereas for the case without mismatch (*A*), no lesion expansion, besides edema, is noted. Also shown for (*B*) are serial FLAIR data in which edema is evident at day 5, whereas the 115-day study shows extensive cavitation and tissue loss.

were observational studies in which the investigators sought to find patterns of DWI and PWI mismatch that predict good outcome after late thrombolytic therapy.[80] Both studies used T_{max} as the perfusion metric and a threshold of greater than or equal to 2 seconds for lesion segmentation. Patients were classified as having a mismatch if (PWI − DWI) was 10 cm^3 or greater and (PWI ÷ DWI × 100) was 120% or greater. DEFUSE found that early reperfusion was associated (*P* = .039) with a favorable outcome in patients with DWI and PWI mismatch, whereas patients without mismatch did not benefit from early reperfusion.[79] DEFUSE identified a malignant pattern associated with severe ICH and poor outcome after reperfusion characterized by either a large DWI lesion volume (>100 cm^3) or large

PWI lesion volume using a threshold of 8 seconds or more (>100 cm^3). EPITHET found that for patients who showed mismatches (N = 80), patients treated with rt-PA tended to have lower infarct growth and increased reperfusion than those given placebo.[80] Trials that used DWI and PWI mismatches for inclusion criteria with varying degrees of success and failure in terms of favorable clinical outcome include the Desmoteplase in Acute Ischemic Stroke Trial (DIAS, N = 57, time window, 3–9 hours),[81] Dose Escalation of Desmoteplase for Acute Ischemic Stroke (DEDAS, N = 37, 3-hour to 9-hour time window),[82] DIAS II (N = 186 treated, 3-hour to 9-hour window),[83] pilot trial of normobaric hyperoxia (N = 16, 0-hour to 12-hour time window),[84] and Flo24 (N = 26, 8-hour to 24-hour time window).[85] Ongoing studies that use admission PWI for patient triage or randomization include Extending the Time for Thrombolysis in Emergency Neurologic Deficits (EXTEND, expected enrollment N = 400, 3-hour to 9-hour time window),[86] and Mechanical Retrieval and Recanalization of Stroke Clots Using Embolectomy (MR RESCUE, N = 120, 0-hour to 8-hour time window).[87] EXTEND is a phase III trial that builds on the results of EPITHET; however, unlike EPITHET, patients are given rt-PA based on PWI and DWI mismatch, using a T_{max} threshold greater than 6 seconds for lesion identification. For MR RESCUE, PWI and DWI mismatch are used for patient randomization based on a computer algorithm, but a mismatch does not need to be present for enrollment. DEFUSE 2 plans to validate the profiles identified by DEFUSE in 100 patients treated for 3 to 8 hours.[88] DIAS3/DIAS4 (N = 400, 3–9 hours)[89] and MR RESCUE[87] use angiographic information requiring the presence of a large-vessel occlusion or high-grade stenosis on CTA or magnetic resonance angiography for patient enrollment.

CLINICAL TRIALS INVOLVING PATIENTS WITH UNWITNESSED STROKE ONSET

With the prevalence of imaging techniques that are sensitive and specific to identifying early stroke duration and potential tissue salvage, several interventional trials in patients with unknown onset time of stroke have been proposed. The designs of the trials vary. One study involving patients who awaken with deficit who can be treated within 2.5 hours of awakening, AWOKE,[90] requires a 20% lesion mismatch based either on CTP (CBV and MTT) or MR PWI (DWI and TTP). The expected number of patients to be enrolled is 20. Inclusion criteria involve patients aged 22 years or older, with an ASPECTS score 7 or higher on DWI or CT-CBV or CTA-SI. Another study involving patients with wake-up stroke is the Wake Stroke Study,[91] which plans to enroll 40 subjects who can be treated within 3 hours of awakening, aged 18 to 80 years, admission NIHSS score 25 or less. Imaging criteria exclude patients presenting with hypodensity greater than one-third MCA territory. MR WITNESS, a phase II safety study, involving 80 patients with wake-up and unclear stroke onset, 18 to 80 years of age, admission NIHSS score 25 or less, presenting with a DWI-positive and FLAIR-negative mismatch who are imaged within 3 hours of symptom discovery (and within 24 hours of last seen well) and who could be treated within 4.5 hours of symptom discovery, has been proposed.[92,93] In addition, FLAIR-positive patients who have a SIR

less than 1.15 may also be enrolled if they meet other inclusion and exclusion criteria. All 3 trials are open-label, single-arm studies in which the primary outcome is safety, as measured by the frequency of sICH. Secondary outcomes for all 3 studies include mRS score at 3 months. Unlike the other 3 studies, a planned trial by Thomalla and colleagues, Wake-UP, is a randomized, double-blind, placebo-controlled trial with 800 patients with wake-up stroke, in which the primary outcome will be favorable outcome at 3 months (Götz Thomalla, MD, Hamburg, Germany, personal communication, January, 2011). Imaging enrollment criteria are expected to be similar to that of MR WITNESS.

SUMMARY

With further refinement and large confirmatory studies, imaging techniques individually or in combination may provide additional insight into tissue injury and salvageability and be used to extend rt-PA to more patients with wake-up stroke and patients with unclear onset who benefit from therapy.

REFERENCES

1. Miniño AM, Xu JQ, Kochanek KD. Deaths: preliminary data for 2008. National Vital Statistics Reports, vol. 59. Hyattsville (MD): National Center for Health Statistics; 2010.
2. Lloyd-Jones D, Adams R, Carnethon M, et al. Heart disease and stroke statistics–2009 update: a report from the American Heart Association Statistics Committee and Stroke Statistics Subcommittee. Circulation 2009;119(3):e21–181.
3. Rymer MM, Thrutchley DE. Organizing regional networks to increase acute stroke intervention. Neurol Res 2005;27(Suppl 1):S9–16.
4. George MG, Tong X, McGruder H, et al. Paul Coverdell National Acute Stroke Registry Surveillance–four states, 2005–2007. MMWR Surveill Summ 2009; 58(7):1–23.
5. Hacke W, Kaste M, Bluhmki E, et al. Thrombolysis with alteplase 3 to 4.5 hours after acute ischemic stroke. N Engl J Med 2008;359(13):1317–29.
6. Barreto AD, Martin-Schild S, Hallevi H, et al. Thrombolytic therapy for patients who wake-up with stroke. Stroke 2009;40(3):827–32.
7. Lago A, Geffner D, Tembl J, et al. Circadian variation in acute ischemic stroke: a hospital-based study. Stroke 1998;29(9):1873–5.
8. Chaturvedi S, Adams HP Jr, Woolson RF. Circadian variation in ischemic stroke subtypes. Stroke 1999; 30(9):1792–5.

9. Serena J, Davalos A, Segura T, et al. Stroke on awakening: looking for a more rational management. Cerebrovasc Dis 2003;16(2):128–33.

10. Marler JR, Price TR, Clark GL, et al. Morning increase in onset of ischemic stroke. Stroke 1989; 20(4):473–6.

11. Marshall J. Diurnal variation in occurrence of strokes. Stroke 1977;8(2):230–1.

12. Argentino C, Toni D, Rasura M, et al. Circadian variation in the frequency of ischemic stroke. Stroke 1990;21(3):387–9.

13. Adams HJ, Bedndixen B, Kappelle J, et al. Classification of subtype of acute ischemic stroke. Definitions for use in a multicenter clinical trial. TOAST. Trial of Org 10172 in Acute Stroke Treatment. Stroke 1993;24:35–41.

14. Elliott WJ. Circadian variation in the timing of stroke onset: a meta-analysis. Stroke 1998;29(5):992–6.

15. Fink JN, Kumar S, Horkan C, et al. The stroke patient who woke up: clinical and radiological features, including diffusion and perfusion MRI. Stroke 2002; 33(4):988–93.

16. Todo K, Moriwaki H, Saito K, et al. Early CT findings in unknown-onset and wake-up strokes. Cerebrovasc Dis 2006;21(5–6):367–71.

17. Silva GS, Lima FO, Camargo EC, et al. Wake-up stroke: clinical and neuroimaging characteristics. Cerebrovasc Dis 2010;29(4):336–42.

18. Iosif C, Oppenheim C, Trystram D, et al. MR imaging-based decision in thrombolytic therapy for stroke on awakening: report of 2 cases. AJNR Am J Neuroradiol 2008;29(7):1314–6.

19. Hellier KD, Hampton JL, Guadagno JV, et al. Perfusion CT helps decision making for thrombolysis when there is no clear time of onset. J Neurol Neurosurg Psychiatry 2006;77(3):417–9.

20. Adams HP Jr, Leira EC, Torner JC, et al. Treating patients with 'wake-up' stroke: the experience of the AbESTT-II trial. Stroke 2008;39(12):3277–82.

21. Adams HP Jr, Effron MB, Torner J, et al. Emergency administration of abciximab for treatment of patients with acute ischemic stroke: results of an international phase III trial: abciximab in emergency treatment of stroke trial (AbESTT-II). Stroke 2008;39(1):87–99.

22. Cho AH, Sohn SI, Han MK, et al. Safety and efficacy of MRI-based thrombolysis in unclear-onset stroke. A preliminary report. Cerebrovasc Dis 2008;25(6): 572–9.

23. NINDS rt-PA Stroke Study Group. Tissue plasminogen activator for acute ischemic stroke. N Engl J Med 1995;333(24):1581–7.

24. del Zoppo GJ, Saver JL, Jauch EC, et al. Expansion of the time window for treatment of acute ischemic stroke with intravenous tissue plasminogen activator: a science advisory from the American Heart Association/American Stroke Association. Stroke 2009;40(8):2945–8.

25. Moseley ME, Cohen Y, Mintorovitch J, et al. Early detection of regional cerebral ischemia in cats: comparison of diffusion and T2 weighted MRI and spectroscopy. Magn Reson Med 1990;14(2): 330–46.

26. Mintorovitch J, Moseley ME, Chileuitt L, et al. Comparison of diffusion- and T2-weighted MRI for the early detection of cerebral ischemia and reperfusion in rats. Magn Reson Med 1991;18(1):39–50.

27. Jiang Q, Zhang ZG, Chopp M, et al. Temporal evolution and spatial distribution of the diffusion constant of water in rat brain after transient middle cerebral artery occlusion. J Neurol Sci 1993; 120(2):123–30.

28. Knight RA, Dereski MO, Helpern JA, et al. Magnetic resonance imaging assessment of evolving focal cerebral ischemia. Comparison with histopathology in rats. Stroke 1994;25(6):1252–61 [discussion: 1261–2].

29. Thomalla G, Rossbach P, Rosenkranz M, et al. Negative fluid-attenuated inversion recovery imaging identifies acute ischemic stroke at 3 hours or less. Ann Neurol 2009;65(6):724–32.

30. Ebinger M, Galinovic I, Rozanski M, et al. Fluid-attenuated inversion recovery evolution within 12 hours from stroke onset: a reliable tissue clock? Stroke 2010;41(2):250–5.

31. Aoki J, Kimura K, Iguchi Y, et al. FLAIR can estimate the onset time in acute ischemic stroke patients. J Neurol Sci 2010;293(1–2):39–44.

32. Petkova M, Rodrigo S, Lamy C, et al. MR imaging helps predict time from symptom onset in patients with acute stroke: implications for patients with unknown onset time. Radiology 2010;257(3):782–92.

33. Barber PA, Hill MD, Eliasziw M, et al. Imaging of the brain in acute ischaemic stroke: comparison of computed tomography and magnetic resonance diffusion-weighted imaging. J Neurol Neurosurg Psychiatry 2005;76(11):1528–33.

34. Universitätsklinikum Hamburg-Eppendorf. Identification of stroke patients ≤3 and ≤4.5 hours of symptom onset by fluid attenuated inversion recovery (FLAIR) imaging and diffusion weighted imaging (DWI) (PRE-FLAIR). In: ClinicalTrials.gov. Bethesda (MD): National Library of Medicine (US); 2000. Available from: http://clinicaltrials.gov/ct2/show/NCT01021319; 2000. NLM Identifier: NCT01021319, Accessed January 4, 2011.

35. Siemonsen S, Mouridsen K, Holst B, et al. Quantitative t2 values predict time from symptom onset in acute stroke patients. Stroke 2009;40(5):1612–6.

36. Jones SC, Kharlamov A, Yanovski B, et al. Stroke onset time using sodium MRI in rat focal cerebral ischemia. Stroke 2006;37(3):883–8.

37. Thulborn KR, Gindin TS, Davis D, et al. Comprehensive MR imaging protocol for stroke management: tissue sodium concentration as a measure of tissue

viability in nonhuman primate studies and in clinical studies. Radiology 1999;213(1):156–66.

38. Hussain MS, Stobbe RW, Bhagat YA, et al. Sodium imaging intensity increases with time after human ischemic stroke. Ann Neurol 2009;66(1):55–62.

39. Tsang A, Stobbe RW, Asdaghi N, et al. Relationship between sodium intensity and perfusion deficits in acute ischemic stroke. J Magn Reson Imaging 2011;33(1):41–7.

40. Jokivarsi KT, Hiltunen Y, Grohn H, et al. Estimation of the onset time of cerebral ischemia using T1rho and T2 MRI in rats. Stroke 2010;41(10):2335–40.

41. Grohn OH, Lukkarinen JA, Silvennoinen MJ, et al. Quantitative magnetic resonance imaging assessment of cerebral ischemia in rat using on-resonance T(1) in the rotating frame. Magn Reson Med 1999;42(2):268–76.

42. Grohn OHJ, Kettunen MI, Makela HI, et al. Early detection of irreversible cerebral ischemia in the rat using dispersion of the magnetic resonance imaging relaxation time, T1rho. J Cereb Blood Flow Metab 2000;20(10):1457–66.

43. Geisler BS, Brandhoff F, Fiehler J, et al. Blood-oxygen-level-dependent MRI allows metabolic description of tissue at risk in acute stroke patients. Stroke 2006;37(7):1778–84.

44. Kohrmann M, Juttler E, Fiebach JB, et al. MRI versus CT-based thrombolysis treatment within and beyond the 3 h time window after stroke onset: a cohort study. Lancet Neurol 2006;5(8):661–7.

45. Schellinger PD, Thomalla G, Fiehler J, et al. MRI-based and CT-based thrombolytic therapy in acute stroke within and beyond established time windows: an analysis of 1210 patients. Stroke 2007;38(10):2640–5.

46. Welch KMA, Windham J, Knight RA, et al. A model to predict the histopathology of human stroke using diffusion and T2-weighted magnetic resonance imaging. Stroke 1995;26(11):1983–9.

47. Helpern JA, Dereski MO, Knight RA, et al. Histopathological correlations of nuclear magnetic resonance imaging parameters in experimental cerebral ischemia. Magn Reson Imaging 1993;11(2):241–6.

48. Jiang Q, Chopp M, Zhang ZG, et al. The temporal evolution of MRI tissue signatures after transient middle cerebral artery occlusion in rat. J Neurol Sci 1997;145(1):15–23.

49. Hajnal JV, Bryant DJ, Kasuboski L, et al. Use of fluid attenuated inversion recovery (FLAIR) pulse sequences in MRI of the brain. J Comput Assist Tomogr 1992;16(6):841–4.

50. Schwamm LH, Koroshetz WJ, Sorensen AG, et al. Time course of lesion development in patients with acute stroke: serial diffusion- and hemodynamic-weighted magnetic resonance imaging. Stroke 1998;29:2268–76.

51. Gaudinski MR, Henning EC, Miracle A, et al. Establishing final infarct volume: stroke lesion evolution past 30 days is insignificant. Stroke 2008;39(10): 2765–8.

52. Fisher M, Feuerstein G, Howells DW, et al. Update of the stroke therapy academic industry roundtable preclinical recommendations. Stroke 2009;40(6): 2244–50.

53. Copen WA, Schwamm LH, Gonzalez RG, et al. Ischemic stroke: effects of etiology and patient age on the time course of the core apparent diffusion coefficient. Radiology 2001;221(1):27–34.

54. Ebinger M, Ostwaldt AC, Galinovic I, et al. Clinical and radiological courses do not differ between fluid-attenuated inversion recovery-positive and negative patients with stroke after thrombolysis. Stroke 2010;41(8):1823–5.

55. Tong DC, Adami A, Moseley ME, et al. Relationship between apparent diffusion coefficient and subsequent hemorrhagic transformation following acute ischemic stroke. Stroke 2000;31(10):2378–84.

56. Oppenheim C, Samson Y, Dormont D, et al. DWI prediction of symptomatic hemorrhagic transformation in acute MCA infarct. J Neuroradiol 2002;29(1):6–13.

57. Fiehler J, Foth M, Kucinski T, et al. Severe ADC decreases do not predict irreversible tissue damage in humans. Stroke 2002;33(1):79–86.

58. Loh PS, Butcher KS, Parsons MW, et al. Apparent diffusion coefficient thresholds do not predict the response to acute stroke thrombolysis. Stroke 2005;36(12):2626–31.

59. Nagesh V, Welch KMA, Windham JP, et al. Time course of ADCw changes in ischemic stroke: beyond the human eye! Stroke 1998;29:1778–82.

60. Miyabe M, Mori S, van Zijl PC, et al. Correlation of the average water diffusion constant with cerebral blood flow and ischemic damage after transient middle cerebral artery occlusion in cats. J Cereb Blood Flow Metab 1996;16(5):881–91.

61. Jones TH, Morawetz RB, Crowell RM, et al. Thresholds of focal cerebral ischemia in awake monkeys. J Neurosurg 1981;54(6):773–82.

62. Fiehler J, Knudsen K, Kucinski T, et al. Predictors of apparent diffusion coefficient normalization in stroke patients. Stroke 2004;35(2):514–9.

63. Kidwell CS, Alger JR, Saver JL. Beyond mismatch: evolving paradigms in imaging the ischemic penumbra with multimodal magnetic resonance imaging. Stroke 2003;34(11):2729–35.

64. Li F, Han SS, Tatlisumak T, et al. Reversal of acute apparent diffusion coefficient abnormalities and delayed neuronal death following transient focal cerebral ischemia in rats. Ann Neurol 1999;46(3):333–42.

65. Marks MP, Tong DC, Beaulieu C, et al. Evaluation of early reperfusion and i.v. tPA therapy using diffusion- and perfusion-weighted MRI. Neurology 1999;52(9): 1792–8.

66. Kidwell CS, Saver JL, Mattiello J, et al. Thrombolytic reversal of acute human cerebral ischemic injury

shown by diffusion/perfusion magnetic resonance imaging. Ann Neurol 2000;47(4):462–9.

67. Dijkhuizen RM, Knollema S, van der Worp HB, et al. Dynamics of cerebral tissue injury and perfusion after temporary hypoxia-ischemia in the rat: evidence for region-specific sensitivity and delayed damage. Stroke 1998;29(3):695–704.

68. van Lookeren Campagne M, Thomas GR, Thibodeaux H, et al. Secondary reduction in the apparent diffusion coefficient of water, increase in cerebral blood volume, and delayed neuronal death after middle cerebral artery occlusion and early reperfusion in the rat. J Cereb Blood Flow Metab 1999;19(12):1354–64.

69. Li F, Silva MD, Liu KF, et al. Secondary decline in apparent diffusion coefficient and neurological outcomes after a short period of focal brain ischemia in rats. Ann Neurol 2000;48(2):236–44.

70. Li F, Liu KF, Silva MD, et al. Acute postischemic renormalization of the apparent diffusion coefficient of water is not associated with reversal of astrocytic swelling and neuronal shrinkage in rats. AJNR Am J Neuroradiol 2002;23(2):180–8.

71. Li F, Han S, Tatlisumak T, et al. A new method to improve in-bore middle cerebral artery occlusion in rats: demonstration with diffusion- and perfusion-weighted imaging. Stroke 1998;29(8):1715–9 [discussion: 1719–20].

72. Rosen B, Belliveau J, Vevea J, et al. Perfusion imaging with NMR contrast agents. Magn Reson Med 1990;14(2):249–66.

73. Williams DS, Detre JA, Leigh JS, et al. Magnetic resonance imaging of perfusion using spin inversion of arterial water. Proc Natl Acad Sci U S A 1992; 89(1):212–6.

74. Sorensen AG, Buonanno FS, Gonzalez RG, et al. Hyperacute stroke: evaluation with combined multi-section diffusion-weighted and hemodynamically weighted echo-planar MR imaging. Radiology 1996;199:391–401.

75. Sorensen AG, Copen WA, Østergaard L, et al. Hyperacute stroke: simultaneous measurement of relative cerebral blood volume, relative cerebral blood flow, and mean tissue transit time. Radiology 1999;210(2):519–27.

76. Warach S, Dashe JF, Edelman RR. Clinical outcome in ischemic stroke predicted by early diffusion-weighted and perfusion magnetic resonance imaging: a preliminary analysis. J Cereb Blood Flow Metab 1996;16(1):53–9.

77. Baird AE, Warach S. Magnetic resonance imaging of acute stroke. J Cereb Blood Flow Metab 1998;18(6): 583–609.

78. Shih LC, Saver JL, Alger JR, et al. Perfusion-weighted magnetic resonance imaging thresholds identifying core, irreversibly infarcted tissue. Stroke 2003;34(6):1425–30.

79. Albers GW, Thijs VN, Wechsler L, et al. Magnetic resonance imaging profiles predict clinical response to early reperfusion: the diffusion and perfusion imaging evaluation for understanding stroke evolution (DEFUSE) study. Ann Neurol 2006;60(5): 508–17.

80. Davis SM, Donnan GA, Parsons MW, et al. Effects of alteplase beyond 3 h after stroke in the Echoplanar Imaging Thrombolytic Evaluation Trial (EPITHET): a placebo-controlled randomised trial. Lancet Neurol 2008;7(4):299–309.

81. Hacke W, Albers G, Al-Rawi Y, et al. The Desmoteplase in Acute Ischemic Stroke Trial (DIAS): a phase II MRI-based 9-hour window acute stroke thrombolysis trial with intravenous desmoteplase. Stroke 2005;36(1):66–73.

82. Furlan AJ, Eyding D, Albers GW, et al. Dose Escalation of Desmoteplase for Acute Ischemic Stroke (DEDAS): evidence of safety and efficacy 3 to 9 hours after stroke onset. Stroke 2006;37(5):1227–31.

83. Hacke W, Furlan AJ, Al-Rawi Y, et al. Intravenous desmoteplase in patients with acute ischaemic stroke selected by MRI perfusion-diffusion weighted imaging or perfusion CT (DIAS-2): a prospective, randomised, double-blind, placebo-controlled study. Lancet Neurol 2009;8(2):141–50.

84. Singhal AB, Benner T, Roccatagliata L, et al. A pilot study of normobaric oxygen therapy in acute ischemic stroke. Stroke 2005;36(4):797–802.

85. CoAxia. Safety and efficacy of NeuroFlo in 8–24 hour stroke patients (Flo 24). In: ClinicalTrials.gov. Bethesda (MD): National Library of Medicine (US); 2000. Available from: http://clinicaltrials.gov/ct2/show/NCT00436592; 2000. NLM Identifier: NCT00436592, Accessed January 9, 2011.

86. National Stroke Research Institute Australia. Extending the Time for Thrombolysis in Emergency Neurological Deficits (EXTEND). In: ClinicalTrials.gov. Bethesda (MD): National Library of Medicine (US); 2000. Available from: http://clinicaltrials.gov/ct2/show/NCT00887328; 2000. NLM Identifier: NCT00887328, Accessed January 9, 2011.

87. University of California Los Angeles. Mechanical Retrieval and Recanalization of Stroke Clots Using Embolectomy (MR RESCUE). In: ClinicalTrials.gov. Bethesda (MD): National Library of Medicine (US); 2000. Available from: http://clinicaltrials.gov/ct2/show/NCT00389467; 2000. NLM Identifier: NCT00389467, Accessed January 9, 2011.

88. National Institute of Neurological Disorders and Stroke. NINDS Awards Recovery Act Funds to Support Neuroimaging Study of Stroke Patients. 2010. Available from: http://www.ninds.nih.gov/recovery/arra-stories/Albers-Defuse.htm. Accessed January 9, 2011.

89. Lundbeck A/S H. Efficacy and Safety Study of Desmoteplase to Treat Acute Ischemic Stroke (DIAS-4).

In: ClinicalTrials.gov. Bethesda (MD): National Library of Medicine (US); 2000. Available from: http://clinicaltrials.gov/ct2/show/NCT00856661; 2000. NLM Identifier:NCT00856661, Accessed January 9, 2011.

90. University of California San Diego. Study for the Use of Alteplase in Patients Who Awaken With Stroke (AWOKE). In: ClinicalTrials.gov. Bethesda (MD): National Library of Medicine (US); 2000. Available from: http://clinicaltrials.gov/ct2/show/NCT01150266; 2000. Identifier:NCT01150266, Accessed January 9, 2011.

91. University of Texas Health Science Center Houston. Safety of Intravenous Thrombolysis for Wake-up Stroke (Wake-Up Stroke). In: ClinicalTrials.gov. Bethesda (MD): National Library of Medicine (US); 2000. Available from: http://clinicaltrials.gov/ct2/show/NCT01183533; 2000. Identifier:NCT01183533, Accessed January 9, 2011.

92. Schwamm LH, Sorensen AG, Wu O, et al. MR WITNESS Investigators. MR WITNESS–Safety Trial of IV rt-PA in Patients With Unwitnessed Stroke Onset. 2010 International Stroke Conference. San Antonio (TX), February 24–26, 2010.

93. Wu O, Song SS, Ritter C, et al. MRI as witness: ready for prime-time? 2011 International Stroke Conference. Los Angeles (CA), Feburary 9–11, 2011.

MR Diffusion Imaging in Ischemic Stroke

Steve H. Fung, MD[a],*, Luca Roccatagliata, MD[b],
R. Gilberto Gonzalez, MD, PhD[c], Pamela W. Schaefer, MD[c]

KEYWORDS

- MR imaging • Diffusion-weighted imaging
- Diffusion tensor imaging • Diffusion kurtosis imaging
- Brain ischemia

Diffusion-weighted imaging (DWI) provides image contrast that is dependent on the molecular motion of water. The method was introduced into clinical practice in the mid-1990s. Because ultrafast MRI sequences such as echo planar imaging (EPI) can be used, DWI is fairly resistant to patient motion, with imaging times ranging from a few seconds to 2 minutes. DWI is the most reliable method for the early detection of cerebral ischemia, for the definition of infarct core, and for the differentiation of acute ischemia from other disease processes that mimic stroke.

Although DWI has been useful in research and clinical management of stroke, diffusion tensor imaging (DTI) and diffusion kurtosis imaging (DKI) may offer additional diagnostic information on the microstructural status of tissue. This is because diffusion in tissue is affected by the presence of semipermeable membranes and oriented microstructures in the intracellular, extracellular, and vascular compartments that result in preferential movement of water parallel to these obstacles. This directional dependence of diffusion is known as anisotropy. In the brain, white matter has relatively high anisotropy because diffusion is much greater parallel than perpendicular to major white matter tracts. Gray matter, alternatively, has relatively low anisotropy. Heterogeneity of the diffusion environment from compartmentalization also results in non-Gaussian probability distribution of

water diffusion, which can be quantified by kurtosis. The purpose of this review is to discuss the development and applications of DWI, DTI, and DKI in acute and chronic ischemia.

BASIC CONCEPTS OF DIFFUSION MR IMAGING

The term, *diffusion*, refers to the general transport of matter whereby molecules or ions mix through normal agitation in a random way. When describing the mixing of different liquids or gases, diffusion is described in terms of a concentration gradient of the diffusing substance. In biologic tissues, the driving force is the motion of water within water, driven by thermal agitation and commonly referred to as Brownian motion. For example, the path of a pollen grain suspended in water provides good visualization of this Brownian motion. After each displacement, there is a collision and then a new random orientation for the next displacement, with a succession of n random displacements. In the case of unrestricted diffusion, the particle wanders freely in all directions throughout the medium (**Fig. 1**A). The root-mean-square distance L traversed by the particle in time t is proportional to the square root of the diffusion coefficient D. Because there is no directional variation in the free D, the diffusion is isotropic. For water at 37°C, D is approximately 3.2×10^{-3} mm²/s.

[a] Neuroradiology Section, Department of Radiology, The Methodist Hospital, Weill Cornell Medical College, 6565 Fannin Street, Houston, TX 77030, USA
[b] Department of Neurosciences, Ophthalmology and Genetics, University of Genoa, Via Antonio De Toni 5, 16132 Genoa, Italy
[c] Neuroradiology Division, Department of Radiology, Massachusetts General Hospital, Harvard Medical School, 55 Fruit Street, Boston, MA 02114, USA
* Corresponding author.
E-mail address: steve_fung@post.harvard.edu

Neuroimag Clin N Am 21 (2011) 345–377
doi:10.1016/j.nic.2011.03.001
1052-5149/11/$ – see front matter © 2011 Elsevier Inc. All rights reserved.

A

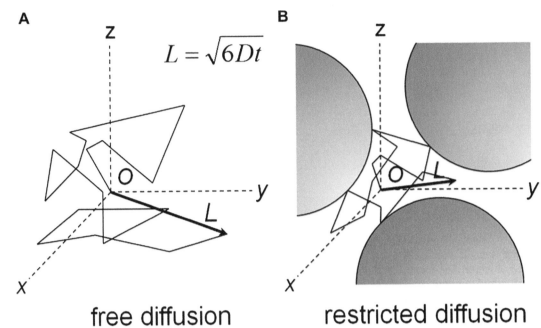

free diffusion   restricted diffusion

Fig. 1. Comparison of a particle with unrestricted or free diffusion (*A*) versus a particle with restricted diffusion (*B*). Biologic structures have barriers that restrict diffusion. For example, white matter tracts have relatively free diffusion along their principal axis and restricted diffusion perpendicular to that axis. This directional diffusion is called anisotropy.

In biologic tissues, water molecules encounter several complex semipermeable structures (see **Fig. 1**B), for example myelin and axonal membranes along white matter tracts, and diffusion through them exhibits directionality, or anisotropy, in the orientation of preferred motion. The measured diffusion is greater parallel to the barriers than perpendicular to them.[1]

In vivo measurement of water diffusion with MR imaging exploits the fact that spins moving through a magnetic field gradient acquire phase at a rate depending on the gradient strength and the velocity of the spins. A basic sequence for measuring diffusion is the Stejskal-Tanner pulse sequence (**Fig. 2**). The method uses a pair of equal but opposite strong gradient pulses placed symmetrically around the 180° refocusing pulse. The effect of the spin echo is to reverse this dephasing (loss of signal due to a fanning out of the spin vectors that do not add coherently) in the interval TE/2 so that an echo, a sum of all spin vectors, is formed at a time TE/2 after the application of the 180° pulse. The effect on the spin system of the first gradient lobe before the 180° pulse is to increase the rate at which the various spin vectors fan out, resulting in a faster signal decay. The gradient lobe after the 180° pulse is polarity reversed relative to the first lobe so that the total gradient dephasing is zero in static tissues.

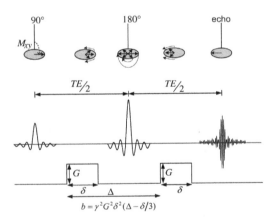

Fig. 2. Stejskal-Tanner diffusion spin-echo sequence. Spins accumulate phase shift during the first gradient pulse. The 180° pulse inverts the phase of all spins. The second gradient lobe induces another phase shift that is opposite to the first gradient pulse. For stationary spins, the phase shifts are identical in magnitude and cancel each other out. For moving spins, the translation of the spins to different locations in time results in incomplete refocusing and attenuation of the resulting echo. γ is the gyromagnetic ratio; and *G* is the magnitude of, δ is the width of, and Δ is the time between the two balanced diffusion gradient pulses.

If the spins are moving, however, during the second gradient pulse, they undergo a different overall phase change because they are in a different magnetic field from where they were during the first pulse. The result is a weaker echo compared with stationary tissue because of the incomplete rephasing of the MR imaging signal. Because spins undergoing diffusion exhibit random motion, each spin within a voxel ends up with a different amount of phase at the end of the second gradient lobe. Because the magnetization vectors of all spins in the voxel are added to form the acquired echo, the spread in spin vectors due to the random motion results in an overall reduction of the echo signal. The measured MR imaging signal loss due to diffusion is given by

$$S = S_0 e^{-bD} \tag{1}$$

where S is the DWI signal intensity, S_0 is the T2-weighted signal with no diffusion gradients applied, b characterizes the diffusion-sensitizing gradient pulses (related to timing, amplitude, shape, and spacing [see **Fig. 2**]), and D is the diffusion coefficient. The DWI signal has a T2-weighted component dependent on the echo time and T2 relaxation time of tissue. The apparent diffusion coefficient (ADC) for a given direction is calculated on a pixel-by-pixel basis by fitting signal intensities to Equation 1 so that

$$D = b \cdot \ln \frac{S_0}{S} \tag{2}$$

where ln is the natural logarithm function. The actual diffusion coefficient (immeasurable) is complicated by other factors, such as variations in anisotropy, choice of parameters in the b-value, inherent perfusion, and inherent motion. The use of single-shot EPI acquisition decreases imaging time and lessens the effects of motion.

Acquiring multiple DWIs for a series of b-value allows the determination of the ADC ($D \approx$ ADC) by pixel-by-pixel least squares fit of Equation 2 (**Fig. 3**) for a specific gradient direction. In the simplest case, 2 images are obtained—one averaged DWI for a specific b-value (for example, diffusion gradients applied along the x-axis) followed by a reference T2-weighted image ($b = 0$) so that ADC_{xx} is obtained from the fit (see **Fig. 3**). The process is repeated to obtain ADC_{yy} and ADC_{zz}.

The DWI, also known as the isotropic image, is calculated as the geometric mean of the 3 DWIs derived from the 3 orthogonal gradient directions (x, y, and z), and is given by

$$DWI_{avg} = \left(DWI_x \cdot DWI_y \cdot DWI_z \right)^{1/3} \tag{3}$$

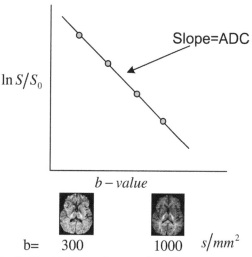

Fig. 3. The ADC for a given gradient direction is calculated on a pixel-by-pixel basis by fitting signal intensities to the diffusion equation for at least 2 DWIs with different b-values.

The resulting DWI has diffusion and T2 contrast. To remove the T2 weighting, the DWI S is divided by the T2-weighted image S_0 ($b = 0$). The exponential image is easily derived from $S = S_0 e^{-bD}$ as

$$EXP = \frac{S}{S_0} = e^{-b \cdot ADC} \tag{4}$$

BASIC MECHANISMS UNDERLYING RESTRICTED DIFFUSION ASSOCIATED WITH ACUTE STROKE

Much of the understanding of the mechanisms underlying DWI changes in acute ischemic stroke is based on experimental animal models of cerebral ischemia. Cerebral ischemia results in decreased diffusion of water molecules within the infarct territory with a rapid decline in ADC values that can be attributed to a combination of complex biophysical factors resulting from disruption of normal cellular metabolism with depletion of ATP (**Box 1**). These processes result in failure of Na^+/K^+ ATPase and other ionic pumps with loss of ionic gradients across cellular membranes. This results in a net shift of water from the extracellular to the intracellular space with a change in the relative volume of these compartments as well as alterations in their microenvironments. Although the physiologic basis for the restricted diffusion associated with acute stroke is still under investigation, 3 major mechanisms have been described: (1) changes in relative volumes of the intracellular and extracellular spaces, (2) increased extracellular space tortuosity, and (3) diminished cytoplasmic

> **Box 1**
> **Mechanisms for decreased diffusion in acute stroke**
>
> 1. Failure of Na^+/K^+ ATPase and other ionic pumps with loss of ionic gradients across membranes, net shift of water from the extracellular to the intracellular space, and changes in the intracellular and extracellular space relative volumes
> 2. Decrease in the size of the extracellular space due to cell swelling with a resultant increase in extracellular space tortuosity
> 3. Diminished energy-dependent intracellular cytoplasmic circulation/microstreaming
> 4. Increased intracellular viscosity and intracellular space tortuosity secondary to breakdown of the cytoskeleton and organelles
> 5. Increased cell membrane permeability
> 6. Temperature decrease

circulation/microstreaming in the intracellular compartment. Some of the key investigations and controversies pertaining to mechanisms of DWI changes are discussed (see **Box 1**).

One widely accepted mechanism for the diffusion changes during cerebral ischemia is that disruption of energy metabolism results in failure of the Na^+/K^+ ATPase pump. This leads to a net shift of water from the extracellular compartment, where the diffusion of water is relatively unrestricted, to the intracellular compartment, where the diffusion of water is relatively restricted.[2] This model is supported by animal studies demonstrating that ischemic infarction is associated with a reduction of Na^+/K^+ ATPase pump activity,[3] that pharmacologic inhibition of the Na^+/K^+ ATPase pump with ouabain results in decreased ADC values,[4,5] and that nonischemic cytotoxic edema secondary to acute hyponatremia is associated with decreased ADC values.[6] Although many experiments support this theory, others dispute it.[7,8]

Several reports have demonstrated that alterations in the extracellular compartment result in changes on diffusion MR imaging.[7–11] Early DWI changes after transient ischemia correlate with shrinkage and re-expansion of the extracellular space.[9] In addition, based on osmotically driven changes in compartment volume in ex vivo rat optic nerve preparations, and assuming that intracellular water and extracellular water constitute approximately 80% and 20% of total water in the brain, respectively, it has been argued that moderate fractional changes in cell volume can result in large changes in the contribution of the extracellular compartment to the ADC.[10] Cellular swelling with associated change in relative compartment volume may result in the decreased ADC seen on MR imaging by increasing the tortuosity of the extracellular space and increasing impedance to diffusion of water molecules.[7,11]

Additional investigations suggest that changes in the intracellular environment contribute to the decreased ADC associated with acute ischemia. In experiments in which 2-[^{19}F]luoro-2-deoxyglucose-6-phosphate (2FDG-6P) was used as a compartment-specific marker for the intracellular and extracellular compartments, the ADC in both compartments was similarly reduced after cerebral ischemia.[7] Furthermore, experiments using diffusion-weighted MR spectroscopy evaluating intracellular metabolites, such as N-acetyl-aspartate and phosphocreatine[12] or the potassium analog cesium,[13] have demonstrated a decrease in the ADC of the intracellular compartment after ischemia. These changes in intracellular ADC may be secondary to disruption of the cytoplasmic motion of molecules or microstreaming.[7] Changes in tissue temperature and membrane permeability may also play a minor role in the diffusion changes observed with acute stroke.[7,14]

DIFFUSION-WEIGHTED IMAGING MAP INTERPRETATION

All DWIs (linearly T2-weighted and exponentially diffusion-weighted) should be reviewed with ADC maps (linearly diffusion-weighted, without a T2 component) and/or exponential images (exponentially diffusion-weighted, without a T2 component) (**Fig. 4**). The use of the ADC map and/or exponential image is essential for proper interpretation of DWIs because both areas of diminished and increased diffusion can appear bright on DWIs. In acute ischemic lesions with restricted diffusion, the T2 and diffusion effects both cause increased signal on DWI, and the DWI has the highest contrast-to-noise ratio. Lesions with restricted diffusion also appear hyperintense on exponential images, but they appear less hyperintense compared with the DWI because there is no T2 effect. Lesions with restricted diffusion appear dark on the ADC map. Conversely, areas of increased diffusion may appear hyperintense, iso-intense, or hypointense to normal brain parenchyma on DWI, depending on the strength of the T2 and diffusion components, but are hyperintense on the ADC map and hypointense on the exponential image (**Fig. 5**). When a lesion is hyperintense on both the DWI and the ADC map and hypointense on the exponential image, the phenomenon is referred to as T2 shine-through and may be seen with late subacute infarcts or chronic ischemic lesions (**Fig. 6**).

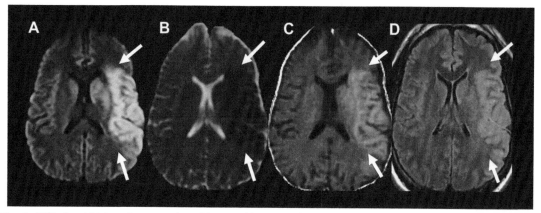

Fig. 4. Diffusion MR imaging maps in a 31-year-old man with an acute left MCA territory infarction (*arrows*), imaged at 6 hours after symptom onset of aphasia and right hemiparesis. The lesion is hyperintense on DWI (*A*), hypointense on the ADC map (*B*), and hyperintense on the exponential map (*C*), due to restricted diffusion secondary to an acute infarction. The lesion is most conspicuous on DWI due to a combination of T2 and diffusion effects. There is mild corresponding hyperintensity on the FLAIR image (*D*).

TIME COURSE OF DWI CHANGES ASSOCIATED WITH ACUTE ISCHEMIA

After the onset of acute ischemia, there is a rapid decrease in water diffusion that is markedly hyperintense on DWI and hypointense on the ADC map (Fig. 7, 6 and 9 hours; Table 1). After the initial ADC decrease, there is a gradual increase in the ADC values secondary to cell lysis and increasing vasogenic edema, with a return to baseline known as pseudonormalization, when the ADC of the nonviable ischemic tissue is similar to normal brain ADC (see Fig. 7, 5 days). In stroke animal models, ADC values are reduced for a short time period and return to baseline at approximately 24 to 48 hours.[15,16] In humans, the ADC nadir occurs between 1 and 4 days with a return to baseline at approximately 1 to 2 weeks from symptom onset.[17-21] The DWI at this stage is typically still hyperintense secondary to T2 effects, whereas on ADC and exponential images the infarct is isointense to normal brain parenchyma. Subsequently, there is a progressive increase in the ADC of an ischemic lesion. This is secondary to gliosis and cavitation that result from breakdown of the normal tissue structure and increase diffusion of water molecules. During the chronic stage, an infarct can be mildly hyperintense, isointense, or hypointense to normal brain parenchyma on DWI depending on the strength of the T2 effects and diffusion components but should be hyperintense on ADC and hypointense on exponential images (see Fig. 7, 3 months).

There is variability in the time course of the DWI and ADC signal changes of evolving infarcts. Several factors, including infarct type, patient age, and reperfusion status, affect the evolution

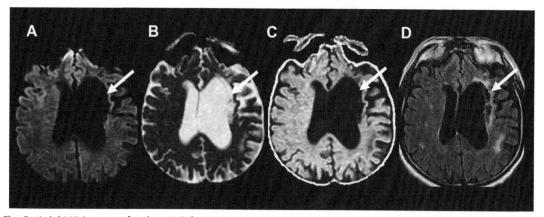

Fig. 5. Axial MR images of a chronic left MCA territory infarction with tissue loss (*arrows*). The lesion is hypointense on DWI (*A*), hyperintense on ADC (*B*), and hypointense on exponential (*C*) images, consistent with elevated diffusion. The infarct appears partially cavitated in FLAIR images (*D*).

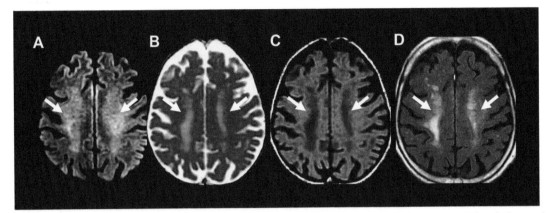

Fig. 6. T2 shine-through. Axial DWI (*A*) demonstrates mild hyperintensity in bilateral centrum semiovale (*arrows*) that raises the possibility of acute ischemia. The lesions are hyperintense on the ADC map (*B*) and hypointense on the exponential map (*C*), however, consistent with elevated diffusion secondary to chronic ischemic changes that are hyperintense on FLAIR images (*D*).

of signal changes on DWI. In one study, the transition from decreasing to increasing ADC values occurred earlier in non-lacunar infarcts than lacunar infarcts.[22] The same study also found a trend toward earlier transition to increasing ADCs of non-lacunar infarcts in patients older than a median age of 66.[22] In another study, there was slightly faster recovery (increase) in ADC values of infarcted gray matter compared with white matter.[20] Early reperfusion after thrombolytic therapy also changes the evolution of diffusion abnormalities (discussed later).

RELIABILITY AND PITFALLS OF DWI IN IDENTIFICATION OF ACUTE ISCHEMIC LESIONS

DWI is highly sensitive (81–100%) and specific (86–100%) for detection of acute ischemia within the first 12 hours after stroke symptom onset,[23–27]

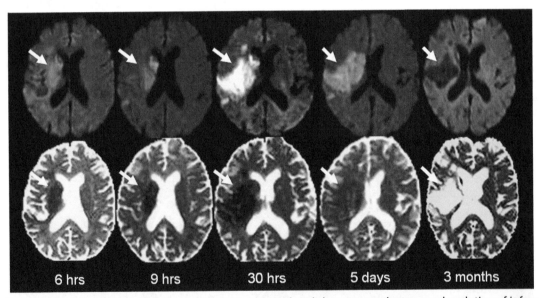

Fig. 7. Axial DWI images (*upper row*) and ADC maps (*second row*) demonstrate the temporal evolution of infarction (*arrows*). At 6 hours, the right MCA territory infarction is mildly hyperintense on DWI and hypointense on ADC maps due to cytotoxic edema. By 30 hours, there is marked DWI hyperintensity and ADC hypointensity due to increased cytotoxic edema at the ADC nadir. By 5 days, the ADC has nearly pseudonormalized due to cell lysis and development of vasogenic edema. The lesion is still hyperintense on DWI because of combined T2 and diffusion components. At 3 months, the chronic infarction is hypointense on DWI and hyperintense on ADC maps because of is increased diffusion secondary to gliosis and tissue cavitation.

Table 1
Evolution of diffusion MR imaging findings in stroke

Pulse Sequence	Hyperacute (0–6 hours)	Acute (6–24 hours)	Early Subacute (1–7 days)	Late Subacute	Chronic
Pathophysiology	Cytotoxic edema	Cytotoxic edema	Cytotoxic edema with small amount of vasogenic edema	Cytotoxic edema and vasogenic edema	Vasogenic edema, then gliosis and neuronal loss
DWI	Hyperintense	Hyperintense	Hyperintense, gyral hypointensity from petechial hemorrhage	Hyperintense (due to T2 component)	Isointense to hypointense
ADC, MD[a]	Hypointense	Hypointense	Hypointense	Isointense	Hyperintense
Low-b T2	Isointense	Hyperintense	Hyperintense, gyral hypointensity from petechial hemorrhage	Hyperintense	Hyperintense
$\lambda_{\parallel}$	Mildly hypointense	Hypointense	Hypointense	Isointense	Hyperintense
$\lambda_{\perp}$	Hypointense	Hypointense	Hypointense	Isointense	Hyperintense
FA[b]	Mildly hyperintense	Mildly hyperintense to hypointense	Hypointense	Hypointense	Hypointense
MK	Hyperintense	Hyperintense	Hyperinense to hypointense	Hypointense	Hypointense
$K_{\parallel}$	Hyperintense	Hyperintense	Hyperinense to hypointense	Hypointense	Hypointense
$K_{\perp}$	Mildly hyperintense	Mildly hyperintense	Hyperinense to hypointense	Hypointense	Hypointense

[a] Early reperfusion accelerates time course of MD with earlier pseudonormalization. Lacunar infarctions have slower time course with longer time to nadir and subsequent pseudonormalization. Younger patients with nonlacunar stroke tend to have earlier pseudonormalization.
[b] Reperfusion results in rapid decrease in FA, reaching a minimum before slowly returning toward baseline.

with sensitivities and specificities in the 90–100% range at specialized stroke centers (**Box 2**). DWI can demonstrate acute ischemic lesions as early as 11 minutes after symptom onset.[28] DWI is superior to conventional MR imaging and CT in the first 6 hours because there is usually insufficient increase in tissue water for reliable detection of hypoattenuation on CT and hyperintensity on T2 and fluid-attenuated inversion recovery (FLAIR) MR images (**Fig. 8**).[23,24,27] In one study, DWI had a sensitivity of 73% and specificity of 92% for identification of ischemic lesions within 3 hours of symptom onset compared with a sensitivity of 12% and specificity of 100% for CT.[23] In another

study, DWI had a sensitivity of 97% and specificity of 100% for identification of acute ischemic lesions within 6 hours of symptom onset compared with 58% and 100%, respectively, for conventional MR imaging sequences and 40% and 92%, respectively, for CT.[27] Although infarcts are usually identifiable on CT, T2, and FLAIR images after 6 hours, DWI can also be valuable at later time points because of its higher contrast-to-noise ratio compared with those sequences. DWI has superior sensitivity for identification of small infarcts that may be overlooked on FLAIR or T2 images. It also enables distinction of small recent white matter infarcts from nonspecific T2 hyperintense white matter lesions, which typically have elevated diffusion and are not hyperintense on DWI (**Fig. 9**).[29,30]

Although false-negative DWI results have been described for different lesion sizes in many cerebral arterial territories, small punctate infarcts, especially those located within the brainstem or deep gray nuclei, have the highest likelihood of a false-negative DWI study (**Fig. 10**).[29,31–38] Among brainstem infarcts, medullary infarcts are the most difficult to detect. Susceptibility artifact from adjacent skull base structures and differences in organization of the normal fiber tracts in this area are likely contributing factors.[31] Obtaining images in the coronal plane or with a higher resolution can improve infarct detection (**Fig. 11**). In addition, there is mildly increased sensitivity for the detection of ischemic lesions at higher b-values (b >2000); however, there is decreased signal-to-noise ratio and increased imaging time, and a clear diagnostic benefit has not been proved.[39–42] Furthermore, in a prospective study comparing 1.5T and 3T acquisitions in 25 patients with clinical symptoms of acute (7/25) or subacute ischemia (18/25), there was increased contrast-to-noise ratio on 3T and a greater number of small ischemic lesions were identified on 3T compared with 1.5T, although all patients with infarcts on 3T had at least one identifiable infarct on their 1.5T images.[43] In any case, a short-term follow-up MR imaging scan within 24 hours should identify most small infarcts not visible on the initial study. Correlation with clinical signs and symptoms that bring into attention regions of potential signal abnormality that would otherwise be dismissed as artifact is essential.

False-positive DWI findings may occur secondary to T2 shine-through (discussed previously), which can be readily distinguished from true restricted diffusion if the DWI images are interpreted in conjunction with the ADC or exponential maps. In addition, a variety of nonischemic lesions can have decreased diffusion and could potentially

---

Box 2
DWI for imaging of acute ischemic stroke: major points

1. DWI is the gold standard for identifying infarct core.
2. DWI has sensitivity and specificity over 95% in high-volume stroke centers with experienced neuroradiologists. Scanning with higher resolution DWI sequences, $b \geq 2000$ s/mm^2, and/or on a 3T scanner increases sensitivity.
3. The rare acute infarcts not detected on DWI (false-negative results) are usually punctate infarcts in the brainstem (especially the medulla) or deep gray nuclei.
4. Single lesions with restricted diffusion thought to represent acute strokes are frequently due to hypoglycemia or demyelinating disease.
5. DWI reversibility (abnormal on initial DWI but normal on follow-up FLAIR or T2 at 1 week or later) is rare. Greater reversibility of DWI-positive lesions has been demonstrated after intravenous (IV) or intra-arterial (IA) recanalization procedures. DWI reversibility is overestimated in some studies due to tissue loss at follow-up imaging at 30 to 90 days. Threshold ADCs for DWI reversibility have not reliably been established.
6. DWI lesion volume correlates with clinical outcome scales and is an independent predictor of outcome in many studies. The correlation depends on lesion location. DWI lesion volume greater than one-third of the expected middle cerebral artery (MCA) territory or 100 mL is associated with poor outcome regardless of reperfusion therapy. Some clinicians use it as an exclusion criteria for thrombolytic therapy.
7. DWI lesion greater than 100 mL is associated with an increased risk of hemorrhagic transformation (HT). Mean ADC $<300 \times 10^{-6}$ mm^2/s in the DWI lesion is predictive of *symptomatic* HT.

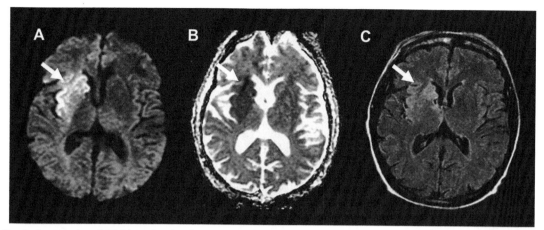

Fig. 8. Superiority of DWI imaging for detecting acute ischemia. Elderly man with acute left hemiparesis, imaged 5 hours after symptom onset. The acute right MCA infarction (*arrows*) is well seen on axial DWI (*A*) and ADC (*B*) images due to restricted diffusion.There is more subtle hyperintensity on FLAIR images (*C*), however, because there is little overall increase in tissue water at this time point.

be mistaken for infarcts (**Table 2**). Most are readily distinguishable from acute infarcts when the DWI findings are considered in conjunction with findings on conventional MR imaging sequences, such as T2, FLAIR, and gadolinium-enhanced T1-weighted images. Hypoglycemia and acute demyelinating disease, however, can present with acute neurologic deficits and a single nonenhancing FLAIR hyperintense lesion with decreased diffusion and are at times misdiagnosed as acute strokes (**Fig. 12**).

REVERSIBILITY OF DWI-POSITIVE LESIONS IN ISCHEMIC STROKE AND USE OF DWI FOR DETERMINATION OF INFARCT CORE

It is widely accepted that DWI is the best method for identifying infarct core or tissue destined to progress to infarction (see **Box 2**). In the absence of early reperfusion in the setting of IV thrombolytic therapy or IA recanalization procedures, reversibility of decreased diffusion (DWI abnormality on the initial scan without a corresponding abnormality on follow-up FLAIR or T2-weighted MR

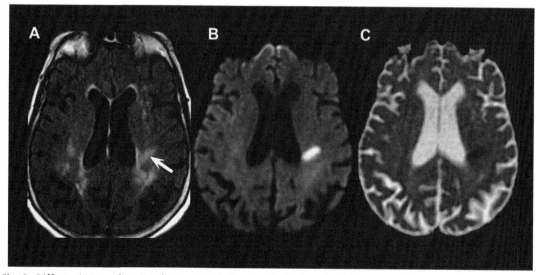

Fig. 9. Differentiation of acute white matter infarction from chronic white matter change. On FLAIR image (*A*), the acute left corona radiata lesion (*arrow*) is indistinguishable from chronic white matter changes. The DWI (*B*) and ADC (*C*) images demonstrate restricted diffusion in the acute infarction and mildly elevated diffusion in the nonspecific white matter changes.

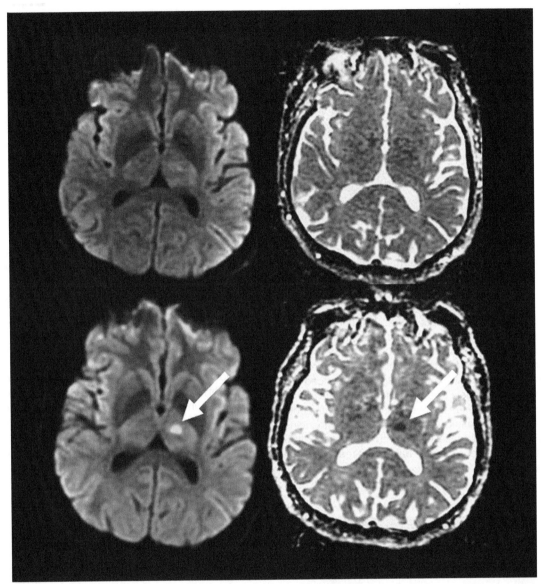

Fig. 10. Thalamic lacune without an acute DWI abnormality. A 45-year-old woman with patent foramen ovale. Initial DWI and ADC images (*upper row*) were interpreted as demonstrating no definite acute infarction. Follow-up DWI and ADC images (*lower row*) demonstrate a 6-mm DWI hyperintense, ADC hypointense left thalamic lacunar infarction (*arrows*).

images) is rare. Frequently, the final infarct volume includes the initial area of diffusion abnormality as well as surrounding ischemic but viable tissues that progress to infarction.[44–46] Much higher rates of partial diffusion reversal have been reported after early reperfusion secondary to thrombolytic therapy.[47–49] In one study of patients treated with IA thrombolysis, 19% had partial reversal of DWI hyperintense regions on follow-up imaging.[49] In another study, 8 of 18 (44%) patients treated with IA or combined IV and IA thrombolytic therapy resulting in recanalization had partial or complete

normalization of diffusion abnormalities on the immediate post-treatment scan; however, in 5 of 8 patients (63%) there was partial or complete reappearance of the lesion on the MR imaging performed on day 7. The investigators called this phenomenon late secondary injury, although permanent injury may already have been present at an earlier time point; animal stroke models have shown transient reversal of MR imaging findings despite histopathologic tissue injury.[50] Persistent normalization of all reversed tissue was seen in 3 of 8 (17% of all patients) on the

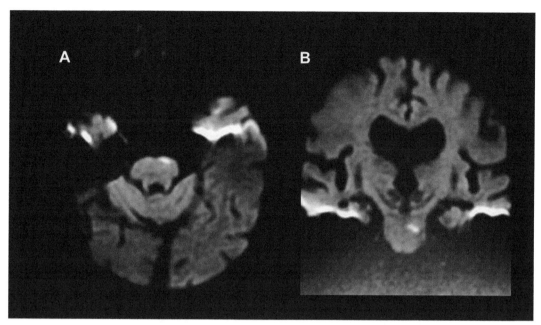

Fig. 11. Acute pontine infarct. (A) Axial DWI image demonstrates mild hyperintensity in the ventral left pontine basis that could represent susceptibility artifact in image. Coronal DWI images (B) unequivocally demonstrates restricted diffusion from a small perforator infarct.

day 7 MR imaging scan. A voxel-by-voxel analysis of the regions of DWI abnormality in all patients combined demonstrated a sustained reversal of 33% in addition to a late reversal of 8% (persistent diffusion abnormality on the immediate post-treatment scan but normal DWI/T2 images on the day 7 scan). A more recent analysis of 32 patients treated with IV tissue plasminogen activator (tPA)

Table 2
Lesions other than acute stroke that may have restricted diffusion on DWI

Entity	Possible Cause of Restricted Diffusion
Cerebral abscess	Increased viscosity
Neoplasms, such as lymphoma and high-grade glial neoplasms	Dense cell packing
Venous infarcts	Cytotoxic edema
Acute demyelinating lesions	Cytotoxic edema and/or inflammatory cell infiltrates, myelin vacuolization
Encephalitides—herpes simplex virus	Cytotoxic edema
Hemorrhage—hyperacute (intracellular oxyhemoglobin) to late subacute (extracellular methemoglobin)	Extracellular space shrinkage with clot retraction, change in hemoglobin conformation, contraction of intact red blood cells, T2 blackout effect
Diffuse axonal injury	Cytotoxic edema, axonal retraction balls
Hypoglycemia	Cytotoxic edema
Hemiplegic migraine	Cytotoxic edema, spreading depression
Seizures	Cytotoxic edema
Transient global amnesia	Cytotoxic edema, spreading depression
Heroin-induced leukoencephalopathy	Myelin vacuolization
Metronidazole toxicity	Cytotoxic edema
Creutzfeldt-Jakob disease	Spongiform change
Osmotic myelinolysis	Cytotoxic edema, myelin vacuolization
Carbon monoxide poisoning	Cytotoxic edema

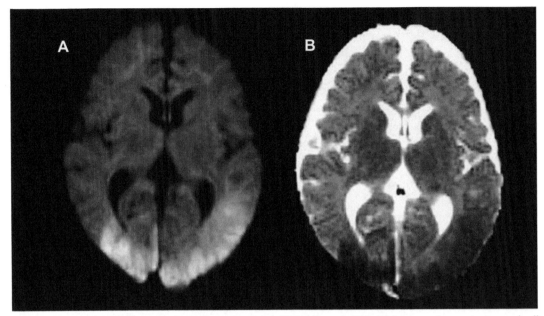

Fig. 12. A 3-month-old boy with hypoglycemia. Axial DWI (*A*) and ADC (*B*) images demonstrate markedly decreased diffusion in the bilateral occipital lobes.

within 3 to 6 hours of symptom onset (DEFUSE trial: *D*iffusion and perfusion imaging *E*valuation *F*or *U*nderstanding Stroke *E*volution), demonstrated a median reversal rate of 43% when comparing final infarct volumes on FLAIR images obtained at day 30 days with the baseline DWI lesion volumes.[51] The DWI reversal rate was higher in patients with early recanalization, normal baseline perfusion, and/or good clinical outcome.

The determination of DWI reversibility is complex. In animal studies, short periods of ischemia can result in a transient decline in ADC with normalization after cessation of the ischemic insult. Despite complete normalization on imaging, there can be neuronal injury on histopathology.[50] Another technical factor that results in overestimation of DWI reversibility is volume loss and tissue retraction on follow-up imaging that results in an underestimation of final infarct volume.

In general, tissues with a higher absolute ADC value have a higher likelihood of reversibility.[52–56] There is a large amount of variation in the reported ADC values of irreversibly damaged ischemic tissue and of DWI reversible tissue, however, and there is much overlap between the two.[52–57] Furthermore, even tissue with severely diminished ADC can recover (**Fig. 13**). Apart from the ADC value, the duration and severity of ischemia and tissue perfusion status are important determinants of final infarct volume in animal and human studies.[48,50,52,55,57,58] Therefore, although tissues

with severely reduced ADC have a higher likelihood of progressing to an irreversible infarct, it is likely that ADC values alone are insufficient for absolute determination of tissue viability.

USE OF DWI FOR PREDICTING HEMORRHAGIC TRANSFORMATION

HT of brain infarcts represents bleeding into ischemic tissue that usually occurs some time after the initial insult (**Fig. 14**). The reported incidence of HT varies widely, in part due to differences in definitions, imaging examinations (CT vs MR imaging with or without gradient-echo images), and timing of follow-up imaging. The incidence is clearly increased, however, after thrombolytic therapy and ranges from 6% up to 44% if susceptibility sensitive MR imaging sequences are used. The incidence of symptomatic HT is significantly lower.[59–67]

Several investigators have assessed the value of initial DWI volume and ADC in predicting HT (see **Box 2**). In one study of 645 patients with anterior circulation strokes treated with IV or IA thrombolytic agents, increasing DWI lesion size was associated with an increase in symptomatic HT.[68] The highest risk for symptomatic HT was 16.1% and was observed in the subgroup with a large DWI abnormality, defined as greater than 100 mL. Another study of 27 patients with acute stroke demonstrated that the mean ADC of ischemic

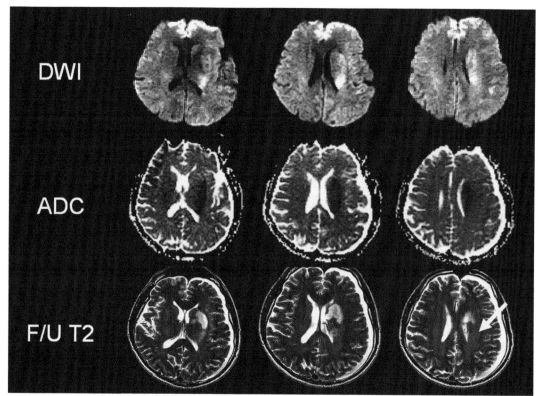

Fig. 13. DWI reversibility. A 68-year-old man with right hemiparesis and dysarthria, who received IA tPA. The initial DWI and ADC images demonstrated restricted diffusion in the left basal ganglia and deep white matter. Most of this region is T2 hyperinense, consistent with infarction. On the follow-up T2-weighted images at 3 days, the left posterior corona radiata (*arrow*) appears normal on follow-up T2-weighted images, consistent with a small region of DWI reversibility.

regions that underwent HT ($510 \pm 140 \times 10^{-6}$ mm²/s) was significantly lower than the mean ADC of all ischemic areas analyzed ($623 \pm 113 \times 10^{-6}$ mm²/s).[69] The investigators also noted that a persistent perfusion deficit within the infarct core on MRIs performed 3 to 6 hours after the baseline scan were associated with a higher risk of HT. A third study of investigation of 29 patients treated with IV thrombolytic therapy demonstrated that the absolute number of voxels with ADC $\leq 550 \times 10^{-6}$ mm²/s correlated with HT.[70] In a fourth study, the investigators concluded that a mean ADC of $< 300 \times 10^{-6}$ mm²/s in the infarct core was predictive of *symptomatic* HT.[71] Despite these studies, other studies have not found a statistically significant difference in the ADC of infarcts that subsequently underwent HT versus those that did not.[67]

More recent work suggests that perfusion MR imaging is important in predicting HT. In an analysis of 91 patients from the *E*cho *P*lanar *I*maging *T*hrombolytic *E*valuation *T*rial (EPITHET), very low cerebral blood volume (<2.5th percentile) was found to predict HT better than DWI lesion volume and thresholded ADC lesion volume ($< 550 \times 10^{-6}$ mm²/s) in receiver operating characteristic curve and logistic regression analysis, although all 3 parameters were significant in univariate analysis.[72] In another study of 184 patients, a large area with a T_{max} of >8 seconds, along with aggressive therapy (endovascular treatment with or without IV tPA) correlated with radiologic HT whereas DWI volume did not.[73] Other imaging parameters associated with an increased risk of HT are increased permeability on dynamic contrast enhanced T1 MRI[74] and early parenchymal enhancement.[75]

Extrapolating from studies using CT scans in which hypoattenuation involving greater than one-third of the MCA territory was associated with an increased risk of HT and poor outcomes after the administration of IV tPA,[76] some clinicians consider a DWI lesion volume greater than one-third of the expected MCA territory a contraindication to the use of IV thrombolytic therapy and/or IA recanalization procedures. There is no widely

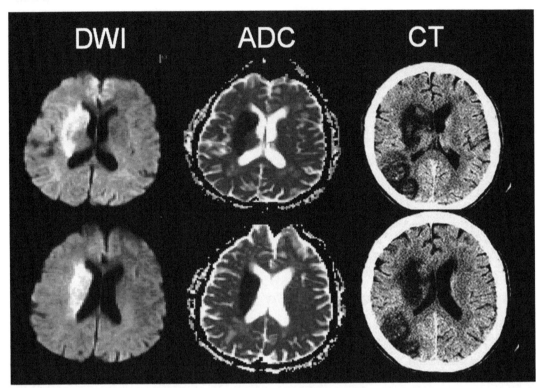

Fig. 14. HT of an acute ischemic stroke. A 76-year-old man treated with IA tPA. DWI and ADC maps demonstrate severely decreased diffusion in the right basal ganglia and deep white matter, consistent with an acute right MCA territory infarction. On follow-up CT there is HT within the infarct bed. There is also extension of the infarction into the right parietal region.

accepted consensus, however, on the use of DWI and other MR imaging parameters for determination of HT risk.

CORRELATION OF DWI LESION VOLUME WITH CLINICAL OUTCOME

Initial DWI and ADC lesion volumes correlate with clinical outcome measured by various acute and chronic neurologic assessment tests, including the National Institutes of Health Stroke Scale, the Glasgow Outcome Scale, the Barthel Index and the Rankin Scale or Modified Rankin Scale (see Box 2).[19,45,46,77–80] Reported correlations range from $r = 0.56$ to $r = 0.73$. Because many of the commonly used clinical scoring systems are weighted toward motor symptoms and language, usually localized to the left hemisphere, lesion location[19,77] can result in a significant discrepancy between total volume of disease and clinical score. For example, a punctate brainstem lesion affecting a motor fiber tract could result in a high clinical score, whereas a punctate lesion in the frontal lobe could be asymptomatic. This may also explain why some studies of posterior fossa

strokes could not find a correlation between DWI volume and clinical outcome.[29]

Nevertheless, there is emerging evidence that patients with a DWI lesion volume greater than approximately 70 mL do poorly regardless of treatment and recanalization status.[81–84] For example, Yoo and colleagues[83] demonstrated that in 54 patients treated mainly with IV tPA or heparin, all patients with a DWI lesion volume greater than 72 mL had a poor outcome (modified Rankin score = 3–6). In addition, in an analysis of 34 patients with anterior circulation strokes who underwent IA reperfusion therapy, the same investigators found that all patients (6/34) with an initial DWI lesion volume greater than 70 mL had poor outcome, in spite of a 50% recanalization rate.[84] In another study analyzing 98 patients from the EPITHET trial, Parsons and colleagues[82] found that although patients with an initial DWI lesion volume of 18 mL had substantially improved chances of a good outcome if treated with IV tPA, the odds of a benefit dropped rapidly at larger volumes and there was little treatment benefit of IV TPA with a DWI lesion volume greater than 25 mL. Similar to the observations by Yoo and colleagues, the investigators from this study found that a large initial DWI lesion volume of greater than 65 mL was strongly associated with a poor outcome.

DIFFUSION TENSOR IMAGING AND DIFFUSION KURTOSIS IMAGING

Although DWI has been useful in the clinical management of stroke, DTI (Table 3) and DKI (Table 4) may offer additional diagnostic information on the microstructural status of tissue because there is directional dependence of diffusion in tissue known as anisotropy. Diffusion in tissue is affected by the presence of semipermeable membranes and oriented structures in the intracellular, extracellular, and vascular compartments that result in preferential movement of water parallel to them. In the brain, white matter has relatively high anisotropy because diffusion is much greater parallel than perpendicular to major white matter tracts. Gray matter has relatively low anisotropy. Heterogeneity of the diffusion environment from compartmentalization also results in non-Gaussian probability distribution of water diffusion, which can be quantified by kurtosis.

THE DIFFUSION TENSOR

Anisotropy can be characterized by the effective diffusion tensor **D**, a second-order tensor with 9 components describing molecular mobility along each direction and correlation between these directions[85]:

$$\mathbf{D} = \begin{bmatrix} D_{xx} & D_{xy} & D_{xz} \\ D_{yx} & D_{yy} & D_{yz} \\ D_{zx} & D_{zy} & D_{zz} \end{bmatrix} \tag{5}$$

Table 3 DTI-derived parameter changes in stroke	
MD	Mean diffusion: overall diffusion in tissue, independent of direction Relatively uniform in GM and WM throughout normal brain MD decreases greater in WM than GM in acute and subacute periods MD increases much more in WM than GM in the chronic period Early reperfusion accelerates time course of MD with earlier pseudonormalization
$\lambda_{\parallel}$	Axial diffusion: diffusion along principal direction, collinear with WM fiber orientation Increased in WM relative to GM in normal brain $\lambda_{\parallel}$ Decreases less than $\lambda_{\perp}$ in WM in hyperacute period $\lambda_{\parallel}$ Decreases more than $\lambda_{\perp}$ in WM in acute and subacute periods
$\lambda_{\perp}$	Radial diffusion: overall diffusion perpendicular to principal direction/WM fiber orientation Decreased in WM relative to GM in normal brain $\lambda_{\perp}$ Decreases more than $\lambda_{\parallel}$ in WM in hyperacute period $\lambda_{\perp}$ Decreases less than $\lambda_{\parallel}$ in WM in acute and subacute periods

FA	Fractional anisotropy: index of anisotropy measuring degree of diffusion differences in different directions
	Increased in WM relative to GM in normal brain
	Correlates with stroke onset time
	Elevated in hyperacute period and then decreases over time
	Correlates inversely with T2 change
	Three temporal stages in stroke evolution
	  Increased FA and decreased MD
	  Decreased FA and decreased MD
	  Decreased FA and increased MD
	FA decreases greater in WM than GM in acute, subacute, and chronic periods
	Reperfusion associated with transient rapid FA reduction reaching a minimum before increasing toward baseline

Fiber tract mapping	Principal direction of diffusion provides information on WM tract orientation Helpful in separating major WM tracts for assessing WM integrity and connectivity Detects antegrade (Wallerian) and retrograde axonal degeneration before conventional images May be useful in predicting motor, language, and cognitive function at outcome

Abbreviations: GM, gray matter; WM, white matter.

Table 4
DKI-derived parameter changes in stroke

MK	Mean kurtosis: qualitative measure of overall diffusional heterogeneity in tissue, independent of direction $MK \neq (K_{\parallel} + 2K_{\perp})/3$, because kurtosis distribution cannot be generally represented by an ellipsoid Increased in WM relative to GM in normal brain MK increases in hyperacute periods with evidence of reversal in regressing infarctions MK increases greater in WM than GM in acute and early subacute periods MK pseudonormalization time earlier than MD pseudonormalization time Evidence of increased MK outside region of infarction with reduced MD, possibly indicate areas of ischemic penumbra or benign oligemia Magnitude of increased MK in acute and early subacute periods may be predictive of eventual tissue outcome in WM
$K_{\parallel}$	Axial diffusion kurtosis: qualitative measure of diffusional heterogeneity along principal direction, collinear with WM fiber orientation Relatively uniform in GM and WM throughout normal brain $K_{\parallel}$ increases more than $K_{\perp}$ in WM in acute and early subacute periods
$K_{\perp}$	Radial diffusion kurtosis: qualitative measure of diffusional heterogeneity perpendicular to principal direction/WM fiber orientation Increased in WM relative to GM in normal brain $K_{\perp}$ increases less than $K_{\parallel}$ in WM in acute and early subacute periods
FA_K	Fractional anisotropy of directional kurtosis: index of anisotropy measuring degree of diffusional heterogeneity differences in different directions Increased in WM relative to GM in normal brain

Abbreviations: GM, gray matter; WM, white matter.

The components of **D** can be estimated by noting the effect of anisotropic diffusion on the MR imaging signal is given by[86]

$$S = S_0 \exp\left(-\sum_{i=x,y,z} \sum_{j=x,y,z} b_{ij} D_{ij} \right) \quad (6)$$

where b_{ij} are components in the **b** matrix, which is equivalent to the b-value used to characterize diffusion-encoding gradient pulses in DWI.[87,88] Because **D** is symmetric, only 6 noncollinear diffusion-encoding gradient directions are necessary in addition to 1 acquisition without diffusion weighting ($b \approx 0$) to determine the effective diffusion tensor fully. With more diffusion-encoding gradient directions, however, data sampling becomes more uniform and less biased to any particular direction with the added benefit of signal-to-noise ratio gain.[89,90] High angular resolution diffusion imaging (HARDI) paradigms are typically obtained by uniform sampling along a sphere, which is particularly important for resolving multiple fiber orientations within a voxel for accurate diffusion fiber tracking.[91,92]

Once the full effective diffusion tensor **D** is determined at each voxel, the following 3 groups of parameters can be calculated that provide information about the underlying tissue microstructure[93,94]:

1. Axial and radial diffusion: By convention, the eigenvalues of **D** are ordered as $\lambda_1 \geq \lambda_2 \geq \lambda_3$. Because diffusion of water is much greater parallel than perpendicular to white matter fiber bundles, the direction of white matter fibers is assumed to be collinear with the eigenvector corresponding to λ_1, known as the principal or axial diffusion and often written as

$$\lambda_{\parallel} = \lambda_1 \quad (7)$$

Because the eigenvectors of **D** are perpendicular, radial diffusion perpendicular to white matter tracts can be inferred to be

$$\lambda_{\perp} = \frac{\lambda_2 + \lambda_3}{2} \quad (8)$$

2. Mean diffusion: A measure of overall diffusion in a voxel is its MD, which is related to the trace of **D** by

$$MD = \frac{Tr(\mathbf{D})}{3} = \frac{D_{xx} + D_{yy} + D_{zz}}{3} = \frac{\lambda_1 + \lambda_2 + \lambda_3}{3} \quad (9)$$

where λ_{ij} are the eigenvalues of **D**. Accurate estimation of MD requires complete determination of the diffusion tensor to calculate its trace because application of a diffusion-encoding gradient pulse sensitive to one direction may also have cross-term contributions from its orthogonal directions.[87,88,95] When calculating MD from the complete diffusion tensor is not practical, for example, in acute stroke assessment, MD can be estimated by

$$MD = \frac{ADC_x + ADC_y + ADC_z}{3} \quad (10)$$

if isotropically-weighted DWI sequences that cancel nondiagonal terms are used.[96–98]

3. Degree of anisotropy: Several commonly used indices of anisotropy are the relative anisotropy (RA), the fractional anisotropy (FA), and the volume ratio (VR), which are all defined by combinations of the eigenvalues λ_1, λ_2, and λ_3 of **D**.[99,100] RA represents the coefficient of variation of the eigenvalues of **D**:

$$RA = \frac{std_\sigma(\lambda)}{mean(\lambda)}$$
$$= \sqrt{\frac{1}{3}} \frac{\sqrt{(\lambda_1 - MD)^2 + (\lambda_2 - MD)^2 + (\lambda_3 - MD)^2}}{MD} \quad (11)$$

FA measures the proportion of **D** that can be assigned to anisotropic diffusion:

$$FA = \frac{std_s(\lambda)}{rms(\lambda)}$$
$$= \sqrt{\frac{3}{2}} \frac{\sqrt{(\lambda_1 - MD)^2 + (\lambda_2 - MD)^2 + (\lambda_3 - MD)^2}}{\sqrt{\lambda_1^2 + \lambda_2^2 + \lambda_3^2}} \quad (12)$$

VR represents the ratio of the volume of an ellipsoid defined by principal axes radii λ_1, λ_2, and λ_3 to the volume of a sphere with radius MD, which is also related to the determinant and trace of **D** by

$$VR = 27 \frac{Det(\mathbf{D})}{Tr(\mathbf{D})^3} = \frac{\lambda_1 \lambda_2 \lambda_3}{MD^3} \quad (13)$$

For perfectly isotropic diffusion, RA = 0, FA = 0, and VR = 1. With infinite anisotropy, RA = $\sqrt{2}$, FA = 1, and VR = 0. White matter tracts generally have FA greater than 0.20. The lattice index, which uses the degree of orientational coherence of neighboring voxels to calculate an intervoxel anisotropy index, is a fourth index of anisotropy,[100] particularly helpful for analyzing noisy DTI data, especially in voxels with multiple fiber orientations.

THE DIFFUSION KURTOSIS TENSOR

In conventional DTI analysis, the probabilistic distribution of water diffusion is assumed to be Gaussian with the standard deviation along each eigenvector direction proportional to the corresponding diffusion coefficient forming a diffusion ellipsoid. Biologic tissues, however, are inherently heterogeneous, with multiple compartments formed by semipermeable membranes and oriented microstructures in the intracellular, extracellular, and vascular domains, which result in non-Gaussian distribution of water diffusion,[101,102] as evidenced by non-monoexponential b-value dependency of diffusion-weighted signal in neural tissues.[103–106]

DKI is a natural extension of DTI that yields standard DTI metrics (described previously) as well as several additional metrics quantifying the degree of non-Gaussian diffusion of water in tissue.[107–110] Mathematically, the kurtosis (K) of an arbitrary probability distribution is related to its standardized fourth central moment and is a dimensionless statistical measure of how peaked ($K>0$) or flat ($K<0$) the distribution is from a normal Gaussian distribution ($K = 0$).[111] From analysis of multiple compartment model, $K \geq 0$ and is proportional to the square of the coefficient of variation for the distribution of compartmental diffusion coefficients,[108] which implies that K is a qualitative measure of diffusional heterogeneity.

It can be shown that the diffusion-weighted signal intensity along a given diffusion direction **n** as a function of b-value is approximated by[108]

$$S(b) = S_0 \exp\left(-bD_\mathbf{n} + \frac{1}{6}b^2 D_\mathbf{n}^2 K_\mathbf{n}\right) \quad (14)$$

where $D_\mathbf{n}$ is the apparent diffusion coefficient and $K_\mathbf{n}$ is the apparent kurtosis coefficient along **n**. To characterize diffusion kurtosis along any arbitrary direction, it is useful to define the kurtosis tensor **W**, which is a fourth-order tensor with $3^4 = 81$ components that is related to Equation 14 by

$$K_\mathbf{n} = \frac{MD^2}{D_\mathbf{n}^2} \sum_{i=x,y,z} \sum_{j=x,y,z} \sum_{k=x,y,z} \sum_{l=x,y,z} n_i n_j n_k n_l W_{ijkl} \quad (15)$$

where n_i is the ith element of the diffusion direction **n**. Because of symmetry, **W** contains only 15 components that are independent. Similar to DTI parameters described previously, the following kurtosis parameters can be calculated once the **W** is determined at each voxel[107,110,112]:

1. Axial and radial kurtosis: Although the kurtosis distribution characterized by **W** is complex and cannot in general be represented by an ellipsoid, K_1, K_2, and K_3 can be defined as kurtosis along eigenvectors of **D** corresponding to λ_1, λ_2, and λ_3. $K_\parallel$ and $K_\perp$ can then be defined as kurtosis parallel and perpendicular to the principal eigen-vector of **D**, respectively, by

$$K_{\parallel} = K_1 \qquad (16)$$

$$K_{\perp} = \frac{K_2 + K_3}{2} \qquad (17)$$

Other definitions of $K_{\perp}$ have been proposed that are qualitatively similar.[107]

2. Mean kurtosis: A measure of overall kurtosis can be estimated by

$$MK = \frac{1}{n} \sum_{i=1}^{n} K_i \qquad (18)$$

where K_i is the apparent kurtosis coefficient along the ith direction, and n is the total number of directions in which diffusion measurements are taken. Unlike MD (Equation 9), MK is not necessarily equal to $(K_{\parallel} + 2K_{\perp})/3$ because the kurtosis distribution cannot in general be represented by an ellipsoid. Other definitions of MK include the isotropic zeroth-order harmonic from spherical harmonic expansion of the kurtosis distribution.[109]

3. Anisotropy of directional kurtosis: Similar to FA in DTI, FA of kurtosis can be defined as

$$FA_K =$$
$$\sqrt{\frac{3}{2}} \frac{\sqrt{(K_1 - MK)^2 + (K_2 - MK)^2 + (K_3 - MK)^2}}{\sqrt{K_1^2 + K_2^2 + K_3^2}}$$
$$(19)$$

In a perfectly isotropic environment, $K_{\parallel} = K_{\perp} = MK$, and $FA_K = 0$. Other measures preserving anisotropy information have been defined, including second-order and fourth-order harmonics from spherical harmonic expansion of the kurtosis distribution.[109]

Although more generalized approaches have been developed, such as q-space imaging and related MR imaging techniques,[91,113–116] which provide more detailed characterization of non-Gaussian behavior of water diffusion by directly estimating the diffusion displacement probability density function, these techniques have high-gradient hardware requirements and need excessively long imaging times that limit many clinical studies. Alternatively, DKI has more modest gradient hardware requirements (maximum b-value of 2000–3000 s/mm² sufficient for brain) and scan times of within 10 minutes on 1.5T and 3T clinical MR imaging systems,[108,109,117] which is more feasible for clinical applications while providing useful information about the underlying tissue microstructure.

Both DTI and DKI parameters have been measured in ischemia and show promise as diagnostic aids in understanding microstructural changes and potentially predicting outcome in ischemia (see **Tables 3** and **4**, respectively).

DTI AND DKI IN THE NORMAL BRAIN

Visual inspection of MD and average ADC maps of the normal adult brain generally shows no significant image contrast between gray matter and white matter, consistent with studies demonstrating relatively uniform average diffusion throughout the developed adult brain.[93] In contrast, white matter tracts are highly anisotropic and easily discriminated from relatively isotropic gray matter on RA, FA, VR, and lattice index maps.[93,100] This is supported by increased diffusional heterogeneity in white matter relative to gray matter on MK maps[108,109] that is even more pronounced in the radial direction perpendicular to white matter tracts as seen on $K_{\perp}$ and FA_K maps.[107,109,112,118] (See DTI and DKI parametric maps of nonischemic regions in **Fig. 15**.)

Although the biophysical basis of anisotropic diffusion in white matter is not completely understood, longitudinally-oriented structures, such as myelin, axonal membranes, and subcellular organelles contained in highly organized fiber bundles, probably all contribute to the overall anisotropy of white matter by acting as barriers to water movement perpendicular to these structures.[119,120] Some experimental evidence suggests that intact axonal membranes may be the dominant source of white matter anisotropy.[120] Nevertheless, modeling white matter as ordered tubes with no significant compartmentalization along its length is an oversimplification because gray matter and white matter exhibit similar $K_{\parallel}$ throughout the brain.[107,112,118] Although myelin plays a major role in accentuating white matter anisotropy by its multiple concentric lipid layers and increasing density of fibers running in parallel, as seen in the developing brain undergoing myelination,[121–123] myelin itself is not a necessary component for anisotropic diffusion in white matter. Diffusion anisotropy has been demonstrated in the nonmyelinated olfactory nerve of the garfish[119] and myelin-deficient rat spinal cord.[124]

DTI is able to detect microstructural changes associated with premyelination modification in white matter, as shown by significant increase in FA within white matter before histologic evidence of myelination.[125,126] In contrast, DKI shows significant differences between white matter and gray matter on MK, $K_{\perp}$, and FA_K maps only after myelination but not during premyelination,[118] which is

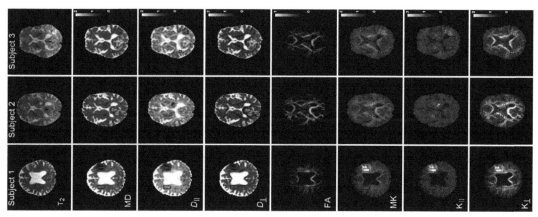

Fig. 15. Parametric maps of DTI and DKI metrics of 3 subjects with acute to early subacute ischemic stroke. Subject 1: a 75-year-old woman imaged 26 hours after onset of stroke in left frontal operculum. Subject 2: a 49-year-old man imaged 24 hours after onset of stroke in left thalamus and posterior limb of left internal capsule. Subject 3: a 61-year-old man imaged 13 hours after onset of stroke in left parietal lobe. Relative change of DTI and DKI metrics in ischemic regions (*red*) are compared with corresponding contralateral nonischemic regions (*blue*). (*Reprinted from* Jensen J, Helpern J. MRI quantification of non-Gaussian water diffusion by kurtosis analysis. NMR Biomed 2010;23:698–710; with permission.)

consistent with the notion that myelination and dense packing of axon fibers contributes significantly to compartmentalization and reduced diffusion in the radial direction.

EVOLUTION OF MEAN DIFFUSION IN ISCHEMIA

Serial longitudinal DTI studies after ischemic stroke demonstrate time course values for MD derived from trace of **D** that are similar to those of ADC.[127–130] One advantage of DTI over conventional DWI is the ability to segment white matter from gray matter based on their differences in anisotropy. No significant difference in MD is observed between gray matter and white matter in hyperacute stroke,[131,132] but several studies have shown a 5% to 20% greater decrease in MD of ischemic white matter relative to gray matter in the acute period ($\leq$24 hours) as well as slightly earlier pseudonormalization of ischemic gray matter relative to white matter.[129,132–134] This finding is not always observed in studies using DWI,[20,135] probably because DTI has a higher signal-to-noise ratio. One explanation for the difference in time course of MD between gray matter and white matter is that gray matter is more vulnerable to acute ischemia. Changes in white matter, however, such as combined oligodendroglial and axonal swelling, periaxonal space enlargement, and reduced bulk water motion from cytoskeletal collapse and disruption of fast axonal transport,

likely also contribute to the different MD changes.[136]

EVOLUTION OF DIFFUSIONAL ANISOTROPY IN ISCHEMIA

Diffusional anisotropy varies widely throughout the brain, including different white matter regions, due to differences in underlying microstructural architecture.[93] Therefore, any alteration in diffusional anisotropy within a particular brain region is always reported relative to the corresponding region in the normal contralateral hemisphere.

In both rats[137] and monkeys,[138] a mild increase in FA up to 20% is observed within minutes after MCA occlusion. FA remains elevated for up to 2 hours in rats and 3 hours in monkeys before progressively declining thereafter. With transient 3-hour MCA occlusion in monkeys, FA drops rapidly after reperfusion and reaches a minimum at 6 hours before slowly climbing back toward baseline afterwards.[138] In a canine study, more severe strokes produced earlier and greater FA elevation in gray matter and showed earlier and shorter periods of transiently increased FA in white matter before subsequently decreasing below normal value.[139]

Human data are more variable, likely due to uncertainty in stroke onset times, heterogeneity of ischemic lesions, differences in reperfusion times and rates, and differences in follow-up imaging time points, among other factors. In general, FA in human ischemia follows a longer time course compared with that observed in animals. FA is mildly elevated relative to normal contralateral tissue for both gray matter and white matter in hyperacute infarction,[131,132] becomes reduced in the late acute period (12–24 hours) and progressively decreases over time thereafter (see **Table 1**).[127–130]

Yang and colleagues[129] describe 3 sequential phases in the relationship between FA and MD (**Fig. 16**). The first phase is marked by elevated FA and reduced MD; the second by reduced FA and reduced MD, and the third by reduced FA and elevated MD. In addition, there is an inverse relationship between relative FA and T2 signal intensity in both gray matter and white matter.[132,140] One plausible explanation for these observed phases is as follows. Elevated FA, reduced MD, and normal T2 occur in hyperacute stroke when cytotoxic edema dominates and there is shifting of water from the extracellular to the intracellular space without a significant change in cell membrane permeability and overall tissue water. Water remaining in the contracted extracellular space is restricted more perpendicular than parallel to white matter fibers, thereby increasing FA. Increasing intracellular water faces diffusion restriction in all directions, thereby decreasing MD. As the infarct progresses into the acute and subacute periods, vasogenic edema develops, resulting in increased tissue water predominantly in the extracellular space while intracellular water remains relatively unchanged due to persisting cytotoxic edema; these changes result in reduced FA, reduced MD, and elevated T2. In the late subacute and chronic periods, the blood-brain barrier is disrupted, vasogenic edema predominates, cells lyse, and gliosis occurs; these changes result in reduced FA, elevated MD, and elevated T2. Other factors,

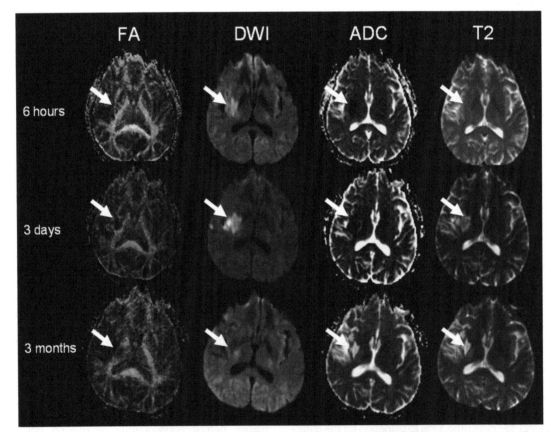

Fig. 16. Evolution of FA changes in acute stroke (*arrows*). 50-year-old man with left hemiparesis examined at 6 hours (*top row*), 3 days (*middle row*), and 3 months (*bottom row*). At 6 hours, the right putamen infarct is hyperintense on the FA and DWI images, hypointense on the ADC map, and not visualized on the T2-weighted image. These findings are consistent with the first stage of FA changes in stroke described by Yang and colleagues.[129] At 3 days, the lesion is hypointense on the FA image, hyperintense on the DWI image, hypointense on the ADC map, and hyperintense on the T2-weighted image. These findings are consistent with the second stage of FA changes in stroke. At 3 months, the lesion is hypointense on the FA and DWI images and hyperintense on the ADC and T2-weighted images. These findings are consistent with the third stage of FA changes in stroke.

such as diminished axonal transport, cellular disruption, and decreasing interstitial fluid flow, likely also contribute to reduced FA over time.

Ischemic lesions are heterogeneous with different temporal rates of FA evolution.[127,129,130,139,141] This may be related to the differential responses of gray and white matter to ischemic injury. In general, the decrease in relative FA is significantly greater in white matter than gray matter ischemic regions.[128,129,134] Although all eigenvalues are reduced in early ischemia, there is greater reduction of $\lambda_\parallel$ relative to $\lambda_\perp$ in white matter,[128] thereby reducing the relative FA of white matter.[142] This suggests that in ischemia, ADC decreases more along the long axis of white matter tracts, which is supported by greater increase in $K_\parallel$ with relatively small elevation in $K_\perp$ in acute and early subacute stroke.[117] The exception is during hyperacute infarction, when there is greater reduction of $\lambda_\perp$ relative to $\lambda_\parallel$ in deep white matter lesions that show elevated relative FA.[132] Because normal gray matter is relatively isotropic, any slight differential reduction in one eigenvalue during ischemia (probably reflecting underlying gray matter microstructure) increases its FA.

DIFFUSIONAL KURTOSIS CHANGES IN ISCHEMIA

Only a few studies have used DKI and related q-space imaging to follow changes in non-Gaussian behavior of water diffusion in human cerebral ischemia. Similar to diffusion anisotropy, diffusional kurtosis varies widely throughout the brain, including different white matter regions, due to differences in underlying microstructural architecture.[109,112] Evolution of DKI parameter changes in ischemic stroke is summarized in **Table 1**.

Peeters and colleagues,[143] in a study using q-space imaging to assess patients with hyperacute infarction, found increasing MK, increasing slow diffusion, decreasing fast diffusion, and other parameters in support of water exchange between fast and slow diffusion compartments (presumably from extracellular to intracellular space, respectively) on initial imaging that continued in this trend over 24 hours in stable or progressive infarctions but reversed in trend with regressing infarctions. Evidence of water exchange between fast and slow diffusion compartments has also been observed in patients with subacute infarctions.[144,145]

Helpern and colleagues,[146] in a study using DKI to follow patients with acute to early subacute infarction, found elevated MK in regions of ischemia coinciding with regions of reduced MD

with some patients showing additional areas of increased MK adjacent to the infarction that do not have corresponding signal changes on other acquired images, possibly indicating areas of ischemic penumbra or benign oligemia.

In another study evaluating patients with acute to early subacute infarction, Lätt and colleagues[147] found elevated MK much greater in white matter (84%) than in gray matter (6%) in regions of ischemia using a short diffusion time of 60 ms. The study also found dependence of MK on diffusion time primarily in the ischemic region with improved conspicuity of the extent of infarction by creating a ΔMK map based on differences in MK between 2 diffusion times (60 ms and 260 ms in the study).

Differential changes in $K_\parallel$ and $K_\perp$ in acute to early subacute infarction has been explored by Jensen and colleagues,[117] who found significant increase in $K_\parallel$ (120%) with relatively small elevation in $K_\perp$ (3%–12%) in regions of infarction comprised mostly of white matter and slightly higher increase in $K_\perp$ (49%) with inclusion of regions with crossing bundles and/or gray matter (see **Fig. 15**). Proposed mechanisms for such increased axial diffusional heterogeneity include formation of axonal beading in ischemia and neuronal injury[148–150] that can result in intracellular more than extracellular contributions in diffusional tortuosity and decreased $\lambda_\parallel$.[151]

By serially following two patients 2, 9, and 90 days after stroke onset, van Westen and colleagues[152] found greater increase in MK on day 2 in ischemic white matter that eventually progresses to gliosis (WM$_{gliosis}$) relative to ischemic white matter that remains normal appearing (WM$_{normal}$) on day 30, indicating initial MK may be useful in predicting ischemic tissue outcome. MK in ischemic white matter becomes progressively reduced with MK pseudonormalization occurring between days 2 and 9 for both WM$_{gliosis}$ and WM$_{normal}$. This is in contrast to the slower time course of observed MD evolution with MD pseudonormalization occurring between days 9 and 90 for WM$_{gliosis}$. The study also found progressively reduced MK in ischemic gray matter that was reduced relative to normal nonischemic gray matter even on day 2.

PREDICTING TISSUE VIABILITY AND CLINICAL OUTCOME

At present, the role of DTI in assessing hyperacute stroke is still uncertain. Although DTI has longer acquisition and postprocessing times than DWI, using a single-shot EPI technique with an efficient diffusion gradient-encoding scheme,[153] the full diffusion tensor can be obtained within minutes.[131,132] FA elevation in hyperacute infarction is at most 20% relative to contralateral normal tissue,[131,132] and the difference is borderline significant at best. Relative changes in other diffusion anisotropy indices, such as RA and VR, are even less apparent,[131] presumably because these indices are more affected by noise. Therefore, reduction in MD, which can be obtained by conventional DWI, remains the most reliable measure for the early detection of hyperacute infarction.

In the acute period, FA may reflect the severity of ischemic injury and may be more helpful in predicting clinical outcome. In one study combining DTI with perfusion-weighted imaging in hyperacute stroke, no tissue with an increase in FA greater than 10% on the initial scan was found normal on follow-up images, although initial FA in penumbral regions was not significantly different from that of the normal contralateral hemisphere.[52] Another study demonstrated statistically significant correlations between relative FA measured within 12 hours of stroke onset and clinical scores measured within 12 hours, in the subacute period (2–10 days), and at outcome (>35 days), with lower FA correlating with worse clinical outcome scores.[129] In contrast, no significant correlation was found between any of the clinical scores and MD or relative FA measured in the subacute and chronic periods, when breakdown of the blood-brain barrier, vasogenic edema, cells lysis, and gliosis lead to increasing tissue heterogeneity.

DTI can also be used to generate directionally encoded color anisotropy maps[154,155] and fiber tractography[156] to delineate major white matter tracts and their relationship to stroke lesions (Fig. 17).[157–160] The corticospinal tract (CST) is the most frequently investigated tract for the following reasons: (1) CST tractography is robust in the posterior limb of the internal capsule and cerebral peduncle because there are few crossing fibers; (2) the CST has well-defined anatomy, and (3) CST motor function can be easily tested on physical examination. In general, the volume of CST involvement by ischemia in the acute to early subacute period correlates directly with motor deficit severity[160] and inversely with motor function recovery.[161] Patients with worsening hemiparesis during the acute and subacute periods often demonstrate enlarging infarctions that involve an increasing amount of the CST on follow-up imaging.[159] In patients with anterior choroidal artery infarctions, a lower intralesional FA measured during the acute to early subacute periods is associated with worse motor outcome at 3 months.[162]

Several animal studies evaluating efficacy of neurorestorative treatment for ischemic stroke, such as neural progenitor cell and erythropoietin therapy, have shown increasing FA in recovery regions along margins of ischemic tissue after treatment that correspond to accelerated white

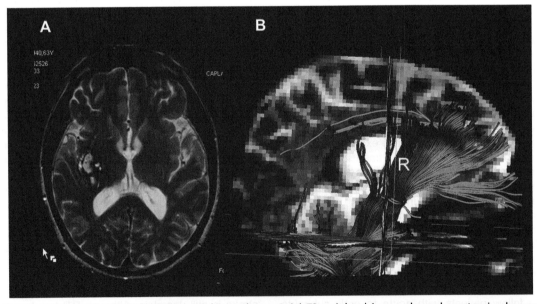

Fig. 17. Elderly patient with hypertensive hemorrhage. Axial T2-weighted image shows hypertensive hemorrhage in the right lentiform nucleus and internal capsule (A). Fiber tractography shows partial disruption of the right CST (B).

matter reorganization with increasing axonal density and myelination on histology.[163–165] White matter reorganization in stroke recovery regions with crossing fibers tracts can also be monitored using generalized FA or similar metrics based on standard deviation of q-ball orientation distribution function that preserve anisotropy information.[166–168]

There is also evidence that DTI may be useful in assessing plasticity of white matter tracts and related structural connectivity changes after rehabilitation therapy after stroke. In a study of nonfluent aphasic patients undergoing intensive melodic intonation speech therapy in the subacute to chronic phase after left hemispheric stroke, comparison of pretreatment and post-treatment fiber tractography identifies significant increase in number and volume of constructed arcuate fasciculus (AF) fiber tracts in the contralateral right hemisphere that correlate with improvement in language outcome measures.[169] Because AF, associated with the larger superior longitudinal fasciculus (SLF), is a major white matter fiber tract reciprocally connecting Wernicke and Broca language areas in the dominant (usually left) hemisphere that is not as well developed in the nondominant hemisphere,[170] these findings suggest intensive speech therapy after left hemispheric stroke may enhance recovery from aphasia by recruiting homologous language regions in the right hemisphere.

SECONDARY WHITE MATTER DEGENERATION

Secondary degeneration of white matter tracts remote from the primary ischemic region can be classified into antegrade (Wallerian) degeneration toward the axonal terminal and retrograde degeneration toward the neuronal body. Histologically, it is characterized by disintegration of axonal structures, myelin degradation, infiltration by macrophages, and gliosis.[171]

DTI has been used to assess Wallerian degeneration of the CST in patients with hemiparesis[172–174] and to distinguish Wallerian degeneration from the primary infarction. Wallerian degeneration can be detected as decreasing anisotropy as early as 2 to 3 weeks after stroke onset before T2 hyperintensity is observed.[175–177] Poor motor recovery is associated with progressive decrease in CST diffusion anisotropy, whereas good recovery is associated with relatively stable diffusion anisotropy with little to no reduction in FA.[175,178] Although chronic infarction is characterized by markedly elevated MD and reduced FA with all eigenvalues (λ_1, λ_2, and λ_3) increased, Wallerian degeneration is characterized by normal to slightly elevated MD and reduced FA with $\lambda_{\parallel}$ decreased and $\lambda_{\perp}$ increased (Fig. 18).[173,174,176] Retrograde degeneration, similar to Wallerian degeneration, demonstrates a progressive decline in FA whereas MD remains relatively unchanged.[179]

Additional white matter tracts have also been studied, such as the SLF and AF connecting Wernicke and Broca language areas in the dominant (usually left) hemisphere. In one study of patients with chronic left MCA territory infarctions, lower FA in the AF was associated with comprehension deficits, and lower FA in the left SLF and AF was associated with decreased ability to repeat spoken language.[180]

In studies assessing patients with subacute to chronic infarctions in the right cerebral hemisphere, fiber tractography of patients with

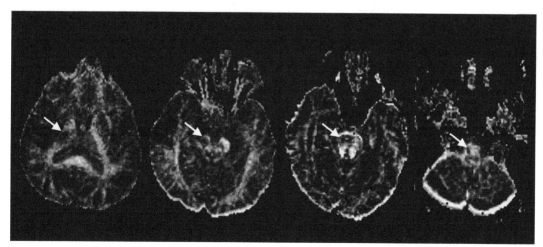

Fig. 18. Wallerian degeneration in the right CST (*arrows*) 3 months after a right MCA territory infarction. FA images demonstrate hypointensity secondary to reduced FA in the right CST.

left hemispatial neglect demonstrates common involvement of the right inferior fronto-occipital fasciculus,[181] involvement of the right anterior AF/SLF, and indeterminate involvement of the right posterior AF.[182] Although not necessary for neglect, involvement of the right optic radiation is associated with worse neglect battery performance.[182] These patients also have significantly decreased FA in the right perisylvian white matter along the course of anterior AF/SLF, internal and external capsules with some areas of reduced FA remote to the infarcted region, presumably from secondary degeneration.[182] These results show that left hemispatial neglect can result from interruptions of associative frontoparietal fiber tracts in the right hemisphere important for spatial attention, arousal, and spatial working memory.

A pitfall of fiber tractography applied to white matter tracts with secondary degeneration is that it may produce anatomically incorrect fiber trajectories in regions with intersecting pathways, such as the rostral pons, where transverse pontine fibers may confound reconstruction of the CST with Wallerian degeneration (Fig. 19).[174] This results from reduced diffusivity parallel to the degenerated fiber tract, whereas diffusivity parallel to the crossing fiber tract is preserved. Consequently, the principal eigenvector with the largest eigenvalue (λ_1) is altered, resulting in a new orientation that is usually parallel to the crossing fiber tract.

PERINATAL HYPOXIC-ISCHEMIC INJURY

MR imaging, including DTI, is becoming the imaging modality of choice for assessing hypoxic-ischemic injury in neonates because of its sensitivity in detecting brain injury and the association of MR imaging findings with neurodevelopmental outcome. The time course of MD in regions of brain injury from perinatal hypoxic-ischemic events in term neonates has been described by several investigators.[183–186] Although MD is decreased in most neonates within 24 hours after injury, the amount of decrease is less than 10% relative to normal tissue, and the extent of injury can be underestimated if patients are scanned in the acute period (Fig. 20).[183,184] This difference in temporal evolution of MD between neonatal brain injury and adult acute stroke is likely due to differences in injury mechanism; oxygenated blood flow almost always occurs immediately after delivery and resuscitation in perinatal ischemic events, whereas reperfusion is usually delayed or does not occur in adult stroke. An alternative explanation is the differential response to ischemia between the developing neonatal brain and the adult brain. MD reaches a minimum of approximately 35% to 40% less than normal at approximately 2 to 5 days, which is the best time to determine the extent of brain injury. In general, pseudonormalization of MD occurs at approximately 1 to 2 weeks. Barkovich and colleagues[184] also note heterogeneity in the time course of MD, particularly in the basal ganglia pattern of injury that usually results from a profound hypoxic-ischemic event. In these patients, the acute scan shows reduced MD in the ventrolateral thalamus with scans on days 3 to 5 showing reduced MD in the putamen, CST, and perirolandic cortex. Subsequently, on days 6 to 7, reduced MD can be seen in the subcortical white

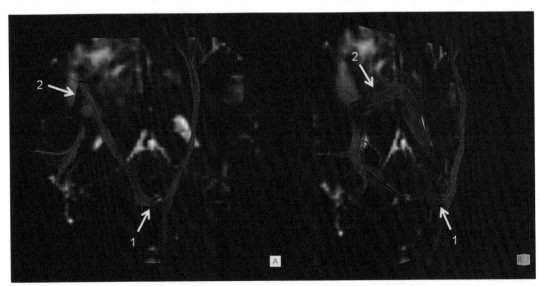

Fig. 19. Nonanatomic fiber trajectories generated from fiber tracking algorithm secondary to Wallerian degeneration of the right CST (1) across intersecting transverse pontine fibers and (2) across intersecting SLF and AF.

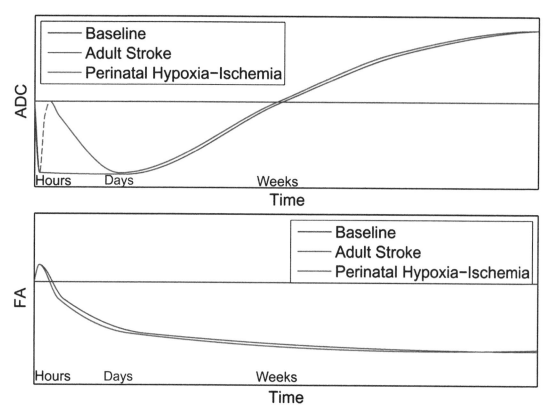

Fig. 20. Schematic diagram showing time course of ADC and FA in perinatal hypoxic-ischemic injury compared with adult stroke with permanent occlusion. ADC and FA are relative to corresponding region in normal age-matched controls. The difference in ADC evolution between perinatal hypoxic-ischemic injury and acute adult stroke is likely due to differences in injury mechanism. Transient hypoxia with immediate resumption of oxygenated blood flow generally occurs after delivery and resuscitation in perinatal ischemic events, whereas reperfusion is usually delayed or does not occur in adult stroke. This explanation is supported by animal studies; transient 30-minute MCA occlusion in rats results in immediate decrease in ADC during occlusion followed by complete recovery at 60 minutes after reperfusion, but declines again 12 to 24 hours after reperfusion (Li and colleagues, 2000).[197] For this reason, neonatal brain injury may be underestimated by DWI if acquired less than 48 hours after the ischemic event.

matter and major white matter tracts, such as the corpus callosum, cingulum, and fronto-occipital fasciculus, whereas pseudonormalization of MD has occurred in the thalamus.

The time course of FA in regions of brain injury from perinatal hypoxic-ischemic events in term neonates is similar to that of adult stroke (see **Fig. 20**).[185,186] In the immediate acute period, FA is mildly elevated in injured white matter relative to normal tissue with greater reduction of $\lambda_\perp$ relative to $\lambda_{\|}$,[185] although this is not observed in all studies even when patients are imaged within 24 hours of birth.[186] FA then progressively declines over time with greater reduction of $\lambda_{\|}$ relative to $\lambda_\perp$. Ward and colleagues[186] have also found in the first week that although FA is decreased in both moderate and severe white matter and basal ganglia patterns of injury as determined by the severity of conventional imaging findings, MD is

decreased only in severe white matter and some severe basal ganglia patterns of injury. Therefore, FA may be more sensitive in confirming injuries in the first week when MD may have pseudonormalized earlier because of tissue heterogeneity.

White matter injury of prematurity is a spectrum of lesions that include cystic periventricular leukomalacia and noncystic white matter abnormalities that demonstrate diffuse excessive high signal intensity (DEHSI) on T2-weighted images,[187] which is thought to be secondary from hypoxia-ischemia and reperfusion injury in premature neonates.[188] Although cystic periventricular leukomalacia is now uncommon in modern neonatal ICUs, DEHSI is seen in up to 21% of premature neonates in the first postnatal week to 79% at term-equivalent age.[187] Studies of premature infants scanned at term-equivalent age demonstrate no significant to mildly elevated MD in white matter with DEHSI,[189–191] whereas diffusion anisotropy is reduced with elevated $\lambda_\perp$ in these lesions.[191–193] The mechanism for these findings is thought to be from microglial activation and reactive oxygen and nitrogen species that result in preoligodendrocyte injury and eventual impairment of myelination.[188] Alteration in fiber diameter, axonal membrane changes, gliosis, and focal areas of necrosis may also contribute to the imaging findings.

There is also evidence from DTI studies that ex utero brain development of premature neonates may be different from in utero brain development of full-term infants. Compared with full-term infants, premature neonates (with normal head ultrasound, no history of asphyxia, normal neurologic examination, and appropriate gestational growth) imaged at term-equivalent age have elevated MD and decreased diffusion anisotropy in their central white matter.[194] Decreased diffusion anisotropy without significant difference in MD is also observed in the posterior limb of the internal capsule, presumably CST, of premature neonates. Furthermore, premature infants with abnormal neurologic examination (including cerebral palsy) but no significant white matter abnormality on conventional MR imaging have more reduced FA in posterior limb of the internal capsule at term-equivalent age compared with that in premature infants with normal neurologic examination.[195] In a long-term follow-up study of premature infants (with no history of neonatal brain injury, normal neonatal head ultrasound, and normal neurologic examination) at 12 years of age, widespread decrease in FA of major association and commissural fibers is observed in premature children relative to full-term children.[196] Decreases in FA of specific white matter tracks are correlated with worsening of specific cognitive, language, and behavioral test scores.

SUMMARY

Diffusion MR imaging has vastly improved evaluation of acute ischemic stroke. It is highly sensitive and specific in the detection of acute ischemic stroke at early time points when CT and conventional MR imaging sequences are unreliable. The initial DWI lesion is thought to represent infarct core and usually progresses to infarction unless there is early reperfusion. The initial DWI lesion volume correlates highly with final infarct volume as well as with acute and chronic neurologic assessment tests. DWI lesion volumes and ADC values may also be useful in determining tissue at risk of undergoing HT after reperfusion therapy. DTI and DKI can delineate the differences in responses of

gray versus white matter to ischemia. FA may be important in determining stroke onset time and tractography provides early detection of Wallerian degeneration that may be important in determining prognosis. DTI is also changing the way perinatal hypoxic-ischemic injury is evaluated and the understanding of white matter injury of prematurity. Further investigation will undoubtedly yield new information that will improve treatment of stroke patients.

REFERENCES

1. Cooper R, Chang D, Young A, et al. Restricted diffusion in biophysical systems. Experiment. Biophys J 1974;14(3):161–77.
2. Goodman JA, Kroenke CD, Bretthorst GL, et al. Sodium ion apparent diffusion coefficient in living rat brain. Magn Reson Med 2005;53(5):1040–5.
3. Mintorovitch J, Yang GY, Shimizu H, et al. Diffusion-weighted magnetic resonance imaging of acute focal cerebral ischemia: comparison of signal intensity with changes in brain water and Na+, K(+)-ATPase activity. J Cereb Blood Flow Metab 1994;14(2):332–6.
4. Benveniste H, Hedlund LW, Johnson GA. Mechanism of detection of acute cerebral ischemia in rats by diffusion-weighted magnetic resonance microscopy. Stroke 1992;23(5):746–54.
5. Veldhuis WB, van der Stelt M, Delmas F, et al. In vivo excitotoxicity induced by ouabain, a Na+/K+-ATPase inhibitor. J Cereb Blood Flow Metab 2003;23(1):62–74.
6. Sevick RJ, Kanda F, Mintorovitch J, et al. Cytotoxic brain edema: assessment with diffusion-weighted MR imaging. Radiology 1992;185(3):687–90.
7. Duong TQ, Ackerman JJ, Ying HS, et al. Evaluation of extra- and intracellular apparent diffusion in normal and globally ischemic rat brain via 19F NMR. Magn Reson Med 1998;40(1):1–13.
8. Babsky AM, Topper S, Zhang H, et al. Evaluation of extra- and intracellular apparent diffusion coefficient of sodium in rat skeletal muscle: effects of prolonged ischemia. Magn Reson Med 2008; 59(3):485–91.
9. Qiao M, Malisza KL, Del Bigio MR, et al. Transient hypoxia-ischemia in rats: changes in diffusion-sensitive MR imaging findings, extracellular space, and Na+-K+ -adenosine triphosphatase and cytochrome oxidase activity. Radiology 2002;223(1): 65–75.
10. Anderson AW, Zhong J, Petroff OA, et al. Effects of osmotically driven cell volume changes on diffusion-weighted imaging of the rat optic nerve. Magn Reson Med 1996;35(2):162–7.
11. van der Toorn A, Sykova E, Dijkhuizen RM, et al. Dynamic changes in water ADC, energy metabolism, extracellular space volume, and tortuosity in

neonatal rat brain during global ischemia. Magn Reson Med 1996;36(1):52–60.

12. van der Toorn A, Dijkhuizen RM, Tulleken CA, et al. Diffusion of metabolites in normal and ischemic rat brain measured by localized 1H MRS. Magn Reson Med 1996;36(6):914–22.

13. Neil JJ, Duong TQ, Ackerman JJ. Evaluation of intracellular diffusion in normal and globally-ischemic rat brain via 133Cs NMR. Magn Reson Med 1996;35(3):329–35.

14. Szafer A, Zhong J, Gore JC. Theoretical model for water diffusion in tissues. Magn Reson Med 1995; 33(5):697–712.

15. Welch KM, Windham J, Knight RA, et al. A model to predict the histopathology of human stroke using diffusion and T2-weighted magnetic resonance imaging. Stroke 1995;26(11):1983–9.

16. Knight RA, Dereski MO, Helpern JA, et al. Magnetic resonance imaging assessment of evolving focal cerebral ischemia. Comparison with histopathology in rats. Stroke 1994;25(6): 1252–61 [discussion: 1261–2].

17. Schlaug G, Siewert B, Benfield A, et al. Time course of the apparent diffusion coefficient (ADC) abnormality in human stroke. Neurology 1997;49(1):113–9.

18. Warach S, Chien D, Li W, et al. Fast magnetic resonance diffusion-weighted imaging of acute human stroke. Neurology 1992;42(9):1717–23.

19. Schwamm LH, Koroshetz WJ, Sorensen AG, et al. Time course of lesion development in patients with acute stroke: serial diffusion- and hemodynamic-weighted magnetic resonance imaging. Stroke 1998;29(11):2268–76.

20. Fiebach JB, Jansen O, Schellinger PD, et al. Serial analysis of the apparent diffusion coefficient time course in human stroke. Neuroradiology 2002; 44(4):294–8.

21. Warach S, Gaa J, Siewert B, et al. Acute human stroke studied by whole brain echo planar diffusion-weighted magnetic resonance imaging. Ann Neurol 1995;37(2):231–41.

22. Copen WA, Schwamm LH, Gonzalez RG, et al. Ischemic stroke: effects of etiology and patient age on the time course of the core apparent diffusion coefficient. Radiology 2001;221(1):27–34.

23. Chalela JA, Kidwell CS, Nentwich LM, et al. Magnetic resonance imaging and computed tomography in emergency assessment of patients with suspected acute stroke: a prospective comparison. Lancet 2007;369(9558):293–8.

24. Gonzalez RG, Schaefer PW, Buonanno FS, et al. Diffusion-weighted MR imaging: diagnostic accuracy in patients imaged within 6 hours of stroke symptom onset. Radiology 1999;210(1): 155–62.

25. Saur D, Kucinski T, Grzyska U, et al. Sensitivity and interrater agreement of CT and diffusion-weighted MR imaging in hyperacute stroke. AJNR Am J Neuroradiol 2003;24(5):878–85.

26. Urbach H, Flacke S, Keller E, et al. Detectability and detection rate of acute cerebral hemisphere infarcts on CT and diffusion-weighted MRI. Neuroradiology 2000;42(10):722–7.

27. Mullins ME, Schaefer PW, Sorensen AG, et al. CT and conventional and diffusion-weighted MR imaging in acute stroke: study in 691 patients at presentation to the emergency department. Radiology 2002;224(2):353–60.

28. Hjort N, Christensen S, Solling C, et al. Ischemic injury detected by diffusion imaging 11 minutes after stroke. Ann Neurol 2005;58(3):462–5.

29. Engelter ST, Wetzel SG, Radue EW, et al. The clinical significance of diffusion-weighted MR imaging in infratentorial strokes. Neurology 2004;62(4): 574–80.

30. Lutsep HL, Albers GW, DeCrespigny A, et al. Clinical utility of diffusion-weighted magnetic resonance imaging in the assessment of ischemic stroke. Ann Neurol 1997;41(5):574–80.

31. Kuker W, Weise J, Krapf H, et al. MRI characteristics of acute and subacute brainstem and thalamic infarctions: value of T2- and diffusion-weighted sequences. J Neurol 2002;249(1):33–42.

32. Oppenheim C, Stanescu R, Dormont D, et al. False-negative diffusion-weighted MR findings in acute ischemic stroke. AJNR Am J Neuroradiol 2000;21(8):1434–40.

33. Ay H, Buonanno FS, Rordorf G, et al. Normal diffusion-weighted MRI during stroke-like deficits. Neurology 1999;52(9):1784–92.

34. Narisawa A, Shamoto H, Shimizu H, et al. [Diffusion-weighted magnetic resonance imaging (MRI) in acute brain stem infarction]. No To Shinkei 2001; 53(11):1021–6 [in Japanese].

35. Etgen T, Grafin von Einsiedel H, Rottinger M, et al. Detection of acute brainstem infarction by using DWI/MRI. Eur Neurol 2004;52(3):145–50.

36. Fitzek S, Fitzek C, Urban PP, et al. Time course of lesion development in patients with acute brain stem infarction and correlation with NIHSS score. Eur J Radiol 2001;39(3):180–5.

37. Linfante I, Llinas RH, Schlaug G, et al. Diffusion-weighted imaging and National Institutes of Health stroke scale in the acute phase of posterior-circulation stroke. Arch Neurol 2001; 58(4):621–8.

38. Toi H, Uno M, Harada M, et al. Diagnosis of acute brain-stem infarcts using diffusion-weighed MRI. Neuroradiology 2003;45(6):352–6.

39. Burdette JH, Elster AD. Diffusion-weighted imaging of cerebral infarctions: are higher B values better? J Comput Assist Tomogr 2002;26(4):622–7.

40. Cihangiroglu M, Citci B, Kilickesmez O, et al. The utility of high b-value DWI in evaluation of ischemic

stroke at 3T. Eur J Radiol 2009. [Epub ahead of print].

41. Kim HJ, Choi CG, Lee DH, et al. High-b-value diffusion-weighted MR imaging of hyperacute ischemic stroke at 1.5T. AJNR Am J Neuroradiol 2005;26(2):208–15.

42. Meyer JR, Gutierrez A, Mock B, et al. High-b-value diffusion-weighted MR imaging of suspected brain infarction. AJNR Am J Neuroradiol 2000;21(10): 1821–9.

43. Kuhl CK, Textor J, Gieseke J, et al. Acute and subacute ischemic stroke at high-field-strength (3.0-T) diffusion-weighted MR imaging: intraindividual comparative study. Radiology 2005;234(2): 509–16.

44. Baird AE, Benfield A, Schlaug G, et al. Enlargement of human cerebral ischemic lesion volumes measured by diffusion-weighted magnetic resonance imaging. Ann Neurol 1997;41(5):581–9.

45. van Everdingen KJ, van der Grond J, Kappelle LJ, et al. Diffusion-weighted magnetic resonance imaging in acute stroke. Stroke 1998;29(9):1783–90.

46. Tong DC, Yenari MA, Albers GW, et al. Correlation of perfusion- and diffusion-weighted MRI with NIHSS score in acute (<6.5 hour) ischemic stroke. Neurology 1998;50(4):864–70.

47. Kidwell CS, Saver JL, Mattiello J, et al. Thrombolytic reversal of acute human cerebral ischemic injury shown by diffusion/perfusion magnetic resonance imaging. Ann Neurol 2000;47(4):462–9.

48. Kidwell CS, Saver JL, Starkman S, et al. Late secondary ischemic injury in patients receiving intraarterial thrombolysis. Ann Neurol 2002;52(6): 698–703.

49. Schaefer PW, Hassankhani A, Putman C, et al. Characterization and evolution of diffusion MR imaging abnormalities in stroke patients undergoing intra-arterial thrombolysis. AJNR Am J Neuroradiol 2004;25(6):951–7.

50. Miyasaka N, Nagaoka T, Kuroiwa T, et al. Histopathologic correlates of temporal diffusion changes in a rat model of cerebral hypoxia/ischemia. AJNR Am J Neuroradiol 2000;21(1):60–6.

51. Olivot JM, Mlynash M, Thijs VN, et al. Relationships between cerebral perfusion and reversibility of acute diffusion lesions in DEFUSE: insights from RADAR. Stroke 2009;40(5):1692–7.

52. Schaefer PW, Ozsunar Y, He J, et al. Assessing tissue viability with MR diffusion and perfusion imaging. AJNR Am J Neuroradiol 2003;24(3): 436–43.

53. Fiehler J, Knab R, Reichenbach JR, et al. Apparent diffusion coefficient decreases and magnetic resonance imaging perfusion parameters are associated in ischemic tissue of acute stroke patients. J Cereb Blood Flow Metab 2001;21(5):577–84.

54. Schlaug G, Benfield A, Baird AE, et al. The ischemic penumbra: operationally defined by diffusion and perfusion MRI. Neurology 1999;53(7): 1528–37.

55. Rohl L, Ostergaard L, Simonsen CZ, et al. Viability thresholds of ischemic penumbra of hyperacute stroke defined by perfusion-weighted MRI and apparent diffusion coefficient. Stroke 2001;32(5):1140–6.

56. Gonen KA, Simsek MM. Diffusion weighted imaging and estimation of prognosis using apparent diffusion coefficient measurements in ischemic stroke. Eur J Radiol 2010;76(2):157–61.

57. Fiehler J, Foth M, Kucinski T, et al. Severe ADC decreases do not predict irreversible tissue damage in humans. Stroke 2002;33(1):79–86.

58. Jones TH, Morawetz RB, Crowell RM, et al. Thresholds of focal cerebral ischemia in awake monkeys. J Neurosurg 1981;54(6):773–82.

59. Calandre L, Ortega JF, Bermejo F. Anticoagulation and hemorrhagic infarction in cerebral embolism secondary to rheumatic heart disease. Arch Neurol 1984;41(11):1152–4.

60. Hakim AM, Ryder-Cooke A, Melanson D. Sequential computerized tomographic appearance of strokes. Stroke 1983;14(6):893–7.

61. Hornig CR, Dorndorf W, Agnoli AL. Hemorrhagic cerebral infarction—a prospective study. Stroke 1986;17(2):179–85.

62. Horowitz SH, Zito JL, Donnarumma R, et al. Computed tomographic-angiographic findings within the first five hours of cerebral infarction. Stroke 1991;22(10):1245–53.

63. Furlan A, Higashida R, Wechsler L, et al. Intra-arterial prourokinase for acute ischemic stroke. The PROACT II study: a randomized controlled trial. Prolyse in Acute Cerebral Thromboembolism. JAMA 1999;282(21):2003–11.

64. Hacke W, Kaste M, Bluhmki E, et al. Thrombolysis with alteplase 3 to 4.5 hours after acute ischemic stroke. N Engl J Med 2008;359(13):1317–29.

65. Intracerebral hemorrhage after intravenous t-PA therapy for ischemic stroke. The NINDS t-PA Stroke Study Group. Stroke 1997;28(11):2109–18.

66. Kim EY, Na DG, Kim SS, et al. Prediction of hemorrhagic transformation in acute ischemic stroke: role of diffusion-weighted imaging and early parenchymal enhancement. AJNR Am J Neuroradiol 2005;26(5):1050–5.

67. Derex L, Hermier M, Adeleine P, et al. Clinical and imaging predictors of intracerebral haemorrhage in stroke patients treated with intravenous tissue plasminogen activator. J Neurol Neurosurg Psychiatry 2005;76(1):70–5.

68. Singer OC, Humpich MC, Fiehler J, et al. Risk for symptomatic intracerebral hemorrhage after thrombolysis assessed by diffusion-weighted magnetic resonance imaging. Ann Neurol 2008;63(1):52–60.

69. Tong DC, Adami A, Moseley ME, et al. Prediction of hemorrhagic transformation following acute stroke: role of diffusion- and perfusion-weighted magnetic resonance imaging. Arch Neurol 2001;58(4): 587–93.

70. Selim M, Fink JN, Kumar S, et al. Predictors of hemorrhagic transformation after intravenous recombinant tissue plasminogen activator: prognostic value of the initial apparent diffusion coefficient and diffusion-weighted lesion volume. Stroke 2002;33(8):2047–52.

71. Oppenheim C, Samson Y, Dormont D, et al. DWI prediction of symptomatic hemorrhagic transformation in acute MCA infarct. J Neuroradiol 2002; 29(1):6–13.

72. Campbell BC, Christensen S, Butcher KS, et al. Regional very low cerebral blood volume predicts hemorrhagic transformation better than diffusion-weighted imaging volume and thresholded apparent diffusion coefficient in acute ischemic stroke. Stroke 2010;41(1):82–8.

73. Kim JH, Bang OY, Liebeskind DS, et al. Impact of baseline tissue status (diffusion-weighted imaging lesion) versus perfusion status (severity of hypoperfusion) on hemorrhagic transformation. Stroke 2010;41(3):e135–42.

74. Kassner A, Roberts T, Taylor K, et al. Prediction of hemorrhage in acute ischemic stroke using permeability MR imaging. AJNR Am J Neuroradiol 2005; 26(9):2213–7.

75. Hjort N, Wu O, Ashkanian M, et al. MRI detection of early blood-brain barrier disruption: parenchymal enhancement predicts focal hemorrhagic transformation after thrombolysis. Stroke 2008;39(3): 1025–8.

76. Adams HP Jr, del Zoppo G, Alberts MJ, et al. Guidelines for the early management of adults with ischemic stroke: a guideline from the American Heart Association/American Stroke Association Stroke Council, Clinical Cardiology Council, Cardiovascular Radiology and Intervention Council, and the Atherosclerotic Peripheral Vascular Disease and Quality of Care Outcomes in Research Interdisciplinary Working Groups: the American Academy of Neurology affirms the value of this guideline as an educational tool for neurologists. Stroke 2007;38(5):1655–711.

77. Lovblad KO, Baird AE, Schlaug G, et al. Ischemic lesion volumes in acute stroke by diffusion-weighted magnetic resonance imaging correlate with clinical outcome. Ann Neurol 1997;42(2): 164–70.

78. Nighoghossian N, Hermier M, Adeleine P, et al. Baseline magnetic resonance imaging parameters and stroke outcome in patients treated by intravenous tissue plasminogen activator. Stroke 2003; 34(2):458–63.

79. Engelter ST, Provenzale JM, Petrella JR, et al. Infarct volume on apparent diffusion coefficient maps correlates with length of stay and outcome after middle cerebral artery stroke. Cerebrovasc Dis 2003;15(3):188–91.

80. Derex L, Nighoghossian N, Hermier M, et al. Influence of pretreatment MRI parameters on clinical outcome, recanalization and infarct size in 49 stroke patients treated by intravenous tissue plasminogen activator. J Neurol Sci 2004;225(1–2):3–9.

81. Sanak D, Nosal V, Horak D, et al. Impact of diffusion-weighted MRI-measured initial cerebral infarction volume on clinical outcome in acute stroke patients with middle cerebral artery occlusion treated by thrombolysis. Neuroradiology 2006;48(9):632–9.

82. Parsons MW, Christensen S, McElduff P, et al. Pretreatment diffusion- and perfusion-MR lesion volumes have a crucial influence on clinical response to stroke thrombolysis. J Cereb Blood Flow Metab 2010;30(6):1214–25.

83. Yoo AJ, Barak ER, Copen WA, et al. Combining acute DWI and MTT lesion volumes with NIHSS score improves the prediction of acute stroke outcome. Stroke 2010;41(8):1728–35.

84. Yoo AJ, Verduzco LA, Schaefer PW, et al. MRI-based selection for intra-arterial stroke therapy: value of pretreatment diffusion-weighted imaging lesion volume in selecting patients with acute stroke who will benefit from early recanalization. Stroke 2009;40(6):2046–54.

85. Stejskal E, Tanner J. Spin diffusion measurements: spin echoes in the presence of a time-dependent field gradient. J Chem Phys 1965;42:288–92.

86. Basser P, Mattiello J, Le Bihan D. Estimation of the effective self-diffusion tensor from the NMR spin echo. J Magn Reson 1994;103:247–54.

87. Mattiello J, Basser P, Le Bihan D. Analytical expressions for the b matrix in NMR diffusion imaging and spectroscopy. J Magn Reson 1994;108:131–41.

88. Mattiello J, Basser P, Le Bihan D. The b-matrix in diffusion tensor echo-planar imaging. Magn Reson Med 1997;37:292–300.

89. Jones D, Horsfield M, Simmons A. Optimal strategies for measuring diffusion in anisotropic systems by magnetic resonance imaging. Magn Reson Med 1999;42:515–25.

90. Papadakis N, Xing D, Huang C, et al. A comparative study of acquisition schemes for diffusion tensor imaging using MRI. J Magn Reson 1999;137:67–82.

91. Frank L. Anisotropy in high angular resolution diffusion-weighted MRI. Magn Reson Med 2001; 45:935–9.

92. Tuch D, Reese T, Wiegell M, et al. High angular resolution diffusion imaging reveals intravoxel white

matter fiber heterogeneity. Magn Reson Med 2002; 48:577–82.

93. Pierpaoli C, Jezzard P, Basser P, et al. Diffusion tensor MR imaging of the human brain. Radiology 1996;201:637–48.

94. Le Bihan D, Mangin J, Poupon C, et al. Diffusion tensor imaging: concepts and applications. J Magn Reson Imaging 2001;13:534–46.

95. Neeman M, Freyer J, Sillerud L. Pulsed-gradient spin-echo studies in NMR imaging. Effects of the imaging gradients on the determination of diffusion gradients. J Magn Reson 1990;90:303–12.

96. Mori S, van Zijl P. Diffusion weighting by the trace of the diffusion tensor within a single scan. Magn Reson Med 1995;33:41–52.

97. Wong E, Cox R, Song A. Optimized isotropic diffusion weighting. Magn Reson Med 1995;34:139–43.

98. Conturo T, McKinstry R, Robinson B. Encoding of anisotropic diffusion with tetrahedral gradients: a general mathematical diffusion formalism and experimental results. Magn Reson Med 1996;35: 399–412.

99. Basser P, Pierpaoli C. Microstructural and physiological features of tissues elucidated by quantitative-diffusion-tensor MRI. J Magn Reson B 1996;111:209–19.

100. Pierpaoli C, Basser P. Toward a quantitative assessment of diffusion anisotropy. Magn Reson Med 1996;36:893–906.

101. Kärger J. Zur bestimmung der diffusion in einem zweibereichsystem mit hilfe von gepulsten feldgradienten. Ann Phys 1969;479:1–4 [in German].

102. Kärger J. NMR self-diffusion studies in heterogeneous systems. Adv Colloid Interface Sci 1985; 23:129–48.

103. Assaf Y, Cohen Y. Non-mono-exponential attenuation of water and N-acetyl aspartate signals due to diffusion in brain tissue. J Magn Reson 1998; 131:69–85.

104. Melhem E, Itoh R, Jones L, et al. Diffusion tensor MR imaging of the brain: effect of diffusion weighting on trace and anisotropy measurements. AJNR Am J Neuroradiol 2000;21:1813–20.

105. Mulkern R, Gudbjartsson H, Westin C, et al. Multi-component apparent diffusion coefficients in human brain. NMR Biomed 1999;12:51–62.

106. Niendorf T, Dijkhuizen R, Norris D, et al. Biexponential diffusion attenuation in various states of brain tissue: implications for diffusion-weighted imaging. Magn Reson Med 1996;36:847–57.

107. Jensen J, Helpern J. MRI quantification of non-Gaussian water diffusion by kurtosis analysis. NMR Biomed 2010;23:698–710.

108. Jensen J, Helpern J, Ramani A, et al. Diffusional kurtosis imaging: the quantification of non-gaussian water diffusion by means of magnetic resonance imaging. Magn Reson Med 2005;53:1432–40.

109. Lu H, Jensen J, Ramani A, et al. Three-dimensional characterization of non-gaussian water diffusion in humans using diffusion kurtosis imaging. NMR Biomed 2006;19:236–47.

110. Wu E, Cheung M. MR diffusion kurtosis imaging for neural tissue characterization. NMR Biomed 2010; 23:836–48.

111. Balanda K, MacGillivray H. Kurtosis: a critical review. Am Stat 1988;42:111–9.

112. Hui E, Cheung M, Qi L, et al. Towards better MR characterization of neural tissues using directional diffusion kurtosis analysis. Neuroimage 2008;42:122–34.

113. Assaf Y, Cohen Y. Structural information in neuronal tissue as revealed by q-space diffusion NMR spectroscopy of metabolites in bovine optic nerve. NMR Biomed 1999;12:335–44.

114. King M, Houseman J, Roussel S, et al. q-Space imaging of the brain. Magn Reson Med 1994;32: 707–13.

115. Tuch D, Reese T, Wiegell M, et al. Diffusion MRI of complex neural architecture. Neuron 2003;40: 885–95.

116. Wedeen V, Hagmann P, Tseng W, et al. Mapping complex tissue architecture with diffusion spectrum magnetic resonance imaging. Magn Reson Med 2005;54:1377–86.

117. Jensen J, Falangola M, Hu C, et al. Preliminary observations of increased diffusional kurtosis in human brain following recent cerebral infarction. NMR Biomed 2010. [Epub ahead of print].

118. Cheung M, Hui E, Chan K, et al. Does diffusion kurtosis imaging lead to better neural tissue characterization? A rodent brain maturation study. Neuroimage 2009;45:286–392.

119. Beaulieu C, Allen P. Determinants of anisotropic water diffusion in nerves. Magn Reson Med 1994; 31:394–400.

120. Beaulieu C. The basis of anisotropic water diffusion in the nervous system—a technical review. NMR Biomed 2002;15:435–55.

121. Rutherford M, Cowan F, Manzur A, et al. MR imaging of anisotropically restricted diffusion in the brain of neonates and infants. J Comput Assist Tomogr 1991;15:188–98.

122. Sakuma H, Nomura Y, Takeda K, et al. Adult and neonatal human brain: diffusional anisotropy and myelination with diffusion-weighted MR imaging. Radiology 1991;180:229–33.

123. Neil J, Shiran S, McKinstry R, et al. Normal brain in human newborns: apparent diffusion coefficient and diffusion anisotropy measured using diffusion tensor MR imaging. Radiology 1998;209:57–66.

124. Gulani V, Webb A, Duncan I, et al. Apparent diffusion tensor measurements in myelin-deficient rat spinal cords. Magn Reson Med 2001;45:191–5.

125. Prayer D, Barkovich A, Kirschner D, et al. Visualization of nonstructural changes in early white matter development on diffusion-weighted MR images: evidence supporting premyelination anisotropy. AJNR Am J Neuroradiol 2001;22:1572–6.

126. Wimberger D, Roberts T, Barkovich A, et al. Identification of "premyelination" by diffusion-weighted MRI. J Comput Assist Tomogr 1995;19:28–33.

127. Armitage P, Bastin M, Marshall I, et al. Diffusion anisotropy measurements in ischaemic stroke of the human brain. MAGMA 1998;6:28–36.

128. Sorensen A, Wu O, Copen W, et al. Human acute cerebral ischemia: detection of changes in water diffusion anisotropy by using MR imaging. Radiology 1999;212:785–92.

129. Yang Q, Tress B, Barber P, et al. Serial study of apparent diffusion coefficient and anisotropy in patients with acute stroke. Stroke 1999;30:2382–90.

130. Zelaya F, Flood N, Chalk J, et al. An evaluation of the time dependence of the anisotropy of the water diffusion tensor in acute human ischaemia. Magn Reson Imaging 1999;17:331–48.

131. Harris A, Pereira R, Mitchell J, et al. A comparison of images generated from diffusion-weighted and diffusion-tensor imaging data in hyper-acute stroke. J Magn Reson Imaging 2004;20:193–200.

132. Bhagat Y, Hussain M, Stobbe R, et al. Elevations of diffusion anisotropy are associated with hyperacute stroke: a serial imaging study. Magn Reson Imaging 2008;26:683–93.

133. Mukherjee P, Bahn M, McKinstry R, et al. Differences between gray matter and white matter water diffusion in stroke: diffusion-tensor MR imaging in 12 patients. Radiology 2000;215:211–20.

134. Munoz Maniega S, Bastin M, Armitage P, et al. Temporal evolution of water diffusion parameters is different in grey and white matter in human ischaemic stroke. J Neurol Neurosurg Psychiatry 2004;75:1714–8.

135. Bastin M, Rana A, Wardlaw J, et al. A study of the apparent diffusion coefficient of grey and white matter in human ischaemic stroke. Neuroreport 2000;11:2867–74.

136. Kuroiwa T, Nagaoka T, Ueki M, et al. Different apparent diffusion coefficient: water content correlations of gray and white matter during early ischaemia. Stroke 1998;29:859–65.

137. Carano R, Li F, Irie K, et al. Multispectral analysis of the temporal evolution of cerebral ischemia in the rat brain. J Magn Reson Imaging 2000;12:842–58.

138. Liu Y, D'Arceuil H, Westmoreland S, et al. Serial diffusion tensor MRI after transient and permanent cerebral ischemia in nonhuman primates. Stroke 2007;38:138–45.

139. Harris A, Andersen L, Kosior R, et al. Evolution of fractional anisotropy in hyperacute ischemic stroke. Proceedings of the 18th Annual Meeting of ISMRM. Stockholm, May 1–7, 2010.

140. Ozsunar Y, Grant P, Huisman T, et al. Evolution of water diffusion and anisotropy in hyperacute stroke: significant correlation between fractional anisotropy and T2. AJNR Am J Neuroradiol 2004; 25:699–705.

141. Ozsunar Y, Koseoglu K, Huisman T, et al. MRI measurements of water diffusion: impact of region of interest selection on ischemic quantification. Eur J Radiol 2004;51:195–201.

142. Green H, Pena A, Price C, et al. Increased anisotropy in acute stroke: a possible explanation. Stroke 2002;33:1517–21.

143. Peeters F, Rommel D, Peeters A, et al. MRI of acute (<6 hours) ischemic stroke patients: a comparison between diffusion-related parameters. Proceedings of the 18th Annual Meeting of ISMRM. Stockholm, May 1–7, 2010.

144. Brugières P, Thomas P, Maraval A, et al. Water diffusion compartmentation at high b values in ischemic human brain. AJNR Am J Neuroradiol 2004;25:692–8.

145. Lätt J, Nilsson M, van Westen D, et al. Diffusion-weighted MRI measurements on stroke patients reveal water-exchange mechanisms in sub-acute ischaemic lesions. NMR Biomed 2009;22:619–28.

146. Helpern J, Lo C, Hu C, et al. Diffusion kurtosis imaging in acute human stroke. Proceedings of the 17th Annual Meeting of ISMRM. Honolulu, April 18–24, 2009.

147. Lätt J, van Westen D, Nilsson M, et al. Diffusion time dependent kurtosis maps visualize ischemic lesions in stroke patients. Proceedings of the 17th Annual Meeting of ISMRM. Honolulu, April 18–24, 2009.

148. Li P, Murphy T. Two-photon imaging during prolonged middle cerebral artery occlusion in mice reveals recovery of dendritic structure after reperfusion. J Neurosci 2008;28:11970–9.

149. Ochs S, Pourmand R, Jersild RJ, et al. The origin and nature of beading: a reversible transformation of the shape of nerve fibers. Prog Neurobiol 1997; 52:391–426.

150. Roediger B, Armati P. Oxidative stress induces axonal beading in cultured human brain tissue. Neurobiol Dis 2003;13:222–9.

151. Budde M, Frank J. Neurite beading is sufficient to decrease the apparent diffusion coefficient after ischemic stroke. Proc Natl Acad Sci U S A 2010; 107:14472–7.

152. van Westen D, Nilsson M, Sjunnesson H, et al. Apparent kurtosis and fractional anisotropy potentially predicts tissue outcome in sub-acute stroke. Proceedings of the 18th Annual Meeting of ISMRM. Stockholm, May 1–7, 2010.

153. Basser P, Pierpaoli C. A simplified method to measure the diffusion tensor from seven MR images. Magn Reson Med 1998;39:928–34.

154. Douek P, Turner R, Pekar J, et al. MR color mapping of myelin fiber orientation. J Comput Assist Tomogr 1991;15:923–9.

155. Pajevic S, Pierpaoli C. Color schemes to represent the orientation of anisotropic tissues from diffusion tensor data: application to white matter fiber tract mapping in the human brain. Magn Reson Med 1999;42:526–40.

156. Mori S, van Zijl P. Fiber tracking: principles and strategies—a technical review. NMR Biomed 2002;15:468–80.

157. Kunimatsu A, Aoki S, Masutani Y, et al. Three-dimensional white matter tractography by diffusion tensor imaging in ischaemic stroke involving the corticospinal tract. Neuroradiology 2003;45:532–5.

158. Lie C, Hirsch J, Rossmanith C, et al. Clinicotopographical correlation of corticospinal tract stroke: a color-coded diffusion tensor imaging study. Stroke 2004;35:86–92.

159. Yamada K, Ito H, Nakamura H, et al. Stroke patients' evolving symptoms assessed by tractography. J Magn Reson Imaging 2004;20:923–9.

160. Konishi J, Yamada K, Kizu O, et al. MR tractography for the evaluation of functional recovery from lenticulostriate infarcts. Neurology 2005;64:108–13.

161. Kunimatsu A, Itoh D, Nakata Y, et al. Utilization of diffusion tensor tractography in combination with spatial normalization to assess involvement of the corticospinal tract in capsular/pericapsular stroke: feasibility and clinical applications. J Magn Reson Imaging 2007;26:1399–404.

162. Nelles M, Gieseke J, Flacke S, et al. Diffusion tensor pyramidal tractography in patients with anterior choroidal artery infarcts. AJNR Am J Neuroradiol 2008;29:488–93.

163. Jiang Q, Alexander D, Ding G, et al. White matter reorganization after stroke measured by Gaussian DTI, q-ball, and PAS MRI. Proceedings of the 15th Annual Meeting of ISMRM. Berlin, May 19–25, 2007.

164. Jiang Q, Zhang Z, Ding G, et al. MRI detects white matter reorganization after neural progenitor cell treatment of stroke. Neuroimage 2006;32:1080–9.

165. Li L, Jiang Q, Ding G, et al. MRI identification of white matter reorganization enhanced by erythropoietin treatment in a rat model of focal ischemia. Stroke 2009;40:936–41.

166. Pourabdillah-Nejed S, Hearshen D, Jiang Q, et al. Application of the diffusion standard deviation map for detection of white matter reorganization after stroke. Proceedings of the 17th Annual Meeting of ISMRM. Honolulu, April 18–24, 2009.

167. Pourabdillah-Nejed S, Jiang Q, Noll D, et al. A statistical approach for creating anisotropy maps of the brain using q-space diffusion weighted images. Proceedings of the 16th Annual Meeting of ISMRM. Toronto, May 3–9, 2008.

168. Tuch D. Q-ball imaging. Magn Reson Med 2004;52:1358–72.

169. Schlaug G, Marchina S, Norton A. Evidence for plasticity in white-matter tracts of patients with chronic Broca's aphasia undergoing intense intonation-based speech therapy. Ann N Y Acad Sci 2009;1169:385–94.

170. Catani M, Mesulam M. The arcuate fasciculus and the disconnection theme in language and aphasia: history and current state. Cortex 2008;44:953–61.

171. Lampert P, Cressman M. Fine-structural changes of myelin sheaths after axonal degeneration in the spinal cord of rats. Am J Pathol 1966;49:1139–55.

172. Wieshmann U, Clark C, Symms M, et al. Anisotropy of water diffusion in corona radiata and cerebral peduncle in patients with hemiparesis. Neuroimage 1999;10:225–30.

173. Werring D, Toosy A, Clark C, et al. Diffusion tensor imaging can detect and quantify corticospinal tract degeneration after stroke. J Neurol Neurosurg Psychiatry 2000;69:269–72.

174. Pierpaoli C, Barnett A, Pajevic S, et al. Water diffusion changes in Wallerian degeneration and their dependence on white matter architecture. Neuroimage 2001;13:1174–85.

175. Wanatabe T, Honda Y, Fujii Y, et al. Three-dimensional anisotropy contrast magnetic resonance axonography to predict the prognosis for motor function in patients suffering from stroke. J Neurosurg 2001;94:955–60.

176. Thomalla G, Glauche V, Koch M, et al. Diffusion tensor imaging detects early Wallerian degeneration of the pyramidal tract after ischemic stroke. Neuroimage 2004;22:1767–74.

177. Thomalla G, Glauche V, Weiller C, et al. Time course of Wallerian degeneration after ischaemic stroke revealed by diffusion tensor imaging. J Neurol Neurosurg Psychiatry 2005;76:266–8.

178. Moller M, Frandsen J, Andersen G, et al. Dynamic changes in corticospinal tracts after stroke detected by fibretracking. J Neurol Neurosurg Psychiatry 2007;78:587–92.

179. Liang Z, Zeng J, Liu S, et al. A prospective study of secondary degeneration following subcortical infarction using diffusion tensor imaging. J Neurol Neurosurg Psychiatry 2007;78:581–6.

180. Breier J, Hasan K, Zhang W, et al. Language dysfunction after stroke and damage to white matter tracts evaluated using diffusion tensor imaging. AJNR Am J Neuroradiol 2008;29:483–7.

181. Urbanski M, Thiebaut de Schotten M, Rodrigo S, et al. Brain networks of spatial awareness: evidence from diffusion tensor imaging tractography. J Neurol Neurosurg Psychiatry 2008;79:598–601.

182. Urbanski M, Thiebaut de Schotten M, Rodrigo S, et al. DTI-MR tractography of white matter damage

in stroke patients with neglect. Exp Brain Res 2011; 208:491–505.

183. McKinstry R, Miller J, Snyder A, et al. A prospective, longitudinal diffusion tensor imaging study of brain injury in newborns. Neurology 2002;59:824–33.

184. Barkovich A, Miller S, Bartha A, et al. MR imaging, MR spectroscopy, and diffusion tensor imaging of sequential studies in neonates with encephalopathy. AJNR Am J Neuroradiol 2006;27:533–47.

185. van Pul C, Buijs J, Janssen M, et al. Selecting the best index for following the temporal evolution of apparent diffusion coefficient and diffusion anisotropy after hypoxic-ischemic white matter injury in neonates. AJNR Am J Neuroradiol 2005;26:469–81.

186. Ward P, Counsell S, Allsop J, et al. Reduced fractional anisotropy on diffusion tensor magnetic resonance imaging after hypoxic-ischemic encephalopathy. Pediatrics 2006;117:e619–30.

187. Maalouf E, Duggan P, Counsell S, et al. Comparison of findings on cranial ultrasound and magnetic resonance imaging in preterm infants. Pediatrics 2001;107:719–27.

188. Volpe J. Cerebral white matter injury of the premature infant - more common than you think. Pediatrics 2003;112:176–80.

189. Huppi P, Murphy B, Maier S, et al. Microstructural brain development after perinatal cerebral white matter injury assessed by diffusion tensor magnetic resonance imaging. Pediatrics 2001;107:455–60.

190. Counsell S, Allsop J, Harrison M, et al. Diffusion-weighted imaging of the brain in preterm infants with focal and diffuse white matter abnormality. Pediatrics 2003;112:1–7.

191. Miller S, Vigneron D, Henry R, et al. Serial quantitative diffusion tensor MRI of the premature brain: development in newborns with and without injury. J Magn Reson Imaging 2002;16:621–32.

192. Counsell S, Shen Y, Boardman J, et al. Axial and radial diffusivity in preterm infants who have diffuse white matter changes on magnetic resonance imaging at term-equivalent age. Pediatrics 2006; 117:376–86.

193. Anjari M, Srinivasan L, Allsop J, et al. Diffusion tensor imaging with tract-based spatial statistics reveals local white matter abnormalities in preterm infants. Neuroimage 2007;35:1021–7.

194. Huppi P, Maier S, Peled S, et al. Microstructural development of newborn cerebral white matter assessed *in vivo* by diffusion tensor magnetic resonance imaging. Pediatr Res 1998;44: 584–90.

195. Arzoumanian Y, Mirmiran M, Barnes P, et al. Diffusion tensor brain imaging findings at term-equivalent age may predict neurologic abnormalities in low birth weight preterm infants. AJNR Am J Neuroradiol 2003;24:1646–53.

196. Constable R, Ment L, Vohr B, et al. Prematurely born children demonstrate white matter microstructural differences at 12 years of age, relative to term control subjects: an investigation of group and gender effects. Pediatrics 2008;121:306–16.

197. Li F, Liu K, Silva M, et al. Transient and permanent resolution of ischemic lesions on diffusion-weighted imaging after brief periods of focal ischemia in rats: correlation with histopathology. Stroke 2000;31:946–54.

Intra-arterial Stroke Therapy: Recanalization Strategies, Patient Selection and Imaging

Daniel P. Hsu, MD*, Gurpreet Sandhu, MD,
Hooman Yarmohammadi, MD, Jeffrey L. Sunshine, MD, PhD

KEYWORDS

• Stroke • Intra-arterial • Thrombolysis • Thrombectomy

With more than 700,000 strokes per year resulting in greater than 160,000 deaths per year, stroke remains the leading cause of disability and third leading cause of death in the United States. Despite an overall decline in stroke mortality over the past 40 years, the total number of stroke deaths continues to increase, suggesting an increase in stroke incidence.[1] The last 20 years of neuroscience advances have moved stroke from a condition that is monitored clinically and imaged serially as it evolves to an entity that can be treated acutely with remarkable alterations in its natural history.

IMAGING TRIAGE

Approval from the US Food and Drug Administration (FDA) for the intravenous (IV) administration of the thrombolytic recombinant tissue plasminogen activator (rt-PA) in the treatment of acute ischemic stroke (AIS) requires exclusion of intracranial hemorrhage (ICH) by imaging. Although nonenhanced computed tomography (NECT) is a widely available modality used to exclude ICH in the treatment of AIS, the FDA approval recommends exclusion of ICH by "CT or other diagnostic imaging method similarly sensitive for the presence of hemorrhage."[2] Similarly, the American Heart Association (AHA) Scientific Statement *Guidelines for the*

Early Management of Adults with Ischemic Stroke[3] gives no single recommendation as to what imaging modality should be used. The AHA Scientific Statement *Recommendations for Imaging of Acute Ischemic Stroke*[4] recommends the use of NECT or magnetic resonance (MR) imaging for evaluation of ICH and frank ischemic changes. Furthermore, in patients presenting within 3 hours, the Guidelines state, "there is a suboptimal detection rate of ischemic changes with NECT alone, and a more definitive diagnosis will be obtained with magnetic resonance – diffusion weighted images (MR-DWI) or CT Angiographic-source images (CTA-SI) … if this does not unduly delay the timely administration of tPA." In addition, a vascular study (CTA, MR angiography, digital subtraction angiography [DSA]) is "probably indicated." For patients beyond 3 hours, MR–diffusion-weighted imaging [DWI] or CTA-SI "should be performed along with vascular imaging and perfusion studies, particularly if mechanical thrombectomy or intra-arterial (IA) thrombolytics therapy is contemplated."

Nonenhanced CT has been used as the sole imaging study in the initial evaluation of patients for AIS treatment in multiple landmark trials[5–7] because it has a historical ability to exclude ICH.[8] MR, specifically gradient-echo sequences, is at least as accurate as NECT in the detection of ICH in patients with acute stroke and has

Department of Radiology, University Hospitals – Case Medical Center, 11100 Euclid Avenue, Cleveland, OH 44106, USA
* Corresponding author.
E-mail address: daniel.hsu@uhhospitals.org

Neuroimag Clin N Am 21 (2011) 379–390
doi:10.1016/j.nic.2011.01.005

a 96% concordance with NECT,[9] although an advantage of NECT is seen when evaluating for subarachnoid hemorrhage. In the National Institute of Neurologic Disorders and Stroke (NINDS) rt-PA Stroke Study, NECT showed 31% specificity for signs of early infarction, which is significantly low given an average National Institute of Health Stroke Scale (NIHSS) score of 14.[6] MR-DWI is clearly the most accurate modality and sequence in the evaluation of AIS,[10] with a significant improvement in sensitivity and specificity in the evaluation of stroke when compared with CT (at 6 hours DWI sensitivity/specificity 91%/95% vs NECT 61%/65%).[11]

NECT has been shown to be of diagnostic and prognostic value when a hyperdense middle cerebral artery sign (HMCAS) is present. Both the presence of a hyperdense middle cerebral artery (MCA) and the expected concurrent high NIHSS score are predictors of poor outcomes in acute stroke treatment.[12] The results of a retrospective analysis suggest that intra-arterial therapy (IAT) is more beneficial than IV thrombolytic therapy in patients with HMCAS on NECT images. HMCAS was observed in 55 patients treated with IAT (n = 268) and 57 patients treated with IV therapy (n = 249). The maximum delay time from symptom onset to IV therapy and IAT was 3 hours and 6 hours, respectively. There was no difference between the 2 groups in terms of baseline stroke severity and patient age. Mean time to treatment was longer in the IAT group (244 ± 63 minutes) than in the IV therapy group (156 ± 21 minutes; $P = .0001$). A favorable outcome (modified Rankin scale [mRS score] ≤2) was more frequently observed after IAT (n = 29, 53%) than after IV therapy (n = 13, 23%; $P = .001$). The mortality was also lower in the IAT (n = 4, 7%) than in the IV therapy group (n = 13, 23%; $P = .022$). Results of multiple regression analysis showed that IAT was associated with a more favorable outcome but similar mortality to IV therapy.[13]

Additional triage with vascular and perfusion imaging has many goals. Normal imaging suggests a resolved vascular or nonvascular cause (such as seizure) for presenting symptoms. In the positive imaging examinations, advanced vascular and perfusion imaging helps select for 2 diverging populations. One is the patient with clear large-vessel occlusion and large infarct (>approximately 100 mL). This population has a poor neurologic outcome regardless of whether IV therapy or IAT results in vessel recanalization. A second group is one that displays vascular stenosis or occlusion with ischemic but not infarcted (or not completely infarcted) tissues that would benefit from endovascular intervention.

MR imaging in the evaluation and triage of patients with AIS has been criticized for limited access and long study time; however, it has been shown that MR imaging can be used rapidly and efficiently, resulting in improved patient evaluation.

Ultrafast MR imaging evaluation of AIS consisting of axial T1, T2, fluid-attenuated inversion recovery, DWI, and contrast-enhanced T1 imaging can be performed and interpreted in 15 minutes or less (as defined by the interval between the patient leaving the emergency department and returning).[14] Review of a group of 97 patients with AIS being evaluated for acute intervention was performed by the same group.[15] After clinical evaluation and NECT was performed, preliminary clinical diagnosis (transient ischemic attack [TIA], small vessel ischemic disease, large-vessel ischemic disease) and prescribed treatment (no treatment, IAT, IV therapy, IV therapy/IAT) were tabulated, the patient was sent for ultrafast MR imaging. Twenty-six percent (25/97) of patients had therapy changed from presumptive plan after CT to definitive plan after MR imaging. Of these patients 52% (13/25) had therapy changed from thrombolytic to non-thrombolytic treatment, 20% (5/25) had therapy changed from planned intra-arterial (IA) intervention to IV rt-PA because of perfusion abnormality confined to the basal ganglia and not the suspected large-vessel occlusion, 4% (1/25) had therapy changed from IV rt-PA to IA intervention, and 12% (3/25) of patients had therapy changed from no treatment to IA intervention.

The usefulness of CT perfusion (CTP) in predicting the final infarct volume and clinical outcomes in patients with acute MCA infarction after intra-arterial thrombolysis has been investigated. Results of a retrospective study involving 22 patients with acute MCA occlusion who had IA thrombolysis showed that baseline CTP (CTA source image) lesion volumes are significantly correlated with the final infarct volume ($P = .0002$) and clinical outcome ($P = .01$). The relationship between the baseline and the final volumes was stronger for those patients who had successful recanalization. A progression of the infarct lesion volume was observed in patients without recanalization. All patients (100%) with a baseline perfusion lesion volume more than 100 mL and without recanalization had a poor outcome (mRS score >3). Conversely, most of the patients (77%) with baseline perfusion lesion volume less than 100 mL and complete recanalization had good or fair functional outcome (mRS score ≤3).[16]

Of great interest to the interventionalist is the difference between the window of intervention based on the absolute time of onset and the physiologic time window. In a retrospective study, the outcomes of IAT during an 8- to 24-hour window in 30 patients with stroke (premorbid mRS score 1; mean NIHSS score 13, range 5–22) identified using CTP imaging were reported. IAT was performed only in those patients who had clinically significant salvageable brain tissue (>30% relative cerebral blood volume values) compared with established core infarct (< one-third of the MCA territory). Patients with established infarct core in larger regions than one-third of the MCA territory were not offered endovascular therapy. IAT was performed using intra-arterial thrombolysis (n = 10), mechanical thrombectomy (n = 21), and balloon angioplasty (n = 14); some patients had a combination of treatments. Successful recanalization (Thrombolysis in Myocardial Infarction [TIMI] score 2/3) and symptomatic ICH were observed in 20 (66.7%) and 3 (10%) of the patients, respectively. Seven (23.3%) patients died during hospitalization as a result of procedural complications, disease progression, or associated morbidities. Mean NIHSS score at discharge was 9.5, representing an overall NIHSS 3.5-point improvement from the baseline values. A total of 10 (33.3%) patients died within 3 months of IAT. The mean mRS score of the survivors after 3 months was 3. The results showed the feasibility and potential usefulness of IAT in a select group of patients with stroke with salvageable brain tissue as identified from CTP images well outside the traditional time from onset (**Fig. 1**).[17]

An application of clinical-diffusion mismatch for triage of patients with AIS has also been studied using MR imaging. In a case series of 11 patients with NIHSS score 8 or greater and limited abnormality on the diffusion-weighted images (smaller than 25 cm) beyond 8 hours of symptom onset, endovascular therapy was performed. All the patients underwent reperfusion therapy after between 12 and 24 hours of symptom onset. A successful recanalization was achieved in 8 patients. The mean NIHSS scores at baseline, 24 hours, and 1 week were 14 ± 4, 11 ± 7 and 6 ± 5, respectively. The mean NIHSS score of those patients who had successful recanalization was 8 ± 5 at 24 hours and 4 ± 3 at 1 week. An improvement of 4 points or greater in NIHSS score was observed in all 8 patients who had successful recanalization. None of the patients in this study had an ICH or worsening of the NIHSS score by 4 points or greater (see **Fig. 1**).[18]

In a comparison study of CTP and MR perfusion (MRP) examining core/penumbra mismatch, 47 patients presenting with acute anterior circulation stroke within 9 hours of onset received both CTP and MRP studies within 3 hours of each other;

they were evaluated for criteria used in trial selection: core infarct less than 100 mL, mean transit time (MTT) lesion greater than 2 cm in diameter, and greater than 20% DWI/MTT mismatch.[19] When excluding for lesions that were inadequately visualized on CTP (because of the limited brain coverage that exists with some CTP packages), the correlation of core/penumbra imaging between CTP and MRP for trial selection showed overall agreement of 97.8%.

As the role of IA intervention expands in AIS so will the role of triage imaging. Other than the need to exclude ICH, the role and modality of imaging has not been uniformly defined. This situation will not likely change in the near future because issues such as hardware availability and operator experience and preference will greatly influence what is done at individual centers.

IAT
Chemical Thrombolysis

There is no drug approved by the FDA for IA chemical thrombolysis. The only FDA-approved drug in the treatment of AIS is the IV administration of rt-PA alteplase. Approved in 1996, its indication is to treat acute stroke within 3 hours of onset of ischemic symptoms.

The Phase II Prolyse in Acute Cerebral Thromboembolism (PROACT) trial was the first randomized, double-blind trial to test the safety and recanalization efficacy of IA-targeted delivery of the plasminogen activator agent recombinant prourokinase (r-proUK) versus saline placebo.[20] Inclusion criteria included randomization and treatment within 6 hours of symptom onset, minimum NIHSS score of 4 (with exception made for aphasia or isolated hemianopsia) and age 18 to 85 years. A total of 105 patients progressed to angiography of 1314 patients screened. Forty-six patients were randomized, and after 6 late exclusions, 40 patients with documented M1 or M2 MCA occlusions (TIMI score 0 or 1) were treated. With a 2:1 treatment/placebo protocol, 26 patients received r-proUK 6 mg IA within the thrombus and 14 received placebo of saline IA. Initially, patients received IV heparin after angiographic verification of thrombus. This high-heparin protocol received by the first 16 patients consisted of a 100-IU/kg bolus followed by continuous infusion of 1000 IU/h for 4 hours. After early analysis of these first 16 patients, 8/11 (73%) of those patients treated with r-proUK showed ICH within 24 hours, and a protocol change consisting of a low-heparin regimen was initiated. This low-heparin protocol gave both treatment arms a heparin bolus of 2000 IU IV and a subsequent drip at 500 IU/h for

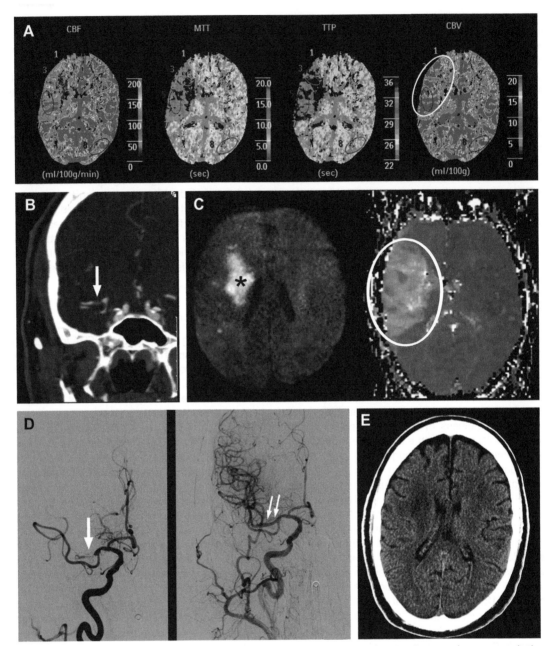

Fig. 1. Patient with 14 hours of partial right MCA syndrome. (*A*) CTP maps showing increased mean transit time (MTT) and time to peak (TTP) and decreased cerebral blood flow within the anterior division of the right MCA territory (*large oval*) and (*B*) CTA showing severe stenosis of the anterior division of the right MCA (*arrow*). Because of comorbid medical conditions, intervention had to be delayed for an additional 12 hours, at which time symptoms abruptly worsened. (*C*) MR-DWI and TTP (now 26 hours after onset of symptoms) show core infarct in the right corona radiata (*) and ischemic penumbra (*oval*). (*D*) DSA images show severely stenotic anterior division right MCA before (*arrow*) and after (*double arrow*) stent placement. (*E*) Three-month follow-up CT scan shows matching gliotic change in region of initial core infarct but preservation of ischemic penumbra with near-complete recovery.

the following 4 hours, although at the price of increased rates of ICH, the concurrent administration of higher-dose IV heparin in PROACT led to increased recanalization rates. Analysis of both

heparin regimens disclosed an overall 42% versus 7% ICH rate favoring placebo, with a reduction to a 15% rate for symptomatic ICH in the combined r-proUK group and no change in the placebo group. Overall recanalization (defined as TIMI score 2 or 3) was 58% for the r-proUK group and 14% for the placebo group. Most importantly, 90-day mortality was reduced from 43% in the placebo group to 27% in the r-proUK arm, and a 10% to 12% absolute increase in excellent neurologic outcome as defined by normal or near normal 90-day functional assessments and NIHSS score.

The use of IA chemical thrombolysis is based largely on the results of the PROACT II trial (Fig. 2).[7] PROACT II was a randomized, controlled trial in which 180 patients (12,323 patients screened) experiencing new, focal neurologic signs in the MCA distribution were randomized to either treatment or control with similar PROACT inclusion criteria. Treatment consisted of the administration of r-proUK 9 mg IA at the site of thrombus over 2 hours. The control patients received no IAT. Both arms received the low-heparin protocol initiated in the PROACT trial.

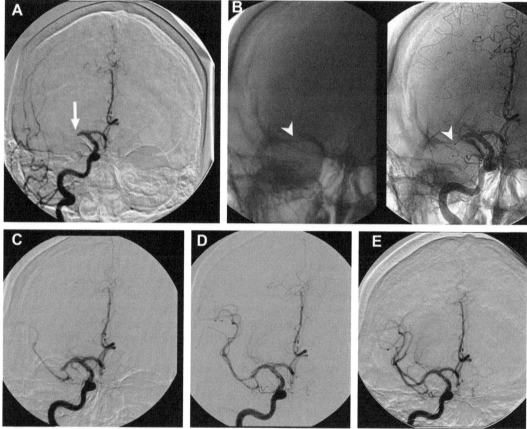

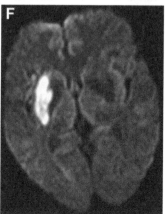

Fig. 2. 37-year-old woman with 1.5 hours of complete right MCA syndrome. (A) DSA right ICA injection with complete M1 occlusion (arrow); (B) microcatheter placed within thrombus (arrowhead). Repeat runs status after placement: (C) 4.5 mg rt-PA, inferior division recanalized; (D) 7 mg rt-PA, middle division recanalized; (E) 12 mg rt-PA, superior division recanalized; (F) MR imaging DWI 48 hours after rt-PA with lentiform nucleus infarction. Patient's neurologic deficits resolved completely within 4 hours of thrombectomy.

Results favored IA treatment with improved recanalization rates (TIMI 2 or 3 flow: 66% treatment, 18% control) and clinical outcome (mRS score 2 or less: 40% treatment, 25% control) but with no significant difference in mortality, which was approximately 25% at 90 days for both groups. In addition, the r-proUK 9 mg IA dose showed improved outcomes compared with the PROACT r-proUK 6 mg dose despite a 4% increase in symptomatic ICH (SICH) when comparing r-proUK-treated PROACT II patients with the low-heparin population in PROACT. The results of PROACT II prompted the AHA Stroke Council to change IA thrombolysis from experimental treatment to an accepted treatment of AIS. The use of r-proUK was widely used until its withdrawal from the US market in 1999.

COMBINED IV THERAPY/IAT

Given that IV lytic therapy can be initiated quickly and in myriad clinical settings, it is not uncommon to have a patient present for IAT with either full or partial dose (0.9 and 0.6 mg/kg, respectively) IV therapy already administered. The Emergency Management of Stroke (EMS) Bridging Trial tested the feasibility, efficacy, and safety of combined IV and IA rt-PA therapy.[21] In this pilot, double-blind, randomized phase I trial, 35 patients presenting with AIS within 3 hours of onset were treated with either IV rt-PA (0.6 mg/kg, 60 mg maximum) or IV placebo. Both groups progressed to cerebral angiography with possible IA rt-PA. Results showed feasibility of combined IV/IA thrombolytic therapy in AIS but failed to show improved clinical outcome.

Proven feasibility but small sample size of the EMS Bridging Trial led to the single-arm, open-label Interventional Management of Stroke (IMS) I and II Studies.[22,23] With the exception of addition of the EKOS microinfusion catheter (EKOS Corporation, Bothell, WA, USA), both trials had identical inclusion criteria of NIHSS score 10 or greater, age 18 to 80 years, and initiation of IV rt-PA within 3 hours of onset. The administration of IV rt-PA in the IMS studies was almost identical to its administration in the EMS trial. After cerebral angiography to confirm occlusion, a microcatheter was placed with its tip distal to clot. rt-PA 2 mg IA was administered followed by an additional 2 mg into the clot itself after catheter repositioning. Through an infusion pump, rt-PA was administered at a rate of 9 mg/h for up to 2 hours with control angiography every 15 minutes, which could be paired with mechanical disruption with the microcatheter. On initial identification of occlusive thrombus, heparin, with a 2000-IU bolus IV and maintenance infusion of 450 IU/h, was administered for the duration of the intervention. IMS I and II enrolled 80 (mean NIHSS score 18) and 81 (mean NIHSS score 18) patients, respectively. Time to initiation of thrombolytic therapy (approximately 140 minutes for both) was longer than the placebo (108 minutes) and IV lytic treatment (90 minutes) arms of the NINDS study, the historical control used as a comparison. Three-month mortality was similar among all groups, although it was numerically lower in IMS I and II. SICH was not statistically significantly different between the IMS I, IMS II, and NINDS treatment arms, although it was numerically higher in IMS II (9.9% vs 6.6% for NINDS IV rt-PA and 1.0% for NINDS placebo). Improved 3-month outcome was seen when IMS treatment arms were compared with the NINDS placebo group. There were no clearly improved outcomes when IMS treatment arms were compared with NINDS rt-PA treatment; however, the odds ratio trended in favor of IMS patients.

A technical note that has come from subset analysis of IMS I and II data is a direct relationship between an increased number of microcatheter injections during IA thrombolysis and ICH.[24]

IMS I and II has evolved to the IMS III trial, which is a phase III trial actively enrolling patients. This randomized, open-label trial will assess standard IV rt-PA therapy alone against combined IV therapy/IAT (chemical and mechanical).[25]

The combined use of IV/IA lytic therapy, with a focus on treatment within 3 hours of symptom onset, has been reported in 3 recent retrospective and prospective case series.[26-28] Although methods for patient selection varied and the IA therapies used varied greatly among the 3 studies and within each study itself, these series showed that IA intervention was feasible within 3 hours and there were improved outcomes in the combined treatment arm. Of the total 186 patients in these studies, improved functional outcomes were seen in a range of 33% to 66% when compared with IV treatment alone. SICH ranged from 0% to 12%.

MECHANICAL THROMBOLYSIS

Mechanical thrombectomy devices, namely the Merci Retrieval System (MRS) (Concentric Medical, Mountain View, CA, USA) and the Penumbra System (PS) (Penumbra, Alameda, CA, USA), have received FDA approval for IA treatment of AIS (Fig. 3).

The MRS was approved by the FDA in August 2004 with an indication to "restore blood flow in the neurovasculature by removing thrombus in patients experiencing AIS. Patients who are

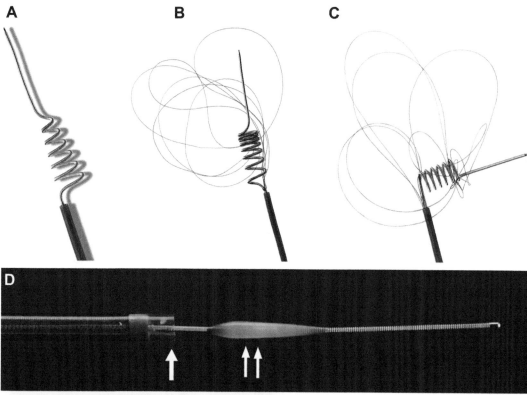

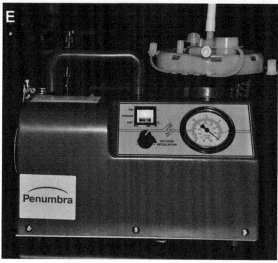

Fig. 3. Merci retrieval devices: (*A*) X, (*B*) L, and (*C*) V series. (*D*) Tip of PS reperfusion catheter (*arrow*) and separator wire (*double arrow*). (*E*) PS aspiration pump.

ineligible for treatment with IV t-PA or who fail IV t-PA are candidates for treatment." An 8-hour time window for treatment was used for initial and subsequent trials; however, a time limit was not included in the FDA approval.

The MRS is a tapered core wire with 5 helical loops at its distal end. The system consists of an 8- or 9-French Merci balloon guide catheter, 2.4-French Merci microcatheter (used to introduce the device), and a Merci Retriever. The

Merci microcatheter is applied through the 8- or 9-French Merci balloon guide catheter and delivered with the tip past the thrombus. The retrieval device is then deployed. The manufacturer recommends deployment of the first 2 to 4 loops of the Merci Retriever approximately 1 to 2 cm distal to the thrombus. The microcatheter and the Merci Retriever are then pulled back along with the thrombus. This procedure is performed under flow reversal achieved by inflating the base balloon occlusion catheter with aspiration performed through the base catheter, which has been placed in the cervical vasculature (Fig. 4). Multiple Merci retrievers are available including the X, L, and V series. The Merci Retriever L and V series differ from the previously cleared X-series devices by the inclusion of a system of arcading filaments attached to a nontapering helical nitinol coil.

The Mechanical Embolus Removal in Cerebral Ischemia (MERCI) trial[29] was a single-arm, multicenter study that consisted of 151 enrolled patients (1809 patients screened) with an NIHSS score of 8 or greater, presenting within 3 to 8 hours or 0 to 3 hours if a contraindication to IV t-PA existed. Treatable vessels in part I of the study were defined by angiography and included the intracranial vertebral artery, basilar artery, intracranial internal carotid artery (ICA) and M1 segment of the MCA, with the addition of the M2 segment of the MCA in Part II. Of the enrolled 151 patients, 10 were excluded for 8 reasons ranging from spontaneous recanalization to anatomy unfavorable for device delivery. Up to 6 passes with the MRS were performed. If TIMI II flow was not restored after the sixth pass of an X-series retriever, it was considered a treatment failure for the device. TIMI II/III flow was established in 46% (69/151) of patients with the embolectomy device. SICH occurred in 7.8% (11/141: 5 subarachnoid hemorrhage [SAH], 6 intraparenchymal hemorrhage) and asymptomatic hemorrhage occurred in an additional 27.7% (39/141). Death, myocardial infarction, or new stroke was seen at 30 days in 40% of all patients (29.9% in those with recanalization, 49.3% not recanalized). Favorable outcome at 90 days with mRS score 2 or less was 27.7% overall (46.0% recanalized, 10.4% not

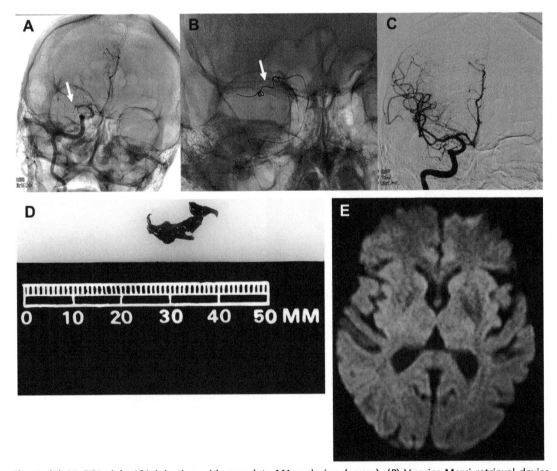

Fig. 4. (A) PA DSA right ICA injection with complete M1 occlusion (arrow). (B) V-series Merci retrieval device deployed across thrombus. Note the distortion of the coil loops surrounding the clot (arrow). (C) Complete thrombectomy and restoration of right MCA flow. (D) Clot removed from patient. (E) 24-hour follow-up MR imaging DWI with no evidence for infarction. The patient had full neurologic recovery at 24 hours.

recanalized) and NIHSS score improvement of 10 points or greater was 32.4% overall (50.0% recanalized, 17.5% not recanalized).

The Multi MERCI trial[30] was designed as an extension of the X-series evaluation performed in the MERCI trial as well as to compare the performance of the newer-generation L series. Although statistical significance was not shown, the overall recanalization rate was higher with the newer-generation when compared with the first-generation retriever and good outcomes trended up, with mortality trending lower.

The PS is a mechanical thrombectomy device that received FDA approval for marketing in 2008 with an indication for use "in the revascularization of patients with AIS secondary to intracranial large-vessel occlusive disease (in the internal carotid, middle cerebral–M1 and M2 segments, basilar and vertebral arteries) within 8 hours of symptom onset."

The PS consists of 3 components: a large-bore reperfusion catheter, a mechanical separator wire, and an aspiration pump. A fourth component, a direct thrombus removal ring, has CE Mark approval in Europe but is not FDA approved. The PS is used by placing the tip of the aspiration catheter within flowing blood at the leading edge of the large-vessel thrombus using a standard microwire technique. After exchange of the microwire for a separator wire, a continuous vacuum supplied by the pump is applied to the aspiration catheter. The separator wire is then continuously advanced and withdrawn through the thrombus as well as the tip of the aspiration catheter. This procedure is performed with the hopes of fragmenting and debulking the thrombus with aspiration into the aspiration pump canister (**Fig. 5**).

The European safety trial for the PS[31] consisted of 23 patients enrolled under an inclusion criteria of clinical signs of ischemic stroke, age 18 years or older, TIMI score of 0 or 1 in a vessel accessible by the PS, and presentation within 8 hours of symptom onset. Twenty-one vessels were treated in 20 patients, with 3 patients not treated because

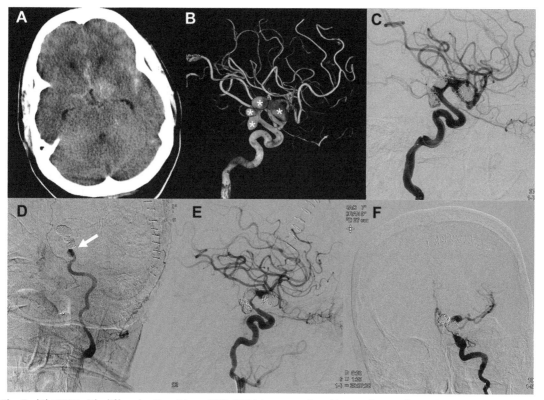

Fig. 5. (*A*) NECT with diffuse basilar cistern SAH. (*B*) Volume-rendered image from a three-dimensional rotational angiogram disclosing 4 saccular aneurysms (*) (fifth aneurysm not identified on this projection) involving the left ICA. (*C*) Status after endovascular treatment of 4 of 5 aneurysms (the fifth could not be treated endovascularly). (*D*) After surgical treatment of the final aneurysm, the patient had right hemiplegia, with emergent angiogram showing complete left ICA occlusion (*arrow*). (*E, F*) Status after PS treatment; flow was restored to the left hemisphere. The PS was felt to be the optimal method for recanalization as a result of recent craniotomy as well as numerous endovascular coil masses in the area of thrombus.

of an inaccessible target vessel. The 20 treated patients had the following demographics before intervention: 8 (40%) were women, mean age 60 ± 18 years, NIHSS score 21± 8, and mRS score of 4.6 ± 0.8. All of the 10 patients who presented within 3 hours of onset were either refractory to or ineligible for IV rt-PA therapy.

In this trial, all patients had successful recanalization to a TIMI score of 2 (48%) or 3 (52%) after use of the PS. Nine patients (45%) did receive adjuvant IA rt-PA after PS use in an attempt to revascularize occlusions distal to the initial thrombus in the patients with a TIMI score of 2.

In the treated patients, 45% (9/20) had either a reduction in NIHSS score of 4 points or greater or an mRS score of 2 or less. A total of 45% (9/20) died within the 30-day follow-up period, with 3 of these 9 experiencing hemorrhagic conversion of infarction and cerebral edema secondary to infarction. SICH (defined as a 4-point deterioration in NIHSS score) occurred in 8 patients. Two procedural adverse events occurred that consisted of a groin hematoma requiring transfusion as well as an arterial perforation that resulted in asymptomatic SAH.

This trial led to the Phase II Penumbra Pivotal Stroke Trial[32] and subsequent FDA approval. Inclusion/exclusion criteria were similar to the preceding safety trial. Of 856 screened patients, 125 were enrolled for treatment and treatment assessment. When compared with the previous safety trial, the patients in the Pivotal trial had a similar age, gender, and mRS profile, but had a slightly less severe mean NIHSS score (17.6 vs 21) as well as a higher percentage of MCA target vessels (70% vs 24%).

After PS intervention, TIMI scores improved from 0 (96%) or 1 (4%) before intervention to a TIMI score of 2 (54%) or 3 (27%) after intervention in 81% of patients. A total of 41.6% achieved an improvement of at least 4 points in NIHSS score and a 30-day mRS score equal to or less than 2. During the course of endovascular treatment, 19 procedural complications were recorded, of which 3 (2.4%) were considered serious. From these serious events, 2 of the patients died. A total of 28% of patients experienced ICH, of whom 14 were symptomatic. At 90 days after treatment, 33% of enrolled patients were dead. Not unlike other studies, predictors of worse outcome included higher baseline NIHSS score, nonrevascularization, and ICA involvement.

STENT PLACEMENT/ANGIOPLASTY FOR STROKE TREATMENT

Despite numerous case reports and retrospective series showing high recanalization rates when using stents for emergency revascularization in AIS (**Fig. 6**),[33,34] there is only 1 FDA-approved trial evaluating stent deployment for the treatment of AIS: the Stent-Assisted Recanalization in Acute Ischemic Stroke (SARIS) trial.[35] Using inclusion criteria that had specific parameters for length of occlusion (<14 mm) as well as parent vessel diameter (<4.5 mm, >2 mm) to account for stent sizing requirements, 20 patients were enrolled (14 women, age 63 ± 18 years, NIHSS score 14 ± 3.8, TIMI score 0: 85%, TIMI score 1: 15%). Nineteen of 20 patients had stents deployed, with 1 patient experiencing recanalization during stent delivery, after control angiography but before stent deployment. Because of the improved flow, the stent and delivery catheter were withdrawn. Of the 19 patients with stents placed (17 with Wingspan Intracranial Stent System [Boston Scientific,

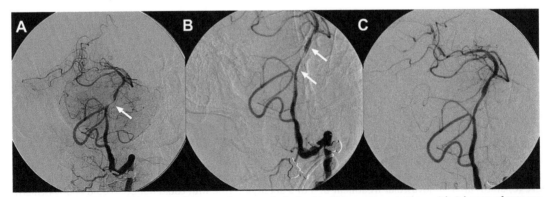

Fig. 6. 52-year-old man with 2-week history of crescendo locked-in TIA now presenting with 2 hours of tetraparesis. (A) Oblique DSA left ventricular artery injection showing a severe basilar artery stenosis (arrow). (B) Status after Wingspan stent placement (arrows showing proximal and distal stent tines). (C) Status after balloon angioplasty.

Fremont, CA, USA], 2 with Enterprise Vascular Reconstruction Devices [Codman Neurovascular, Raynham, MA, USA]), 1 patient had a trial of MER-CI retrieval before definitive stent placement, and 12 patients received additional IATs after stent placement, including antiplatelet agent administration, angioplasty, and thrombolytics.

After intervention, 100% of patients achieved TIMI 2 or 3 flow (40% and 60%, respectively). One-month follow-up showed improved NIHSS score of 4 points or more in 13 (65%) patients, mRS score of 3 or less in 12 patients, and a 25% (5 patients) mortality. Despite maintenance of antiplatelet agents after stent placement, 3 patients experienced ICH, of whom 1 (5%) was symptomatic.

The use of temporary vascular reconstruction devices, which are partially deployed across a thrombus to restore flow and are subsequently retrieved, has been described.[36] In the United States, the use of these devices as well as the use of any off-label humanitarian use device is subject to Humanitarian Device Exemption, FDA Emergency Use Only, and Institutional Review Board regulations.

SUMMARY

The options of and roles for intra-arterial therapies in AIS have grown significantly in recent years. Multiple trials are enrolling patients and many new devices are under FDA review for the treatment of stroke. With the aging US population, there will be no shortage of patients who will benefit from these medical and technological advances in the foreseeable future.

REFERENCES

1. Goldstein LB, Adams R, Alberts MJ, et al. Primary prevention of ischemic stroke: a guideline from the American Heart Association/American Stroke Association Stroke Council: cosponsored by the Atherosclerotic Peripheral Vascular Disease Interdisciplinary Working Group; Cardiovascular Nursing Council; Clinical Cardiology Council; Nutrition, Physical Activity, and Metabolism Council; and the Quality of Care and Outcomes Research Interdisciplinary Working Group: the American Academy of Neurology affirms the value of this guideline. Stroke 2006;37: 1583–633.

2. Available at: http://www.fda.gov/Drugs/Development ApprovalProcess/HowDrugsareDevelopedandApproved/ ApprovalApplications/TherapeuticBiologicApplications/ ucm080430.htm. Accessed June 18, 1996.

3. Adams HP Jr, del Zoppo G, Alberts MJ, et al. Guidelines for the early management of adults with ischemic stroke: a guideline from the American Heart

Association/American Stroke Association Stroke Council, Clinical Cardiology Council, Cardiovascular Radiology and Intervention Council, and the Atherosclerotic Peripheral Vascular Disease and Quality of Care Outcomes in Research Interdisciplinary Working Groups: the American Academy of Neurology affirms the value of this guideline as an educational tool for neurologists. Stroke 2007;38:1655–711.

4. Latchaw RE, Alberts MJ, Lev MH, et al. Recommendations for imaging of acute ischemic stroke: a scientific statement from the American Heart Association. Stroke 2009;40:3646–78.

5. Hacke W, Kaste M, Fieschi C, et al. Intravenous thrombolysis with recombinant tissue plasminogen activator for acute hemispheric stroke. The European Cooperative Acute Stroke Study (ECASS). JAMA 1995;274:1017–25.

6. Tissue plasminogen activator for acute ischemic stroke. The National Institute of Neurological Disorders and Stroke rt-PA Stroke Study Group. N Engl J Med 1995;333:1581–7.

7. Furlan A, Higashida R, Wechsler L, et al. Intra-arterial prourokinase for acute ischemic stroke. The PROACT II study: a randomized controlled trial. Prolyse in Acute Cerebral Thromboembolism. JAMA 1999;282:2003–11.

8. Jacobs L, Kinkel WR, Heffner RR Jr. Autopsy correlations of computerized tomography: experience with 6,000 CT scans. Neurology 1976;26:1111–8.

9. Kidwell CS, Chalela JA, Saver JL, et al. Comparison of MRI and CT for detection of acute intracerebral hemorrhage. JAMA 2004;292:1823–30.

10. Perkins CJ, Kahya E, Roque CT, et al. Fluid-attenuated inversion recovery and diffusion- and perfusion-weighted MRI abnormalities in 117 consecutive patients with stroke symptoms. Stroke 2001;32:2774–81.

11. Fiebach JB, Schellinger PD, Jansen O, et al. CT and diffusion-weighted MR imaging in randomized order: diffusion-weighted imaging results in higher accuracy and lower interrater variability in the diagnosis of hyperacute ischemic stroke. Stroke 2002; 33:2206–10.

12. Tomsick T, Brott T, Barsan W, et al. Prognostic value of the hyperdense middle cerebral artery sign and stroke scale score before ultraearly thrombolytic therapy. AJNR Am J Neuroradiol 1996;17: 79–85.

13. Mattle HP, Arnold M, Georgiadis D, et al. Comparison of intraarterial and intravenous thrombolysis for ischemic stroke with hyperdense middle cerebral artery sign. Stroke 2008;39:379–83.

14. Sunshine JL, Tarr RW, Lanzieri CF, et al. Hyperacute stroke: ultrafast MR imaging to triage patients prior to therapy. Radiology 1999;212:325–32.

15. Heidenreich JO, Hsu D, Wang G, et al. Magnetic resonance imaging results can affect therapy

decisions in hyperacute stroke care. Acta Radiol 2008;49:550–7.

16. Lev MH, Segal AZ, Farkas J, et al. Utility of perfusion-weighted CT imaging in acute middle cerebral artery stroke treated with intra-arterial thrombolysis: prediction of final infarct volume and clinical outcome. Stroke 2001;32:2021–8.

17. Natarajan SK, Snyder KV, Siddiqui AH, et al. Safety and effectiveness of endovascular therapy after 8 hours of acute ischemic stroke onset and wake-up strokes. Stroke 2009;40:3269–74.

18. Janjua N, El-Gengaihy A, Pile-Spellman J, et al. Late endovascular revascularization in acute ischemic stroke based on clinical-diffusion mismatch. AJNR Am J Neuroradiol 2009;30:1024–7.

19. Schaefer PW, Barak ER, Kamalian S, et al. Quantitative assessment of core/penumbra mismatch in acute stroke: CT and MR perfusion imaging are strongly correlated when sufficient brain volume is imaged. Stroke 2008;39:2986–92.

20. del Zoppo GJ, Higashida RT, Furlan AJ, et al. PROACT: a phase II randomized trial of recombinant pro-urokinase by direct arterial delivery in acute middle cerebral artery stroke. PROACT Investigators. Prolyse in Acute Cerebral Thromboembolism. Stroke 1998;29:4–11.

21. Lewandowski CA, Frankel M, Tomsick TA, et al. Combined intravenous and intra-arterial r-TPA versus intra-arterial therapy of acute ischemic stroke: Emergency Management of Stroke (EMS) bridging trial. Stroke 1999;30:2598–605.

22. IMS Study Investigators. Combined intravenous and intra-arterial recanalization for acute ischemic stroke: the Interventional Management of Stroke Study. Stroke 2004;35:904–11.

23. IMS II Trial Investigators. The interventional management of stroke (IMS) II study. Stroke 2007;38:2127–35.

24. Khatri P, Broderick JP, Khoury JC, et al. Microcatheter contrast injections during intra-arterial thrombolysis may increase intracranial hemorrhage risk. Stroke 2008;39:3283–7.

25. Khatri P, Hill MD, Palesch YY, et al. Methodology of the interventional management of stroke III trial. Int J Stroke 2008;3:130–7.

26. Sugiura S, Iwaisako K, Toyota S, et al. Simultaneous treatment with intravenous recombinant tissue plasminogen activator and endovascular therapy for acute ischemic stroke within 3 hours of onset. AJNR Am J Neuroradiol 2008;29:1061–6.

27. Burns TC, Rodriguez GJ, Patel S, et al. Endovascular interventions following intravenous thrombolysis may improve survival and recovery in patients with acute ischemic stroke: a case-control study. AJNR Am J Neuroradiol 2008;29:1918–24.

28. Mathews MS, Sharma J, Snyder KV, et al. Safety, effectiveness, and practicality of endovascular therapy within the first 3 hours of acute ischemic stroke onset. Neurosurgery 2009;65:860–5 [discussion: 865].

29. Smith WS, Sung G, Starkman S, et al. Safety and efficacy of mechanical embolectomy in acute ischemic stroke: results of the MERCI trial. Stroke 2005;36:1432–8.

30. Smith WS, Sung G, Saver J, et al. Mechanical thrombectomy for acute ischemic stroke: final results of the Multi MERCI trial. Stroke 2008;39:1205–12.

31. Bose A, Henkes H, Alfke K, et al. The Penumbra System: a mechanical device for the treatment of acute stroke due to thromboembolism. AJNR Am J Neuroradiol 2008;29:1409–13.

32. Penumbra Pivotal Stroke Trial Investigators. The penumbra pivotal stroke trial: safety and effectiveness of a new generation of mechanical devices for clot removal in intracranial large vessel occlusive disease. Stroke 2009;40:2761–8.

33. Sauvageau E, Samuelson RM, Levy EI, et al. Middle cerebral artery stenting for acute ischemic stroke after unsuccessful Merci retrieval. Neurosurgery 2007;60:701–6 [discussion: 706].

34. Levy EI, Mehta R, Gupta R, et al. Self-expanding stents for recanalization of acute cerebrovascular occlusions. AJNR Am J Neuroradiol 2007;28:816–22.

35. Levy EI, Siddiqui AH, Crumlish A, et al. First Food and Drug Administration-approved prospective trial of primary intracranial stenting for acute stroke: SARIS (stent-assisted recanalization in acute ischemic stroke). Stroke 2009;40:3552–6.

36. Kelly ME, Furlan AJ, Fiorella D. Recanalization of an acute middle cerebral artery occlusion using a self-expanding, reconstrainable, intracranial microstent as a temporary endovascular bypass. Stroke 2008;39:1770–3.

Noninvasive Carotid Artery Imaging with a Focus on the Vulnerable Plaque

V.E.L. Young, MRCS, MPhil*, U. Sadat, MRCS, MPhil,
J.H. Gillard, MD, FRCR, MBA

KEYWORDS

- Carotid • Atherosclerosis • Vulnerable plaque
- Noninvasive imaging

Stroke is the third most common cause of death in the United States, with approximately 795,000 new or recurrent events occurring every year, of which 87% are ischemic.[1] Cerebrovascular events impose a significant health, social, and economic burden, with stroke being a major cause of long-term disability that will account for an estimated $73.7 billion of direct and indirect costs in 2010.[1] Carotid atherosclerosis is a significant risk factor for stroke and transient ischemic attack (TIA), with the annual stroke risk from asymptomatic disease being approximately 1.3% and from symptomatic disease (major stroke) being approximately 9.0%.[2] Therefore, investigation of carotid atherosclerosis, as a treatable and preventable cause of stroke, is important in the reduction of this burden.

Current practice in carotid atherosclerosis is to treat either medically or surgically based on the degree of stenosis present and the symptoms. In symptomatic individuals, 3 large randomized controlled trials (North American Symptomatic Carotid Endarterectomy Trial [NASCET], European Carotid Surgery Trial [ESCT], and the Veteran Affairs Cooperative Program Trial) have shown the benefit of carotid endarterectomy compared with medical management in patients with high-grade stenosis (70%–99%).[3–5] In patients with mild degrees of stenosis (<50% NASCET) the risk/benefit ratio was in favor of medical management. It has also been shown that there is no benefit of operating on individuals who have near occlusive disease.[6] Some benefit for operative intervention in symptomatic individuals with moderate stenosis (50%–69%) was seen.[3,4,6] The risk of recurrent events following TIA has been shown to be as high as 9% within the first 7 days, which has led to a more aggressive surgical strategy, designed to treat individuals with operative disease within 2 weeks of symptom onset.[7]

For those patients with asymptomatic carotid disease the decision on when to operate is less clear. The Asymptomatic Carotid Atherosclerosis Study (ACAS) and the Asymptomatic Carotid Surgery Trial (ACST) randomized patients between medical therapy and carotid endarterectomy (>60% stenosis in ACAS, >70% in ACST) with a similar lower rate of stroke/death in the surgical cohort.[8,9] A more recent review of more than 5000 cases of carotid endarterectomy for asymptomatic disease showed a similar stroke rate between medical therapy and carotid endarterectomy, with no definite advantage of surgery.[10]

Interest in imaging of carotid atheroma is now shifting from focusing on luminal stenosis to identification of the vulnerable plaque. This shift is

Funding: Research studies in this department are supported by a National Institute of Health Research Cambridge Biomedical Research Centre grant.
Conflicts of interests: Professor Gillard acts as a consultant for Glaxo-Smith Kline, Bayer Schering and Guerbet.
University Department of Radiology, Addenbrookes Hospital, Box 218, Hills Road, Cambridge CB2 0QQ, UK
* Corresponding author.
E-mail address: vy207@cam.ac.uk

Neuroimag Clin N Am 21 (2011) 391–405
doi:10.1016/j.nic.2011.01.006
1052-5149/11/$ – see front matter © 2011 Elsevier Inc. All rights reserved.

a result of the greater understanding of the pathogenesis of the disease and the acknowledgment that strokes can still occur in populations not considered suitable for surgical management in the previously mentioned studies (eg, 30%–49% stenosis).[6] Also, some patients identified as appropriate surgical candidates using the criteria of degree of stenosis may have clinically/pathologically stable disease. This concept of a vulnerable plaque is not new, with the phrase having been originally introduced by Muller and colleagues[11] in 1985 in relation to studies of coronary artery disease. This concept has been applied to other vascular territories affected with atherosclerosis, but it is only recently that noninvasive imaging of plaque has become possible, and the carotid artery is far more amenable to this than the coronary artery.

LUMINAL IMAGING

Although digital subtraction angiography (DSA) is still the gold standard for assessing the degree of stenosis in carotid atherosclerosis, because of the risks associated with an interventional procedure,[12] most patients are now investigated and managed based on noninvasive methods that have compared well with DSA.[13–15]

Ultrasound

The most widely available and used method for assessing carotid disease is ultrasound (US). It is an established and inexpensive technique with proven accuracy.[14] Two methods of US are commonly used for assessment of carotid disease (B-mode and Doppler ultrasound [DUS]), and these are often combined. B-mode US allows visualization of the lumen and the vessel wall so that luminal diameters may be assessed (**Fig. 1**). DUS relies on measurement of blood velocity in the vessel to calculate the degree of stenosis (**Fig. 2**). Although studies have shown the accuracy of DUS, there are limitations to the technique: it is operator dependent,[16] subject to artifacts in calcified disease (see **Fig. 1**), and inaccurate in distinguishing near occlusion.[17] However, even with these limitations, sensitivities and specificities compare well with the other imaging modalities.[18] It is particularly useful as an exclusionary examination before proceeding onto more costly imaging modalities.[19]

Computed Tomography Angiography

Computed tomography angiography (CTA) is a popular noninvasive method of carotid imaging. It allows for rapid imaging and a large anatomic coverage, from the arch of the aorta to the circle of Willis. It is also minimally invasive, requiring only peripheral venous injection of iodinated contrast media. Axial source images can be postprocessed in several ways (eg, maximal intensity projections [MIPs], multiplanar reformatting) to produce a three-dimensional (3D) angiogram. CTA is well tolerated as an investigation by patients, but there are some disadvantages. CTA involves ionizing radiation, which means it is less desirable for repeated/follow-up examinations. CTA is highly specific, but is arguably the least sensitive of the noninvasive methods for assessing luminal stenosis compared with DSA[14]; however, comparisons have shown a good level of agreement with DUS.[20] Another issue can be the method of measurement. For example, when stenotic measurements taken as diameters from DSA were compared with area measurements from CTA, CTA tended to underestimate the degree of stenosis.[21] There can also be issues with heavy calcification where assessment of the degree of stenosis is obscured by the calcification, although image processing methods may alleviate this problem (**Fig. 3**).[22] CTA can also be used to detect other plaque features such as ulceration, which is evidence of vulnerable disease.[23]

Magnetic Resonance Angiography

Contrast-enhanced magnetic resonance angiography (CE-MRA) is gaining in popularity because of the high sensitivity and specificity that has been shown compared with DSA; it is arguably the best of the noninvasive modalities,[14] and the multimodal approach of DUS and CE-MRA

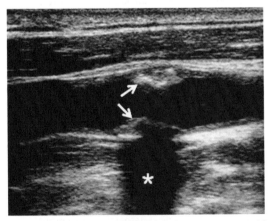

Fig. 1. B-mode US image of the right common carotid artery in longitudinal section showing plaque in the vessel wall encroaching on the lumen and causing a nonsignificant degree (<50%) of stenosis (*white arrows*). The plaque is calcified causing hypoechoic shadows (*white asterisk*).

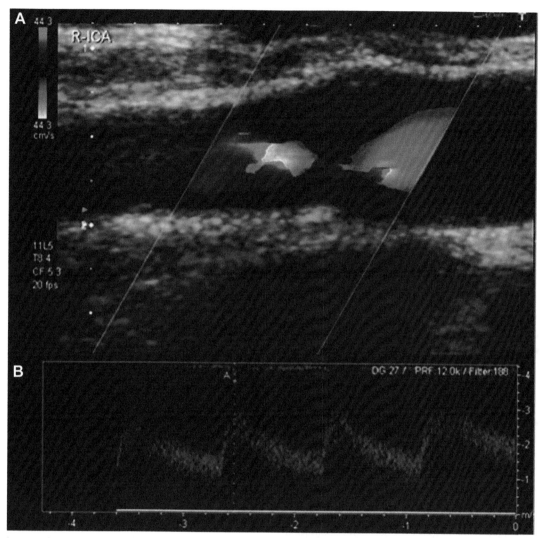

Fig. 2. Color DUS of the right internal carotid artery illustrating a stenosis of greater than 85%. The color Doppler shows a velocity of 375 cm/s (*A*) and a damped Doppler waveform (*B*).

enhances the already high sensitivity/specificity.[24] Combined with this good diagnostic performance, the cost-effectiveness compared with DSA makes it an attractive imaging option.[25] However, in some centers, because magnetic resonance (MR) is not as accessible as US or CTA, it is not the imaging method of choice. Several different methods have been used in different clinical trials for measuring degree of stenosis. When comparing these methods for CE-MRA and DSA, the NASCET criteria performed most consistently between the 2 examinations and therefore is the most appropriate method of assessing CE-MRA images.[26] Like CTA, this is a minimally invasive technique that produces high-quality images with a large anatomic coverage (Fig. 4), with the added advantage of no ionizing radiation.

Unenhanced MRA can also be performed, usually as time-of flight (TOF) imaging, which can be either a two-dimensional (2D) slice or 3D volumetric acquisition. Both acquisitions can be viewed in a slice or a MIP format. Although this method has the benefit of no contrast administration, there are issues with the diagnostic quality of this technique. In general, unenhanced TOF MRA has shown better diagnostic accuracy than CTA compared with DSA but has a tendency to overestimate the degree of stenosis.[27] Furthermore, it cannot reliably distinguish near occlusion from occlusion when there is no flow-related enhancement within the internal carotid artery.[28] In addition, T1 hyperintense thrombus can give the appearance of luminal patency, although on 3D TOF imaging it has been proposed that the halo sign

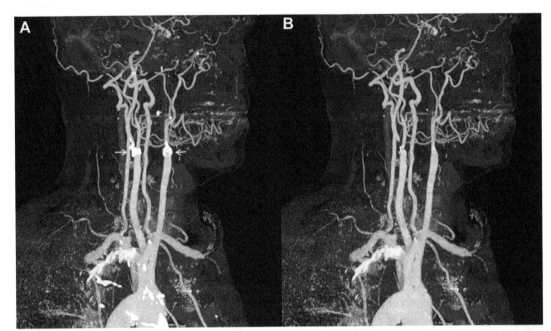

Fig. 3. Patient with severe (>70%) right internal carotid artery stenosis and an occluded left internal carotid artery with overlying heavily calcified plaque at both carotid bifurcations shown on the computer tomography angiogram. The images have been processed to show the stenosis with (A) (arrow) and without the calcification (B).

may indicate the presence of wall thrombus.[29] Flow artifacts can also affect the diagnostic quality of the images.

PLAQUE IMAGING

As the understanding of atherosclerosis as a disease process has evolved, the focus has moved from simple measurement of stenosis to considering the importance of plaque composition, biologic markers, and biomechanical properties. These factors are key to the concept of vulnerable plaque versus stable disease and are all believed to be linked to developing disease and eventual translation from subclinical to symptomatic disease.

Morphologic Imaging

Pathologic studies have shown that atheromatous disease can undergo outward remodeling that can lead to a significant disease burden being present with limited luminal compromise.[30] Other features that have been identified as making a plaque more vulnerable are a large, lipid-rich necrotic core; a thin or ruptured fibrous cap; plaque ulceration; and the presence of intraplaque hemorrhage.[31,32] In the coronary artery, the presence of calcified nodules is an accepted criterion for vulnerable disease.[33] In contrast, in the carotid artery, it is not the presence of calcification that is believed to affect

plaque but its location within the plaque, with calcium deposits within a thin fibrous cap increasing maximal plaque wall stresses compared with deposits at other locations that have little effect.[34,35]

US

US has been used in 3 different ways to try to assess plaque vulnerability: assessment of plaque echogenicity, measurement of intima media thickness (IMT), and contrast-enhanced US. Contrast-enhanced US is used to assess pathologic processes and is discussed later.

Carotid plaque echolucency on B-mode US, using a method called median gray scale (GSM), has been related to both clinically symptomatic disease and the presence of cerebral infarction on CT.[36–38] Comparison with histologic specimens has shown that plaques that have a low GSM on US histologically have high-risk features such as high lipid and hemorrhage content.[39] Echogenicity seems to be a risk factor for symptoms independently of the degree of stenosis present[40] and seems to be an indicator of risk in individuals who have experienced silent nonlacunar cerebral infarcts.[41] Low GSM (<25) has also been linked to increased risk of stroke with carotid stenting procedures.[42,43] IMT, an early measure of carotid atherosclerotic disease, has been correlated with the presence of plaque, but the direct link to stroke/TIA is not as clear.[43,44] However, recent

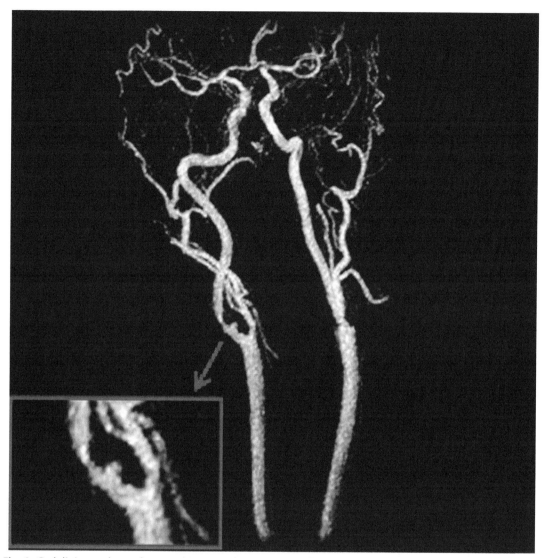

Fig. 4. Gadolinium-enhanced magnetic resonance angiogram of carotid and cerebral arteries showing ulcerated atheromatous plaque affecting the right internal carotid artery. The enlarged section (*arrow*) demonstrates the ulcerated plaque distal to the carotid bifurcation.

work in patients with coronary disease undergoing carotid assessment has indicated that the combination of both IMT and echogenicity of the internal carotid artery could be of value in prediction of coronary risk.[45] Furthermore, IMT in the common carotid artery and Framingham Risk Score independently predicted carotid artery atherosclerotic plaque formation at 5 years, in initially disease-free internal, external, or common carotid arteries, in a population-based longitudinal study of 1922 patients.[46]

High-resolution magnetic resonance imaging
High-resolution magnetic resonance imaging (MRI) has been used to show plaque features with favorable comparison with histology.

Angiographic TOF images are acquired to localize the disease-affected section of the vessel, then multicontrast imaging (T1-weighted, T2-weighted, and proton density–weighted images) are acquired through this segment at matched slice locations (**Fig. 5**). Short tau inversion recovery (STIR) images can also provide a benefit in plaque characterization by showing a distinct signal difference between fibrous cap and lipid core. Review of these images then allows the plaque morphology to be identified (**Table 1**),[47,48] and a modified version of the American Heart Association (AHA) plaque classification has been created for MRI.[49] Morphologic imaging has allowed plaque characteristics to be assessed in mild (<50% stenosis)

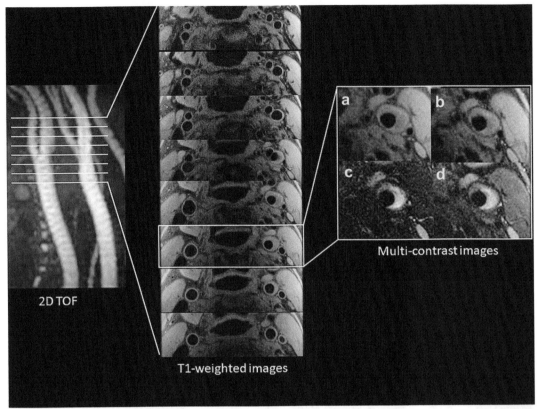

Fig. 5. A 2D TOF MR angiogram (*left of image*) has been used to prescribe high-resolution axial T1-weighted images (*middle*) through the carotid bifurcations that show a 50% carotid stenosis in the left common and internal carotid arteries. Multicontrast MRI, shown for 1 slice location, illustrate that this is a mainly fibrotic plaque, so most of the plaque, particularly on the luminal side, is isointense on T1-weighted (a) and proton density–weighted (b) images and hyperintense on T2-weighted (c) and STIR images (d), and is therefore likely to be stable disease.

to moderate (50%–69% stenosis) disease, for which previously there was little information because surgical intervention is not offered.[50] At this earlier stage of disease, hemorrhage and larger lipid core have been independently shown to be associated with thin/ruptured fibrous caps, all markers of vulnerable disease.[51] The rate of vulnerable lesions (AHA type VI) at mild levels of stenosis seems to be much higher than was generally appreciated (29.8% prevalence in arteries with a stenosis of 49% or less, increasing with degree of stenosis).[52] The advantages of this method of MRI have been exploited to perform longitudinal assessments of disease progression and to assess

Table 1
MR classification of plaque components

		T1-Weighted	T2-Weighted	Proton Density–Weighted	STIR	Contrast-enhanced T1-Weighted
Lipid-rich Necrotic Core		—	—/↑	—/↓	—/↑	↓	↓
Fibrous Tissue		—	—/↑	—	—	↑	↑
Hemorrhage	Fresh	↑	↓	↓	↓	—
	Recent	↑	↑	↑	↑	—
Calcification		—	↓	↓	↓	↓	↓

evolution of disease characteristics such as hemorrhage,[53] as well as to monitor responses to pharmacologic intervention.[54] Multiple features of vulnerability, as detected by high-resolution imaging, have been linked to symptoms, compared with asymptomatic counterparts: presence of thrombus, large lipid core, thin/ruptured fibrous cap, and type VI lesions.[55,56]

Addition of other sequences can aid plaque characterization. One sequence proposed to aid in the diagnosis of vulnerable plaque is a gradient echo sequence termed direct thrombus imaging, which has been used to show high signal in symptomatic disease compared with contralateral asymptomatic vessels, suggesting that it may be a method of identifying vulnerable plaque.[57] Diffusion-weighted imaging (DWI) is another method that has been proposed to aid the delineation of plaque components in unenhanced imaging. Ex vivo imaging indicated that DWI provided the best method for separating lipid from other tissue types.[58] The first in vivo carotid study has shown promising results for using apparent diffusion coefficient (ADC) values derived from DWI for distinguishing lipid (lower ADC) and fibrous tissue.[59]

The addition of gadolinium contrast media greatly enhances the differentiation of fibrous tissue (more enhancement) and lipid on morphologic MRI.[60] By using this technique, one study found that the incidence of vulnerable plaque was significantly higher in nonoperable disease (by stenosis criteria) than in the severely stenotic lesions.[61] One of the issues that has kept plaque MRI in the research rather than clinical setting has been the lengthy imaging times. Comparison of the number of sequences needed for classification found that there was good agreement between plaque classification using 3 sequences (T1-weighted, contrast-enhanced T1-weighted, and TOF) and 5 sequences (T1-weighted, contrast-enhanced T1-weighted, T2-weighted, proton density–weighted, TOF), which would reduce the imaging time.[62]

Imaging of Pathologic Processes

Further risk stratification for future clinical sequelae from carotid atherosclerosis can be made by imaging the pathophysiology of the disease. Two disease processes with the potential to be imaged are plaque neovascularization and inflammation. Initially lipoproteins aggregate in the vessel wall and become oxidized, triggering the production of endothelial molecules and activation of endothelial receptors, causing monocytes to be recruited into the vessel wall.[63] The monocytes develop into activated macrophages

that ingest the lipoproteins and then transform into foam cells, creating the lipid-rich necrotic core.[64] This process provides the inflammatory component of atherosclerosis. As the plaque expands, the oxygen demand increases, leading to the formation of neovessels from the vasa vasorum extending into the plaque. This process has been linked to inflammation and may be a route by which inflammatory cells enter.

Neovascularization

Both MRI and contrast-enhanced ultrasound (CEUS) have been used to image this process. CEUS uses gas-filled microbubbles injected intravenously, which have a different echogenicity to soft tissue. Their general structure consists of a hydrophilic microbubble shell (commonly albumin or lipid) with an echogenic gas core such as perfluorocarbon or nitrogen.

Several studies have been conducted in the past few years using CEUS to examine plaque neovascularization. Comparison of imaging with histologic specimens from subjects who underwent carotid endarterectomy showed that those plaques with enhancement had a significantly higher vasa vasorum density than those without an enhancement pattern; the plaques that enhanced the most were also more echolucent.[65,66] It has been suggested that CEUS could be used as a method for plaque risk stratification because it has been found that symptomatic plaques enhanced significantly more than asymptomatic plaques (n = 104, 35 symptomatic).[67]

MRI using gadolinium chelates provides information on plaque neovascularization in addition to plaque composition and luminal information. MRI can be used to image neovascularization in 1 of 2 ways: delayed[60] or dynamic imaging.[68] Areas of plaque that strongly enhance on delayed T1-weighted imaging have a good correlation with the histologic presence of neovascularization.[60]

The feasibility of dynamic contrast-enhanced MRI (DCE-MRI) for human carotid imaging was first proposed in 1999[69] and later pursued further, imaging with dedicated phased array coils, using a spoiled gradient echo sequence without cardiac gating, giving a temporal resolution of 15 seconds.[68] Fractional blood volume was used to assess the images, and measurements were higher in the areas that correlated to the presence of microvessels on histology. Later work used K^{Trans} and Vp as metrics of neovascularization derived from the DCE-MR.[70] These metrics are widely used in the main application of DCE, namely tumors. K^{Trans} and Vp measurements correlated not only with the presence of neovascularization on histology but also macrophages, suggesting a link between neovascularization and inflammation.[70,71] K^{Trans} was also found to correlate with clinical parameters, with measurements being higher in smokers than nonsmokers,[70] and K^{Trans} being significantly higher in patients requiring carotid endarterectomy than in those with moderate stenosis.[71] Several different gadolinium agents are available and comparison of 2 indicated that, although measurements are similar, K^{Trans} values do differ between agents, and this should be considered when comparing results.[72]

Inflammation

Three different methods have been used to image inflammation: CEUS, positron emission tomography (PET), and MRI. The microbubbles used for CEUS are phagocytosed by monocytes but remain acoustically active for up to 30 minutes. Therefore, late-phase US imaging has been used to assess whether microbubbles can potentially detect inflammation in vivo. Greater enhancement was seen in symptomatic compared with asymptomatic plaques but no histology was available to determine whether inflammation was present.[73]

PET using ^{18}F-fluorodeoxyglucose (FDG) has been widely used for showing inflammation. It uses radiolabeled glucose to highlight areas of increased glucose consumption, such as inflammation. However, this is nonspecific because it shows all areas of increased glucose uptake. The other disadvantage of PET imaging is that it has a low resolution; so images need to be coregistered to CT or MRI to accurately identify the anatomic site of tracer uptake.[74] However, using combined FDG-PET/CT imaging has shown good detection of vascular inflammation compared with histology,[75] with good reproducibility.[76] It has also shown that symptomatic lesions had a higher level of inflammation compared with contralateral asymptomatic disease (n = 6).[75] FDG-PET of recently symptomatic patients (TIA), examining target lesions identified at angiography, found that the suspicious lesion identified at angiography may not always be the lesion that causes symptoms. For 3/12 cases, the target lesions had low uptake, but other nonstenotic lesions in the appropriate territory for the symptoms had high uptake, suggesting that these vulnerable plaques were more likely causative lesions.[77] PET/CT combined with multicontrast MRI has correlated the findings of inflammatory change with lipid burden within carotid plaque, a previously mentioned vulnerable feature.[78]

MRI for inflammation uses ultrasmall paramagnetic iron oxides (USPIOs). USPIOs have been used both in animal and human studies to show the presence of macrophages, and thereby inflammation, within carotid plaque.[79–82] USPIOs are nanoparticles (typically approximately 50 nm in diameter, containing iron oxide particles within a dextran or siloxane coat) that become incorporated within the macrophages that are then taken up into the inflammatory atherosclerotic plaque. To allow time for this process and maximize the uptake within the plaque, imaging after contrast administration is delayed to an optimal time window; one study showed this to be 24 to 48 hours in human carotid MRI for ferumoxtran-10.[83] On postcontrast imaging, USPIOs act as a negative contrast medium by decreasing T2 relaxation and creating areas of signal loss on T2- and T2*-weighted imaging.

Examination of plaque inflammation, as shown by USPIO uptake, and degree of luminal stenosis found no correlation between the 2 measurements, suggesting that they are likely to be independent risk factors for stroke.[84] From a morphologic point of view, USPIO uptake was detected in most (27/36) of the plaques that had ruptured or were rupture prone, but in only 1 of the 14 plaques that had a stable morphologic configuration, suggesting a relationship between inflammation and vulnerability.[85] In a comparison of symptomatic and asymptomatic disease, USPIO uptake was significantly higher in symptomatic plaques, suggesting that symptomatic disease was more inflammatory and asymptomatic disease more stable.[86] However, inflammation was still seen in the contralateral, asymptomatic side of individuals who had experienced carotid-related symptoms even though generally the inflammation was to a lesser extent and the stenosis was to a lower degree,[87] similar to the findings of the PET studies.[75,88] Comparison of contralateral asymptomatic disease, in symptomatic individuals, with truly asymptomatic disease, found that even truly asymptomatic disease showed inflammation, although to a lesser extent than other disease, but this evidence suggests that there may be a case for monitoring and treating asymptomatic disease.[89]

The use of USPIO imaging has taken the application of carotid imaging a stage further by monitoring the short-term response to therapy in the ATHEROMA study.[90] Forty-seven patients with carotid stenosis underwent USPIO-enhanced MRI and were randomized to high- or low-dose atorvastatin (80 or 10 mg). A significant reduction in plaque inflammation, as shown by signal loss with USPIO, was seen at 12 weeks, showing that this type of imaging can be used to assess response to therapy in a short time period (Fig. 6).

PET and MRI use different methodologies but a good concordance has been shown between

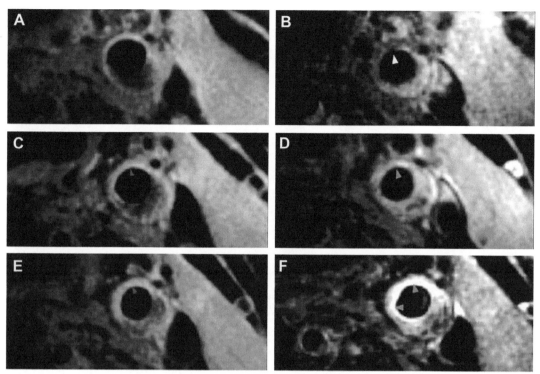

Fig. 6. Example of a patient from the ATHEROMA study who was receiving a high dose and was imaged 3 times with USPIO at 0 (*A, B*), 6 (*C, D*) and 12 (*E, F*) weeks. T_2*-weighted imaging of a left common carotid artery before (*A, C, E*) and after (*B, D, F*) USPIO infusion clearly show USPIO uptake in the plaque at baseline (*yellow arrowhead in B*) with no residual USPIO remaining before reimaging (*red arrowhead in C and E*). The plaque begins to enhance at 6 weeks (*blue arrowhead in D*) and at 12 weeks there is no evidence of signal voids (*blue arrowheads in F*), indicating little USPIO uptake and therefore minimal inflammation. (*Reprinted from* Tang TY, Howarth SP, Miller SR, et al. The ATHEROMA (Atorvastatin therapy: effects on reduction of macrophage activity) study. Evaluation using ultrasmall superparamagnetic iron oxide-enhanced magnetic resonance imaging in carotid disease. J Am Coll Cardiol 2009;53(22):2046, copyright 2009; with permission from Elsevier.)

the two modalities for detecting inflammation (**Fig. 7**).[91] Both PET and USPIO imaging have shown that inflammatory disease is associated with a higher microemboli count to the brain (a surrogate marker of cerebrovascular disease), as detected by transcranial DUS compared with noninflammatory disease, indicating that inflammatory disease may be associated with a higher risk of future events.[90,92] The administration of high-dose, short-term (12 weeks) statin therapy reduced the microemboli counts in inflammatory disease, as detected by USPIO on MRI, compared with baseline counts, suggesting that statin therapy may, even in such a short time, not only reduce plaque inflammation, but also lead to some degree of plaque stabilization.[90]

Biomechanics and Imaging

An application of imaging that is becoming more widely accepted in the assessment of vulnerable plaque is biomechanical modeling of plaque stresses. The opportunity to apply this idea in vivo to individuals arose with the information provided by MRI. Two types of stresses have been proposed as being important in atherosclerosis: mechanical stress and wall shear stress, both of which can be derived from MR imaging.[93,94] Although it has been suggested that shear stress may have a role in initiation of atherosclerosis and plaque development, modeling-based MRI of plaque morphology and flow indicates that mechanical stress is more likely to play a role in plaque rupture.[93] Stresses on the fibrous caps of ruptured plaques (defined on MRI) are higher than those on the fibrous caps of unruptured plaques.[95] The location of calcification within the plaque also affects the stresses, with calcification that is within the fibrous cap causing the maximal plaque stress.[34] Furthermore, MRI-based modeling has shown that maximal predicted plaque stresses in symptomatic patients are higher than those in asymptomatic patients, suggesting that plaques with higher stresses may be more rupture prone.[96,97] Inflammation may also

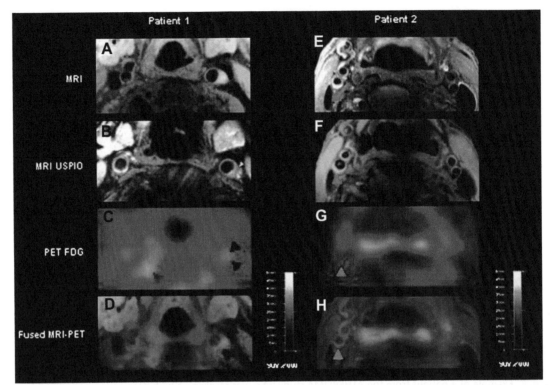

Fig. 7. Axial MRI and PET images of patients with and without carotid artery inflammation. Patient 1 shows signal loss on MRI after USPIO administration (*yellow arrowheads* in *B*) with matching high uptake of FDG into the plaque (*blue arrows in C* and *D*) consistent with carotid wall inflammation, and there is also contralateral vertebral artery inflammation (*purple arrows* in *C* and *D*). In patient 2, no change of MRI signal and no increased FDG uptake are seen (*green arrows* in *E–H*), therefore there is no evidence of inflammatory disease. (*Reprinted from* Tang TY, Moustafa RR, Howarth SP, et al. Combined PET-FDG and USPIO-enhanced MR imaging in patients with symptomatic moderate carotid artery stenosis. Eur J Vasc Endovasc Surg 2009;36(1):54, copyright 2008; with permission.)

add to this complex picture, leading to plaque rupture; imaging with USPIO of carotid atheroma combined with biomechanical modeling has shown that maximal stresses are congruent with sites of inflammation in the plaque.[98] Furthermore, biomechanical stress simulations have been used to study plaque evolution in patients with TIA; fresh plaque hemorrhage was associated with 30% higher maximum critical stress than chronic plaque hemorrhage in one study.[99]

FUTURE DEVELOPMENTS

As more is understood about the pathogenesis of atherosclerosis, the future strategy will be to target imaging at a much earlier stage of the pathogenesis. This method is being explored with both PET and MRI in the form of molecular imaging. Several parts of the atherosclerotic pathway have been suggested as possible targets for vulnerable disease, but most potential agents are still being explored in animal models.[100] Some

of the many potential targets include adhesion molecules (VCAM-1 and E-selectin),[101,102] high-density lipoprotein,[103] macrophages,[104] apoptosis,[105] collagen,[106] thrombus,[107] and matrix metalloproteases.[108]

As well as development of future agents, application of the previously mentioned techniques on a larger scale is required. The BioImage Study is attempting to image subclinical carotid, coronary, and aortic disease with CTA, PET, and CE-MRI.[109]

SUMMARY

Current treatment guidelines are based on assessing carotid atherosclerosis for degree of luminal stenosis, which can be done to a high degree of sensitivity and specificity noninvasively, negating the need for invasive imaging in most cases. US provides a good exclusionary test, with CTA and MRA providing a more accurate measure to guide definitive management. Imaging is now evolving to provide an assessment of plaque characteristics to aid in the risk stratification of patients following the introduction of the concept of the vulnerable plaque. Future imaging developments are attempting to target the disease in a more specific way and at an earlier stage of pathogenesis.

ACKNOWLEDGMENTS

We are grateful to Tjun Tang, Martin Graves, Dr Elizabeth Warburton, Dr Peter Martin, Peter Kirkpatrick, Rikin Trivedi, Dr Nagui Antoun, Dr Justin Cross, Dr Nicholas Higgins, Ilse Joubert, Iain Sellars, and Dr Zhi-Yong Li for their help and collaboration.

REFERENCES

1. Association AH. Heart disease and stroke statistics - 2010 Update. Dallas (TX): American Heart Association; 2010.

2. Wilterdink JL, Easton JD. Vascular event rates in patients with atherosclerotic cerebrovascular disease. Arch Neurol 1992;49(8):857–63.

3. Beneficial effect of carotid endarterectomy in symptomatic patients with high-grade carotid stenosis. North American Symptomatic Carotid Endarterectomy Trial Collaborators. N Engl J Med 1991;325(7):445–53.

4. MRC European Carotid Surgery Trial: interim results for symptomatic patients with severe (70–99%) or with mild (0–29%) carotid stenosis. European Carotid Surgery Trialists' Collaborative Group. Lancet 1991;337(8752):1235–43.

5. Mayberg MR, Wilson SE, Yatsu F, et al. Carotid endarterectomy and prevention of cerebral ischemia in symptomatic carotid stenosis. Veterans Affairs Cooperative Studies Program 309 Trialist Group. JAMA 1991;266(23):3289–94.

6. Rothwell PM, Gutnikov SA, Warlow CP. Reanalysis of the final results of the European Carotid Surgery Trial. Stroke 2003;34(2):514–23.

7. Ois A, Gomis M, Rodriguez-Campello A, et al. Factors associated with a high risk of recurrence in patients with transient ischemic attack or minor stroke. Stroke 2008;39(6):1717–21.

8. Halliday A, Mansfield A, Marro J, et al. Prevention of disabling and fatal strokes by successful carotid endarterectomy in patients without recent neurological symptoms: randomised controlled trial. Lancet 2004;363(9420):1491–502.

9. Moore WS, Young B, Baker WH, et al. Surgical results: a justification of the surgeon selection process for the ACAS trial. The ACAS Investigators. J Vasc Surg 1996;23(2):323–8.

10. Woo K, Garg J, Hye RJ, et al. Contemporary results of carotid endarterectomy for asymptomatic carotid stenosis. Stroke 2010;41(5):975–9.

11. Muller JE, Stone PH, Turi ZG, et al. Circadian variation in the frequency of onset of acute myocardial infarction. N Engl J Med 1985;313(21):1315–22.

12. Dawkins AA, Evans AL, Wattam J, et al. Complications of cerebral angiography: a prospective analysis of 2,924 consecutive procedures. Neuroradiology 2007;49(9):753–9.

13. Heiserman JE, Dean BL, Hodak JA, et al. Neurologic complications of cerebral angiography. AJNR Am J Neuroradiol 1994;15(8):1401–7 [discussion: 8–11].

14. Wardlaw JM, Chappell FM, Best JJ, et al. Non-invasive imaging compared with intra-arterial angiography in the diagnosis of symptomatic carotid stenosis: a meta-analysis. Lancet 2006;367(9521): 1503–12.

15. Barth A, Arnold M, Mattle HP, et al. Contrast-enhanced 3-D MRA in decision making for carotid endarterectomy: a 6-year experience. Cerebrovasc Dis 2006;21(5–6):393–400.

16. Mathiesen EB, Joakimsen O, Bonaa KH. Intersonographer reproducibility and intermethod variability of ultrasound measurements of carotid artery stenosis: the Tromso Study. Cerebrovasc Dis 2000; 10(3):207–13.

17. Lubezky N, Fajer S, Barmeir E, et al. Duplex scanning and CT angiography in the diagnosis of carotid artery occlusion: a prospective study. Eur J Vasc Endovasc Surg 1998;16(2):133–6.

18. Blakeley DD, Oddone EZ, Hasselblad V, et al. Noninvasive carotid artery testing. A meta-analytic review. Ann Intern Med 1995;122(5):360–7.

19. Saleem MA, Sadat U, Walsh SR, et al. Role of carotid duplex imaging in carotid screening programmes - an overview. Cardiovasc Ultrasound 2008;6:34.

20. Saba L, Sanfilippo R, Montisci R, et al. Correlation between US-PSV and MDCTA in the quantification of carotid artery stenosis. Eur J Radiol 2010; 74(1):99–103.

21. Zhang Z, Berg M, Ikonen A, et al. Carotid stenosis degree in CT angiography: assessment based on luminal area versus luminal diameter measurements. Eur Radiol 2005;15(11):2359–65.

22. Thomas C, Korn A, Ketelsen D, et al. Automatic lumen segmentation in calcified plaques: dual-energy CT versus standard reconstructions in comparison with digital subtraction angiography. AJR Am J Roentgenol 2010;194(6):1590–5.

23. U-King-Im JM, Fox AJ, Aviv RI, et al. Characterization of carotid plaque hemorrhage: a CT angiography and MR intraplaque hemorrhage study. Stroke 2010;41(8):1623–9.

24. U-King-Im JM, Trivedi RA, Graves MJ, et al. Contrast-enhanced MR angiography for carotid disease: diagnostic and potential clinical impact. Neurology 2004;62(8):1282–90.

25. U-King-Im JM, Hollingworth W, Trivedi RA, et al. Contrast-enhanced MR angiography vs intra-arterial

digital subtraction angiography for carotid imaging: activity-based cost analysis. Eur Radiol 2004;14(4):730–5.

26. U-King-Im JM, Trivedi RA, Cross JJ, et al. Measuring carotid stenosis on contrast-enhanced magnetic resonance angiography: diagnostic performance and reproducibility of 3 different methods. Stroke 2004;35(9):2083–8.

27. Magarelli N, Scarabino T, Simeone AL, et al. Carotid stenosis: a comparison between MR and spiral CT angiography. Neuroradiology 1998; 40(6):367–73.

28. Nederkoorn PJ, van der Graaf Y, Eikelboom BC, et al. Time-of-flight MR angiography of carotid artery stenosis: does a flow void represent severe stenosis? AJNR Am J Neuroradiol 2002;23(10): 1779–84.

29. Yim YJ, Choe YH, Ko Y, et al. High signal intensity halo around the carotid artery on maximum intensity projection images of time-of-flight MR angiography: a new sign for intraplaque hemorrhage. J Magn Reson Imaging 2008;27(6):1341–6.

30. Glagov S, Weisenberg E, Zarins CK, et al. Compensatory enlargement of human atherosclerotic coronary arteries. N Engl J Med 1987; 316(22):1371–5.

31. Naghavi M, Libby P, Falk E, et al. From vulnerable plaque to vulnerable patient: a call for new definitions and risk assessment strategies: part I. Circulation 2003;108(14):1664–72.

32. Saam T, Hatsukami TS, Takaya N, et al. The vulnerable, or high-risk, atherosclerotic plaque: noninvasive MR imaging for characterization and assessment. Radiology 2007;244(1):64–77.

33. Granada JF, Kaluza GL, Raizner AE, et al. Vulnerable plaque paradigm: prediction of future clinical events based on a morphological definition. Catheter Cardiovasc Interv 2004;62(3):364–74.

34. Li ZY, Howarth S, Tang T, et al. Does calcium deposition play a role in the stability of atheroma? Location may be the key. Cerebrovasc Dis 2007;24(5): 452–9.

35. Xu X, Ju H, Cai J, et al. High-resolution MR study of the relationship between superficial calcification and the stability of carotid atherosclerotic plaque. Int J Cardiovasc Imaging 2010;26(Suppl 1): 143–50.

36. Biasi GM, Sampaolo A, Mingazzini P, et al. Computer analysis of ultrasonic plaque echolucency in identifying high risk carotid bifurcation lesions. Eur J Vasc Endovasc Surg 1999;17(6): 476–9.

37. Pedro LM, Pedro MM, Goncalves I, et al. Computer-assisted carotid plaque analysis: characteristics of plaques associated with cerebrovascular symptoms and cerebral infarction. Eur J Vasc Endovasc Surg 2000;19(2):118–23.

38. Mathiesen EB, Bonaa KH, Joakimsen O. Echolucent plaques are associated with high risk of ischemic cerebrovascular events in carotid stenosis: the Tromso study. Circulation 2001;103(17):2171–5.

39. El-Barghouty NM, Levine T, Ladva S, et al. Histological verification of computerised carotid plaque characterisation. Eur J Vasc Endovasc Surg 1996; 11(4):414–6.

40. Cave EM, Pugh ND, Wilson RJ, et al. Carotid artery duplex scanning: does plaque echogenicity correlate with patient symptoms? Eur J Vasc Endovasc Surg 1995;10(1):77–81.

41. Sabetai MM, Tegos TJ, Clifford C, et al. Carotid plaque echogenicity and types of silent CT-brain infarcts. Is there an association in patients with asymptomatic carotid stenosis? Int Angiol 2001; 20(1):51–7.

42. Biasi GM, Froio A, Diethrich EB, et al. Carotid plaque echolucency increases the risk of stroke in carotid stenting: the Imaging in Carotid Angioplasty and Risk of Stroke (ICAROS) study. Circulation 2004;110(6):756–62.

43. Kalogeropoulos A, Terzis G, Chrysanthopoulou A, et al. Risk for transient ischemic attacks is mainly determined by intima-media thickness and carotid plaque echogenicity. Atherosclerosis 2007;192(1): 190–6.

44. Hallerstam S, Carlstrom C, Zetterling M, et al. Carotid atherosclerosis in relation to symptoms from the territory supplied by the carotid artery. Eur J Vasc Endovasc Surg 2000;19(4):356–61.

45. Hirano M, Nakamura T, Kitta Y, et al. Assessment of carotid plaque echolucency in addition to plaque size increases the predictive value of carotid ultrasound for coronary events in patients with coronary artery disease and mild carotid atherosclerosis. Atherosclerosis 2010;211(2):451–5.

46. von Sarnowski B, Ludemann J, Volzke H, et al. Common carotid intima-media thickness and Framingham Risk Score predict incident carotid atherosclerotic plaque formation: longitudinal results from the study of health in Pomerania. Stroke 2010;41(10):2375–7.

47. Trivedi RA, U-King-Im J, Graves MJ, et al. Multisequence in vivo MRI can quantify fibrous cap and lipid core components in human carotid atherosclerotic plaques. Eur J Vasc Endovasc Surg 2004;28(2):207–13.

48. Yuan C, Kerwin WS, Yarnykh VL, et al. MRI of atherosclerosis in clinical trials. NMR Biomed 2006;19(6):636–54.

49. Cai JM, Hatsukami TS, Ferguson MS, et al. Classification of human carotid atherosclerotic lesions with in vivo multicontrast magnetic resonance imaging. Circulation 2002;106(11):1368–73.

50. Kwee RM, van Oostenbrugge RJ, Prins MH, et al. Symptomatic patients with mild and moderate

carotid stenosis: plaque features at MRI and association with cardiovascular risk factors and statin use. Stroke 2010;41(7):1389–93.

51. Ota H, Yu W, Underhill HR, et al. Hemorrhage and large lipid-rich necrotic cores are independently associated with thin or ruptured fibrous caps: an in vivo 3T MRI study. Arterioscler Thromb Vasc Biol 2009;29(10):1696–701.

52. Saam T, Underhill HR, Chu B, et al. Prevalence of American Heart Association type VI carotid atherosclerotic lesions identified by magnetic resonance imaging for different levels of stenosis as measured by duplex ultrasound. J Am Coll Cardiol 2008; 51(10):1014–21.

53. Wang Q, Wang Y, Cai J, et al. Differences of signal evolution of intraplaque hemorrhage and associated stenosis between symptomatic and asymptomatic atherosclerotic carotid arteries: an in vivo high-resolution magnetic resonance imaging follow-up study. Int J Cardiovasc Imaging 2010; 26(Suppl 2):323–32.

54. Boussel L, Arora S, Rapp J, et al. Atherosclerotic plaque progression in carotid arteries: monitoring with high-spatial-resolution MR imaging–multicenter trial. Radiology 2009;252(3):789–96.

55. U-King-Im JM, Tang TY, Patterson A, et al. Characterisation of carotid atheroma in symptomatic and asymptomatic patients using high resolution MRI. J Neurol Neurosurg Psychiatry 2008;79(8):905–12.

56. Sadat U, Weerakkody RA, Bowden DJ, et al. Utility of high resolution MR imaging to assess carotid plaque morphology: a comparison of acute symptomatic, recently symptomatic and asymptomatic patients with carotid artery disease. Atherosclerosis 2009;207(2):434–9.

57. Murphy RE, Moody AR, Morgan PS, et al. Prevalence of complicated carotid atheroma as detected by magnetic resonance direct thrombus imaging in patients with suspected carotid artery stenosis and previous acute cerebral ischemia. Circulation 2003;107(24):3053–8.

58. Clarke SE, Hammond RR, Mitchell JR, et al. Quantitative assessment of carotid plaque composition using multicontrast MRI and registered histology. Magn Reson Med 2003;50(6):1199–208.

59. Young VE, Patterson AJ, Sadat U, et al. Diffusion-weighted magnetic resonance imaging for the detection of lipid-rich necrotic core in carotid atheroma in vivo. Neuroradiology 2010;52(10):929–36.

60. Yuan C, Kerwin WS, Ferguson MS, et al. Contrast-enhanced high resolution MRI for atherosclerotic carotid artery tissue characterization. J Magn Reson Imaging 2002;15(1):62–7.

61. Gao T, Zhang Z, Yu W, et al. Atherosclerotic carotid vulnerable plaque and subsequent stroke: a high-resolution MRI study. Cerebrovasc Dis 2009; 27(4):345–52.

62. Zhao X, Underhill HR, Yuan C, et al. Minimization of MR contrast weightings for the comprehensive evaluation of carotid atherosclerotic disease. Invest Radiol 2010;45(1):36–41.

63. Libby P, Ridker PM, Maseri A. Inflammation and atherosclerosis. Circulation 2002;105(9):1135–43.

64. Libby P. Inflammation in atherosclerosis. Nature 2002;420(6917):868–74.

65. Coli S, Magnoni M, Sangiorgi G, et al. Contrast-enhanced ultrasound imaging of intraplaque neovascularization in carotid arteries: correlation with histology and plaque echogenicity. J Am Coll Cardiol 2008;52(3):223–30.

66. Giannoni MF, Vicenzini E, Citone M, et al. Contrast carotid ultrasound for the detection of unstable plaques with neoangiogenesis: a pilot study. Eur J Vasc Endovasc Surg 2009;37(6):722–7.

67. Xiong L, Deng YB, Zhu Y, et al. Correlation of carotid plaque neovascularization detected by using contrast-enhanced US with clinical symptoms. Radiology 2009;251(2):583–9.

68. Kerwin W, Hooker A, Spilker M, et al. Quantitative magnetic resonance imaging analysis of neovasculature volume in carotid atherosclerotic plaque. Circulation 2003;107(6):851–6.

69. Aoki S, Aoki K, Ohsawa S, et al. Dynamic MR imaging of the carotid wall. J Magn Reson Imaging 1999;9(3):420–7.

70. Kerwin WS, O'Brien KD, Ferguson MS, et al. Inflammation in carotid atherosclerotic plaque: a dynamic contrast-enhanced MR imaging study. Radiology 2006;241(2):459–68.

71. Kerwin WS, Oikawa M, Yuan C, et al. MR imaging of adventitial vasa vasorum in carotid atherosclerosis. Magn Reson Med 2008;59(3):507–14.

72. Kerwin WS, Zhao X, Yuan C, et al. Contrast-enhanced MRI of carotid atherosclerosis: dependence on contrast agent. J Magn Reson Imaging 2009;30(1):35–40.

73. Owen DR, Shalhoub J, Miller S, et al. Inflammation within carotid atherosclerotic plaque: assessment with late-phase contrast-enhanced US. Radiology 2010;255(2):638–44.

74. Okane K, Ibaraki M, Toyoshima H, et al. 18F-FDG accumulation in atherosclerosis: use of CT and MR co-registration of thoracic and carotid arteries. Eur J Nucl Med Mol Imaging 2006; 33(5):589–94.

75. Rudd JH, Warburton EA, Fryer TD, et al. Imaging atherosclerotic plaque inflammation with [18F]-fluorodeoxyglucose positron emission tomography. Circulation 2002;105(23):2708–11.

76. Rudd JH, Myers KS, Bansilal S, et al. Atherosclerosis inflammation imaging with 18F-FDG PET: carotid, iliac, and femoral uptake reproducibility, quantification methods, and recommendations. J Nucl Med 2008;49(6):871–8.

77. Davies JR, Rudd JH, Fryer TD, et al. Identification of culprit lesions after transient ischemic attack by combined 18F fluorodeoxyglucose positron-emission tomography and high-resolution magnetic resonance imaging. Stroke 2005;36(12): 2642–7.

78. Silvera SS, Aidi HE, Rudd JH, et al. Multimodality imaging of atherosclerotic plaque activity and composition using FDG-PET/CT and MRI in carotid and femoral arteries. Atherosclerosis 2009;207(1): 139–43.

79. Corot C, Petry KG, Trivedi R, et al. Macrophage imaging in central nervous system and in carotid atherosclerotic plaque using ultrasmall superparamagnetic iron oxide in magnetic resonance imaging. Invest Radiol 2004;39(10):619–25.

80. Kawahara I, Nakamoto M, Kitagawa N, et al. Potential of magnetic resonance plaque imaging using superparamagnetic particles of iron oxide for the detection of carotid plaque. Neurol Med Chir (Tokyo) 2008;48(4):157–61 [discussion: 161–2].

81. Trivedi RA, Mallawarachi C, U-King-Im JM, et al. Identifying inflamed carotid plaques using in vivo USPIO-enhanced MR imaging to label plaque macrophages. Arterioscler Thromb Vasc Biol 2006;26(7):1601–6.

82. Trivedi RA, U-King-Im JM, Graves MJ, et al. In vivo detection of macrophages in human carotid atheroma: temporal dependence of ultrasmall superparamagnetic particles of iron oxide-enhanced MRI. Stroke 2004;35(7):1631–5.

83. Tang TY, Patterson AJ, Miller SR, et al. Temporal dependence of in vivo USPIO-enhanced MRI signal changes in human carotid atheromatous plaques. Neuroradiology 2009;51(7):457–65.

84. Tang TY, Howarth SP, Miller SR, et al. Correlation of carotid atheromatous plaque inflammation using USPIO-enhanced MR imaging with degree of luminal stenosis. Stroke 2008;39(7):2144–7.

85. Kooi ME, Cappendijk VC, Cleutjens KB, et al. Accumulation of ultrasmall superparamagnetic particles of iron oxide in human atherosclerotic plaques can be detected by in vivo magnetic resonance imaging. Circulation 2003;107(19): 2453–8.

86. Howarth SP, Tang TY, Trivedi R, et al. Utility of USPIO-enhanced MR imaging to identify inflammation and the fibrous cap: a comparison of symptomatic and asymptomatic individuals. Eur J Radiol 2009;70(3):555–60.

87. Tang T, Howarth SP, Miller SR, et al. Assessment of inflammatory burden contralateral to the symptomatic carotid stenosis using high-resolution ultrasmall, superparamagnetic iron oxide-enhanced MRI. Stroke 2006;37(9):2266–70.

88. Font MA, Fernandez A, Carvajal A, et al. Imaging of early inflammation in low-to-moderate carotid stenosis by 18-FDG-PET. Front Biosci 2009;14: 3352–60.

89. Tang TY, Howarth SP, Miller SR, et al. Comparison of the inflammatory burden of truly asymptomatic carotid atheroma with atherosclerotic plaques contralateral to symptomatic carotid stenosis: an ultra small superparamagnetic iron oxide enhanced magnetic resonance study. J Neurol Neurosurg Psychiatry 2007;78(12):1337–43.

90. Tang TY, Howarth SP, Miller SR, et al. The ATHEROMA (Atorvastatin Therapy: Effects on Reduction of Macrophage Activity) Study. Evaluation using ultrasmall superparamagnetic iron oxide-enhanced magnetic resonance imaging in carotid disease. J Am Coll Cardiol 2009;53(22): 2039–50.

91. Tang TY, Moustafa RR, Howarth SP, et al. Combined PET-FDG and USPIO-enhanced MR imaging in patients with symptomatic moderate carotid artery stenosis. Eur J Vasc Endovasc Surg 2008;36(1):53–5.

92. Moustafa RR, Izquierdo-Garcia D, Fryer TD, et al. Carotid plaque inflammation is associated with cerebral microembolism in patients with recent TIA or stroke: a pilot study. Circ Cardiovasc Imaging 2010;3(5):536–41.

93. Li ZY, Taviani V, Tang T, et al. The mechanical triggers of plaque rupture: shear stress vs pressure gradient. Br J Radiol 2009;82(Spec No 1):S39–45.

94. Sui B, Gao P, Lin Y, et al. Assessment of wall shear stress in the common carotid artery of healthy subjects using 3.0-tesla magnetic resonance. Acta Radiol 2008;49(4):442–9.

95. Li ZY, Howarth S, Trivedi RA, et al. Stress analysis of carotid plaque rupture based on in vivo high resolution MRI. J Biomech 2006;39(14):2611–22.

96. Li ZY, Howarth SP, Tang T, et al. Structural analysis and magnetic resonance imaging predict plaque vulnerability: a study comparing symptomatic and asymptomatic individuals. J Vasc Surg 2007; 45(4):768–75.

97. Trivedi RA, Li ZY, U-King-Im J, et al. Identifying vulnerable carotid plaques in vivo using high resolution magnetic resonance imaging-based finite element analysis. J Neurosurg 2007;107(3): 536–42.

98. Tang TY, Howarth SP, Li ZY, et al. Correlation of carotid atheromatous plaque inflammation with biomechanical stress: utility of USPIO enhanced MR imaging and finite element analysis. Atherosclerosis 2008;196(2):879–87.

99. Sadat U, Teng Z, Young VE, et al. Impact of plaque haemorrhage and its age on structural stresses in atherosclerotic plaques of patients with carotid artery disease: an MR imaging-based finite element simulation study. Int J Cardiovasc Imaging 2010:1–6. DOI:10.1007/s10554-010-9679-z.

100. Young VEL, Tang TY, Sadat U, et al. Molecular MRI of atherosclerosis. Curr Cardiovasc Imaging Rep 2010;3:4–11.

101. Radermacher KA, Beghein N, Boutry S, et al. In vivo detection of inflammation using pegylated iron oxide particles targeted at E-selectin: a multimodal approach using MR imaging and EPR spectroscopy. Invest Radiol 2009;44(7): 398–404.

102. Nahrendorf M, Jaffer FA, Kelly KA, et al. Noninvasive vascular cell adhesion molecule-1 imaging identifies inflammatory activation of cells in atherosclerosis. Circulation 2006;114(14):1504–11.

103. Cormode DP, Chandrasekar R, Delshad A, et al. Comparison of synthetic high density lipoprotein (HDL) contrast agents for MR imaging of atherosclerosis. Bioconjug Chem 2009;20(5): 937–43.

104. Ronald JA, Chen JW, Chen Y, et al. Enzyme-sensitive magnetic resonance imaging targeting myeloperoxidase identifies active inflammation in experimental rabbit atherosclerotic plaques. Circulation 2009; 120(7):592–9.

105. Smith BR, Heverhagen J, Knopp M, et al. Localization to atherosclerotic plaque and biodistribution of biochemically derivatized superparamagnetic iron oxide nanoparticles (SPIONs) contrast particles for magnetic resonance imaging (MRI). Biomed Microdevices 2007;9(5):719–27.

106. Cyrus T, Abendschein DR, Caruthers SD, et al. MR three-dimensional molecular imaging of intramural biomarkers with targeted nanoparticles. J Cardiovasc Magn Reson 2006;8(3):535–41.

107. Spuentrup E, Botnar RM, Wiethoff AJ, et al. MR imaging of thrombi using EP-2104R, a fibrin-specific contrast agent: initial results in patients. Eur Radiol 2008;18(9):1995–2005.

108. Amirbekian V, Aguinaldo JG, Amirbekian S, et al. Atherosclerosis and matrix metalloproteinases: experimental molecular MR imaging in vivo. Radiology 2009;251(2):429–38.

109. Muntendam P, McCall C, Sanz J, et al. The BioImage Study: novel approaches to risk assessment in the primary prevention of atherosclerotic cardiovascular disease–study design and objectives. Am Heart J 2010;160(1):49–57 e1.

ASPECTS and Other Neuroimaging Scores in the Triage and Prediction of Outcome in Acute Stroke Patients

Bijoy K. Menon, MD[a], Volker Puetz, MD[b],
Puneet Kochar, MD[c], Andrew M. Demchuk, MD, FRCPC[d],*

KEYWORDS

- ASPECTS • Acute stroke • Neuroimaging scores
- Intra-arterial thrombolysis

Brain imaging has revolutionized the treatment of patients with acute ischemic stroke. With the visual differentiation of hemorrhagic from ischemic stroke, thrombolytic therapy became feasible. The effort since then has been to use imaging techniques to help determine which patients would benefit most with thrombolytic therapy. With the availability of endovascular techniques capable of opening an occluded artery faster than intravenous (IV) recombinant tissue plasminogen activator (rtPA), imaging techniques have also been used to tailor therapy appropriate to a patient. This review summarizes current knowledge on the Alberta Stroke Program Early CT Score (ASPECTS) and other neuroimaging scores that help a clinician determine prognosis and decide on appropriate therapy in patients presenting with acute ischemic strokes.

ASPECTS

In the National Institute of Neurological Disorders and Stroke (NINDS) rtPA Stroke Study, computed tomography (CT) was used as a screening tool to exclude intracranial hemorrhage (ICH) before rtPA administration. The extent of early ischemic changes (EIC) on the baseline CT scan did not influence patient eligibility.[1] Initial EIC definition was based on edema and mass effect. A total of 5.2% patients had evidence of such findings. Their presence was associated with a higher risk of symptomatic intracranial hemorrhage (sICH); however, no treatment-modifying effect was demonstrated.[2] A more detailed re-review of the NINDS rtPA Stroke Study scans resulted in a higher prevalence of EIC (31%), largely due to a differing

Conflicts of interest disclosure: The authors report no conflicts of interest.
Financial disclosure: A.M.D. received salary support from Alberta Heritage Foundation for Medical Research.
a Calgary Stroke Program, Department of Clinical Neurosciences, University of Calgary, 29 Street NW, Calgary T2N2T9, Canada
b Department of Neurology, Dresden University Stroke Centre, University of Technology Dresden, Fetscherstrausse 74, Dresden 01307, Germany
c Department of Radiology, Foothills Medical Centre, University of Calgary, Calgary, Canada
d Calgary Stroke Program, Department of Clinical Neurosciences, Foothills Medical Centre, University of Calgary, Room 1162, 29 Street NW, Calgary T2N2T9, Canada
* Corresponding author.
E-mail address: ademchuk@ucalgary.ca

appreciation and definition of EIC.[3] However, again no EIC-by-treatment interaction was statistically demonstrated.

The European Cooperative Acute Stroke Study (ECASS-1) pioneered the importance of assessing EIC to predict benefit from thrombolysis and introduced the "one-third" rule.[4] A post hoc analysis suggested that the extent of EIC is an important predictor of the response to IV thrombolysis.[5] In patients with a small ($\leq$1/3 of the middle cerebral artery [MCA] territory) hypoattenuating area, thrombolysis increased the chance of good functional outcome (odds ratio [OR] 3.43; 95% confidence interval [CI] 1.61–7.33). The benefit was less clear for patients with absence of EIC (OR 1.27, 95% CI 0.82–1.95) or hypoattenuation involving greater than one-third of the MCA territory (OR 0.41, 95% CI 0.06–2.70). Increased risk for sICH was confirmed in secondary analysis of the ECASS-2 CT scans.[6] However, despite evidence that the one-third MCA rule was a good prognostic marker, no statistical evidence of treatment effect modification was proven. In addition, volume estimation with the one-third rule was found in routine practice not to be reliable.[7,8]

Given the difficulties with the reliability of the one-third MCA rule, the Calgary Stroke Program developed ASPECTS as a simple, reliable, and systematic approach to assessing EIC on noncontrast CT (NCCT). Early Ischemic Changes (EIC) on cerebral NCCT were initially defined as: (1) parenchymal hypoattenuation (gray-white indistinction or decreased density of brain tissue relative to attenuation of other parts of the same structure or of the contralateral hemisphere); and (2) focal swelling or mass effect (any focal narrowing of the cerebrospinal fluid spaces as a result of compression by adjacent structures).[1]

Because isolated cortical swelling is associated with differential tissue outcomes and may represent actual penumbral tissue, EIC contributing to ASPECTS are defined as parenchymal hypoattenuation only.[9–11] Parenchymal hypoattenuation can be focal hypodensity and/or loss of gray-white matter differentiation. Regions with isolated cortical swelling, that is, focal swelling without associated hypoattenuation on NCCT, do not contribute to ASPECTS.

Methodology

ASPECTS allots the MCA territory 10 regions of interest, which are weighted based on functional importance (Fig. 1). Equal weighting is given to smaller structures (such as the internal capsule, basal ganglia, and caudate nucleus) as is given to larger cortical areas. ASPECTS methodology includes assessment of all axial cuts of the brain CT scan in two standardized levels of the MCA territory. The boundary of these two levels is the caudate head (see Fig. 1). Any ischemic lesion on axial CT cuts at the level of the caudate head or below is adjudicated to a ganglionic ASPECTS region (M1–M3, insula, caudate nucleus, lentiform nucleus, internal capsule); ischemic lesions above the level of the caudate head are adjudicated to a supraganglionic ASPECTS region (M4–M6). The caudate nucleus is assessed in both the ganglionic level (head of caudate) and supraganglionic level (body and tail of caudate) (see Fig. 1).

To compute the ASPECTS, a single point is subtracted from 10 for evidence of EIC in each of the 10 ASPECTS regions (see Fig. 1). A score of 10 reflects a normal CT scan, a score of 0 diffuse ischemic involvement throughout the complete MCA territory. To allow visualization of all ASPECTS regions in more than one slice, axial cuts with 4- to 5-mm slice thickness should be used. EIC should be visible on at least 2 adjacent cuts to ensure that a lesion is truly abnormal rather than a partial-volume effect. In addition, great care should be taken when comparing left and right hemispheres when patients are not adequately positioned in the CT scanner. Head tilt, motion artifact, and bone artifact are 3 of the commonest reasons for false-positive regional scoring with ASPECTS. The rule of thumb is that if there is doubt about a region, do not call it abnormal. Examples of typical ASPECTS patterns in patients with MCA M1- or M2-segment occlusions are presented in Figs. 2 and 3.

Does ASPECTS on NCCT at Baseline Predict Clinical Outcome in Patients with Acute Ischemic Strokes?

In the original ASPECTS study on patients thrombolyzed within 3 hours from symptom onset, a baseline ASPECTS value of 7 or below sharply discriminated patients who were highly unlikely to achieve an independent functional outcome.[12] Since then, several studies have confirmed the prognostic value of ASPECTS in a 0- to 3-hour[10,13,14] and 0- to 6-hour time window.[15,16]

The prognostic information of ASPECTS was reproduced in the Canadian Alteplase for Stroke Effectiveness Study (CASES).[17] Among 936 patients, the baseline NCCT ASPECTS score was a strong predictor of outcome, with lower scores implying a lower probability of an independent functional outcome (OR 0.81, 95% CI 0.75–0.87, per point ASPECTS decrease). However, with the larger number of patients

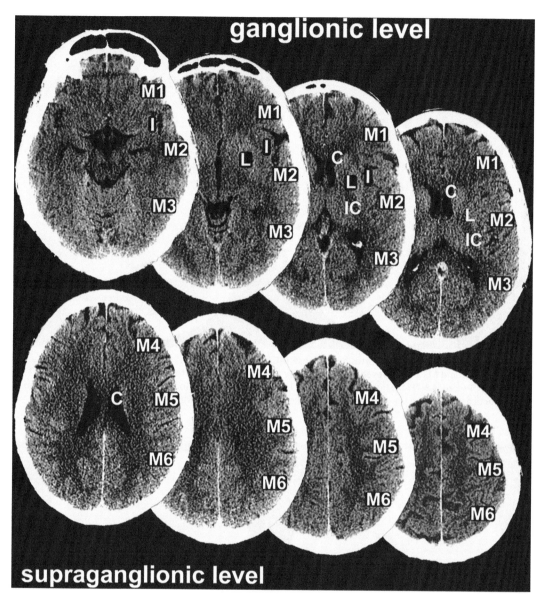

Fig. 1. ASPECTS scoring scheme. The upper row demonstrates axial CT cuts of the ganglionic ASPECTS level (M1–M3, insula [I], lentiform nucleus [L], caudate nucleus [C], posterior limb of the internal capsule [IC]). The lower row demonstrates CT cuts of the supraganglionic ASPECTS level (M4–M6). As illustrated in the figure, the authors prefer to use cuts in the inferior orbitomeatal line (rather than superior orbitomeatal line). All axial cuts are reviewed for ASPECTS scoring. EIC in the caudate nucleus are scored in the ganglionic level (head of caudate) and supraganglionic level (body and tail of caudate). (*From* Puetz V, Dzialowski I, Hill MD, et al. The Alberta Stroke Program Early CT Score in clinical practice: what have we learned? Int J Stroke 2009; 4(5):354–64; with permission.)

studied in CASES, the prognostic information from ASPECTS was not dichotomous (as noticed in the smaller ASPECTS study), but near linear. In subsequent analysis, ASPECTS predicted functional outcome in a graded fashion, with a linear relationship for ASPECTS scores 6 through 10 and an ill-defined pattern for ASPECTS 0 through 5.[18] With ASPECTS values 6 to 10, about 50% of

patients experienced an independent functional outcome. By contrast, with an ASPECTS score of 0 to 3 the chance for an independent functional outcome was very low (about 15%). However, the ability of ASPECTS to discriminate individual outcomes was only modest (c-statistic = 0.63; 95% CI 0.59–0.67) and less than that of the baseline National Institutes of Health Stroke

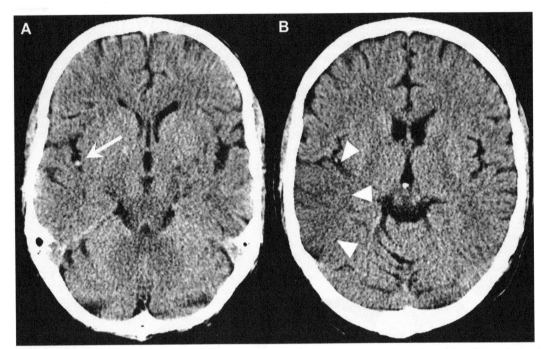

Fig. 2. Baseline NCCT (*A*) demonstrates hyperdense MCA branch "dot sign" in the right Sylvian fissure (*arrow*). The ASPECTS M2 and M3 territories show hypodensity and loss of gray-white matter differentiation (*arrowheads*, *B*). The ASPECT score is 8. (*From* Puetz V, Dzialowski I, Hill MD, et al. The Alberta Stroke Program Early CT Score in clinical practice: what have we learned? Int J Stroke 2009;4(5):354–64; with permission.)

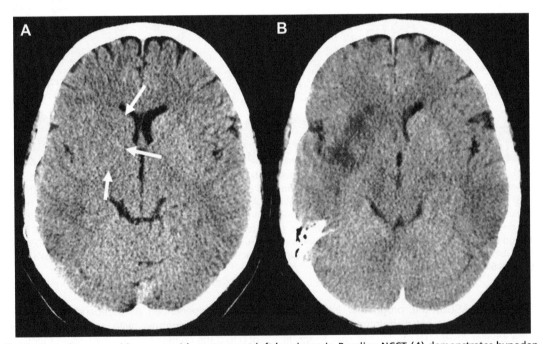

Fig. 3. Forty-four-year-old woman with acute-onset left hemiparesis. Baseline NCCT (*A*) demonstrates hypodensities in the right lentiform nucleus and caudate nucleus (*arrows*) with an ASPECT score of 8. The patient had right MCA occlusion that was successfully recanalized with combined IV-IA thrombolysis. Follow-up NCCT (*B*) reveals infarction with minor hemorrhagic transformation in the same territory. (*From* Puetz V, Dzialowski I, Hill MD, et al. The Alberta Stroke Program Early CT Score in clinical practice: what have we learned? Int J Stroke 2009; 4(5):354–64; with permission.)

Scale (NIHSS) score (c-statistic = 0.71; 95% CI 0.67–0.74).

In an analysis of the Penumbra Pivotal Stroke Trial,[19] good clinical outcome (modified Rankin Scale 0–2) was significantly greater in the ASPECTS >7 group when compared with the ASPECTS ≤7 group (risk ratio [RR] 3.3, 95% CI 1.6–6.8). No patient with an ASPECTS score of 4 or less had good clinical outcome.[20]

Does ASPECTS on NCCT at Baseline Predict Response to Thrombolysis?

Although the extent of infarcted brain at baseline is a known prognostic factor in acute ischemic stroke,[12] proof of treatment effect modification by imaging in acute ischemic stroke has been limited. This discrepancy between the proven role of baseline imaging as a prognostic factor and the inability to show effect modification with treatment is a central problem in our field. An oft-quoted explanation for this discrepancy is that the range of variation in patient outcome due to treatment effect is quite small when compared with the effect of imaging as a prognostic factor. Although this is true for large lesions where the prognosis is so poor that the effect of treatment may be negligible, it does not explain the lack of treatment effect modification in patients with small cores and large penumbra. Lack of uniformity in measurement is another possible explanation, and has plagued the technique of perfusion

imaging and the mismatch hypothesis. There is, however, some data to suggest that such an interaction may exist with ASPECTS on NCCT (Table 1).

Intravenous thrombolysis

In a post hoc analysis of the NINDS rtPA Stroke Study, ASPECTS on baseline NCCT dichotomized into greater than 7 versus 7 or less did not have a treatment-modifying effect on favorable functional outcome. However, higher ASPECTS values (ASPECTS 8–10) were associated with a greater extent of benefit from IV thrombolysis (absolute risk reduction 19.5% [10.2–28.8]; number needed to treat [NNT] = 5) and a trend toward reduced mortality. Mean final infarct volumes were also half as large in rtPA compared with placebo patients (7.8 mL vs 15.2 mL, respectively). Patients with a moderate extent of EIC (ASPECTS 3–7) still benefited from IV thrombolysis (absolute risk reduction 13.3% [0.3–26.3]; NNT = 8) but no mortality difference was seen. Final infarct volumes were 30% smaller in rtPA-treated patients (51.1 mL vs 66 mL, respectively). In the low ASPECTS group (ASPECTS 0–2) with extensive EIC no benefit of rtPA could be demonstrated. These patients had large mean final infarct volumes exceeding 200 mL. This extensive EIC group represented only 16 of 608 patients (2.6%) in the NINDS trial, thus limiting the group's clinical relevance.[10]

Effect modification of IV thrombolysis in a 0- to 6-hour time window has been addressed by

---

Table 1
Major results of ASPECTS applied to NCCT scans from clinical trials

Study	Treatment Modality	Patient Selection Criteria	Main Findings
NINDS	IV, ≤3 h	No ICH on NCCT	Larger amount of benefit with higher ASPECTS values No thrombolysis effect modification
ECASS-2	IV, ≤6 h	No ICH on NCCT EIC <1/3 MCA	Increased PH rate with ASPECTS ≤7 vs >7 No thrombolysis effect modification
PROACT-II	IA, ≤6 h	No ICH on NCCT M1 or M2 occlusion on DSA	Treatment effect modification by dichotomized ASPECTS (>7 vs ≤7) NNT = 3 with ASPECTS >7
IMS-1	IV-IA, ≤3 h	No ICH on NCCT EIC <1/3 MCA	Treatment effect modification by dichotomized ASPECTS (>7 vs ≤7)
Penumbra Pivotal Stroke Trial	IA alone or refractory to IV, <8 h	No ICH on CT, EIC <1/3 MCA, NIHSS ≥8	Onset to recanalization time by dichotomized ASPECTS (>7 vs ≤7) effect modification

Abbreviations: DSA, digital subtraction cerebral angiography; EIC, early ischemic changes; IA, intra-arterial; ICH, intracranial hemorrhage; IV, intravenous; MCA, middle cerebral artery; NNT, number needed to treat; PH, parenchymal hematoma.

applying ASPECTS to the ECASS-2 brain CT scans.[15] The analysis also did not reveal a multiplicative thrombolysis-by-ASPECTS treatment interaction on functional outcome ($P = .29$ for the interaction term). Moreover, this lack of a multiplicative thrombolysis-by-ASPECTS interaction was consistent for the 0- to 3-hour ($P = .89$) and 3- to 6-hour ($P = .22$) time window subgroups.

An inability to show treatment effect modification in these large IV thrombolytic trials could be because a large proportion of subjects had an ASPECTS of 10 and therefore possibly no occlusion or distal occlusions, EICs may not be sensitive enough within an early (3-hour) time window, and because the studies are underpowered to show such an effect.

Intra-arterial thrombolysis

In a post hoc analysis of the Prourokinase Acute Cerebral Infarct Trial II (PROACT-II) scans reevaluated for EIC using ASPECTS, a clear treatment interaction was identified.[21] PROACT-II patients represented a fairly homogeneous cohort of patients with angiographically proven MCA M1- or M2-segment occlusions.[22] Patients in the active treatment group received intra-arterial (IA) thrombolysis infusion with prourokinase proximal to the thrombus within 6 hours from symptom onset. Specifically, the reanalysis demonstrated that patients treated with IA prourokinase did better than controls only with a baseline ASPECTS greater than 7. The magnitude of benefit for these patients was large, with an NNT of 3 to yield functional independence at 90 days. Moreover, the benefit of IA thrombolysis progressively increased from ASPECTS 8 through 10 (RR 3.2 [95% CI 1.2–9.1] for ASPECTS >7; 7.5 [95% CI 1.1–51.4] for ASPECTS >8; and infinite for ASPECTS >9). In contrast, on average, patients with a baseline ASPECTS value ≤ 7 did not benefit from IA thrombolysis (RR 1.2, 95% CI 0.5–2.7).

CT scans of the Reevaluation of the Interventional Management of Stroke (IMS-1) study sought to determine whether ASPECTS could predict which patients would particularly benefit from combined IV-IA thrombolysis.[23] IMS-1 used a safety and futility design, comparing historical control subjects from the NINDS rtPA Stroke Study. In IMS-1, a total of 80 patients were treated with IV rtPA (0.6 mg/kg) within 3 hours from symptom onset. At angiography, 62 received additional IA rtPA to a maximum dose of 22 mg.[24] Patients with an ASPECTS score of greater than 7 were more likely to benefit from the combined IV-IA approach than from IV rtPA alone (based on matched subjects from the NINDS rtPA study ASPECTS analysis), with a NNT of 10. Patients with an ASPECTS score of less than 8 were less likely to benefit from combined IV-IA than from IV thrombolysis, and more likely to be harmed by interventional therapy. These data are evidence of both a qualitative and quantitative interaction effect.

Does ASPECTS Predict sICH Risk?

Numerous studies have demonstrated the association between the extension of EIC on NCCT and risk of hemorrhagic transformation after thrombolysis.[6,12,15,25] However, a consistent EIC-by-thrombolysis interaction on sICH risk has not been established. In the original ASPECTS study, the authors found a 14-fold (95% CI 1.8–117) increased odds for sICH with ASPECTS scores of 7 or less versus greater than 7.[12] In the secondary analysis of the NINDS-stroke trial, ASPECT scores of more than 7 and 3 to 7 carried a similar sICH rate of 5% and 4.5%, respectively. Only patients with very extensive EICs (ASPECTS 0–2) showed a trend toward increased sICH risk (20%; 95% CI 1.6–38.3). In secondary analysis of ECASS-2 with ASPECTS, an effect modification by ASPECTS greater than 7 versus 7 or less in predicting radiologically defined parenchymal hematoma but not sICH was demonstrated. When dichotomized ASPECTS was applied to the PROACT-II CT scans, ASPECTS 7 or less was associated with doubled risk for treatment-related sICH compared with scores of more than 7 (15.4% vs 7.7%, respectively). However, no IA-thrombolysis-by-ASPECTS interaction on sICH risk was demonstrated.[21]

The extent of EIC using ASPECTS is associated with the risk for thrombolysis-related hemorrhagic transformation. From current data, dichotomized ASPECTS modifies the risk for thrombolysis-related radiologically defined parenchymal hematoma but not clinically defined sICH.

Does ASPECTS on NCCT at Baseline Help Predict the Time Window Available for Recanalization?

Time has been shown to be an important modifier of intravenous thrombolytic treatment effect in randomized trials. In an updated pooled analysis of ECASS, ATLANTIS, NINDS, and EPITHET trials, Lees and colleagues[26] show benefit with IV tPA in patients treated within 4.5 hours of symptom onset. By demonstrating an effect of "onset to treatment time" on clinical outcomes in the treatment group vis-a-vis placebo, they show the time-dependent nature of treatment benefit and risk. This makes biologic sense, as progression to irreversible infarction in the penumbra is a time-dependent phenomenon and early treatment aimed at recanalization should modify this process. This penumbral hypothesis raises the possibility that patients with smaller areas of infarction at baseline imaging would benefit most, and as infarct core increases in size the time window available shrinks rapidly. This interaction between baseline CT scan and onset to recanalization time is particularly appealing given our understanding of modern imaging.

A post hoc analysis of the IMS-1 study failed to show an interaction between ASPECTS on NCCT at baseline and time to treatment.[23] However, an analysis of data from the Penumbra Pivotal Stroke Trial[19] (a prospective, single-armed 125-patient study designed to assess the safety and efficacy of the "Penumbra" system for removing thrombi in acute ischemic strokes) showed that in the ASPECTS >7 group, 62.5% of patients with onset to recanalization time of 300 minutes or less had good clinical outcome when compared with 45.5% patients with either onset to recanalization time of longer than 300 minutes or nonrecanalizers. In the ASPECTS ≤7 group, the corresponding figures were 33.3% with onset to recanalization time of 300 minutes or less versus 7.9% in the >300 minutes or nonrecanalizer group (Fig. 4). After adjusting for baseline stroke severity, there was evidence of an ASPECTS-by-onset to recanalization time interaction ($P = .066$) in the multivariable model. The direction of interaction was such that among patients with ASPECTS greater than 7, the relative effect of onset to recanalization time (≤300 minutes or >300 minutes) in predicting outcome was small. Among patients with ASPECTS of 7 or less, only those with an onset to recanalization time of 300 minutes or less had some chance of achieving a good functional outcome. Patients with an unfavorable scan (ASPECTS ≤7), with late recanalization, did poorly. At any treatment time point, if there are extensive changes on CT scan (ASPECTS ≤4), endovascular therapy simply does not help.[20]

Reliability of ASPECTS Compared with the One-Third Rule

The original ASPECTS study compared reliabilities of the one-third rule and ASPECTS. ASPECTS dichotomized at >7 versus ≤7 consistently demonstrated higher agreement (κ = 0.71–0.89) as compared with the one-third rule (κ = 0.52–0.64) among stroke neurologists, radiology trainees, and experienced neuroradiologists.[12,27] ASPECTS was also reliable in real time when stroke neurologists and stroke fellows prospectively recorded NCCT ASPECT scores in the emergency department.[28]

However, Mak and colleagues[29] found a higher reliability with the one-third rule (κ = 0.49) compared with dichotomized ASPECTS (κ = 0.34) among reviewers from different specialties. The investigators attributed this result, in part, to

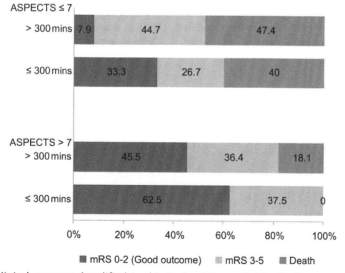

ASPECTS ≤ 7

> 300 mins | 7.9 | 44.7 | 47.4
≤ 300 mins | 33.3 | 26.7 | 40

ASPECTS > 7

> 300 mins | 45.5 | 36.4 | 18.1
≤ 300 mins | 62.5 | 37.5 | 0

0%   20%   40%   60%   80%   100%

■ mRS 0-2 (Good outcome)   ■ mRS 3-5   ■ Death

Fig. 4. Unadjusted clinical outcome (modified Rankin Scale at 3 months) in the 2 groups ASPECTS >7 and ≤7, stratified by onset-to-recanalization time <300 minutes and ≥300 minutes in a post hoc analysis of the Penumbra Pivotal Stroke Trial. (*Data from* Goyal M, Menon BK, Coutts SB, et al. Effect of baseline CT scan appearance and time to recanalization on clinical outcomes in endovascular thrombectomy of acute ischemic strokes. Stroke 2010;42(1):93–7.)

a more systematic approach to the one-third rule by applying the worksheet from the ATLANTIS/CT summit criteria.[30] When experienced stroke neurologists used a more systematic approach to the one-third rule with the ICE method (Idealize the MCA territory; Close a geometric figure around the areas of hypodensities; Estimate the ratio of the 2 geometric figures), kappa statistics were similar for the one-third rule and dichotomized ASPECTS ($\kappa = 0.7$ for both).[31,32]

A more systematic approach may improve reliability of the one-third rule.[30,31] Such systematic approaches are essentially the same as ASPECTS. In fact, dichotomized ASPECTS and the one-third rule may provide similar information.[15,32] An ASPECTS cutoff of 6 or less had 94% sensitivity and 98% specificity, respectively, to estimate MCA infarction greater than one-third.[32] In the ECASS-2 study baseline CTs independently scored to have EIC in more than one-third of the MCA territory, the median ASPECTS score was 4.[15] Thus, the authors have recommended that an ASPECTS of less than 5 is equivalent to more than one-third MCA infarction. A major advantage of ASPECTS is its increased sensitivity for EIC in the MCA territory.[10,15,29]

ASPECTS on CT Angiography Source Image

Hypoattenuation on NCCT brain is caused by a shift in brain tissue water content secondary to significant ischemia (brain parenchyma with blood flow <12 ml/100 g/min).[33] Animal experiments suggest that a 1% increase in brain tissue water content results in a drop of 1.8 Hounsfield Unit in attenuation.[34] For hypoattenuation to be visible to the human eye, there has to be a large shift in water uptake in ischemic tissue. This process is dependent on time and degree of ischemia and therefore is better appreciated at later time intervals from stroke onset.[35] On the other hand, hypoattenuation on CT angiography source image (CTA-SI) (if image is in the venous phase) is an indicator of reduced cerebral blood volume in the area of ischemia and is not as time dependent as ischemia on NCCT.[36] Areas of hypoattenuation on CTA-SI correlate well with lesions on diffusion-weighted imaging (DWI) and final infarcts.[36,37] Applied on ASPECTS, CTA-SI has improved the prediction of final infarct size and clinical outcome compared with NCCT (Fig. 5).[38,39]

ASPECTS on Multimodal CT and Magnetic Resonance Imaging

Although ASPECTS was originally designed for use with NCCT, recent studies indicate its practicability with perfusion CT (CTP) and multimodal magnetic resonance (MR) imaging with DWI and perfusion-weighted imaging (PWI). MR) with diffusion-weighted sequences is more sensitive for EIC than NCCT, particularly in patients presenting with minor symptoms.[40] ASPECTS on DWI may therefore overestimate EIC with prognostic relevance. As a consequence, the authors do not advocate use of ASPECTS on DWI in patients with transient ischemic attack or minor stroke. However, in patients presenting with disabling symptoms within 6 hours from symptom onset, the ASPECTS differences between NCCT and DWI in visualizing early infarction were small.[16] Consequently, ASPECTS applied to DWI was

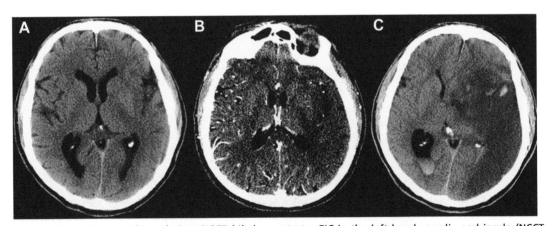

Fig. 5. Patient with carotid-T occlusion. NCCT (*A*) demonstrates EIC in the left basal ganglia and insula (NCCT ASPECTS 7). CTA-SI (*B*) demonstrates extensive hypocontrast in most of the left hemisphere (CTA-SI ASPECTS 3). Follow-up NCCT (*C*) demonstrates malignant middle cerebral artery infarction.

a reliable tool for predicting poor outcome in patients thrombolyzed within 3 hours from symptom onset in a recent study, with a DWI ASPECTS of 5 or less being an independent predictor of poor functional outcome (OR 33.4; 95% CI 2.7–410.8; $P = .0062$).[41] In a large IV tPA registry, a pretreatment ASPECTS of 7 or more on DWI was related to good clinical outcome (OR 1.85; 95% CI 1.07–3.24) when compared with an ASPECTS of 4 or less, which was related to death (OR 3.61; 95% CI 1.23–9.91), and ASPECTS 5 or less, related to symptomatic ICH (OR 4.74; 95% CI 1.54–13.64).[42]

Efforts to use the penumbral hypothesis to identify a subgroup of patients who would benefit with thrombolysis has not yielded expected results. Lack of uniformity in measurement of perfusion parameters is an explanation.[43] In clinical practice, rapid and reliable assessment tools to define a CTP- or MR imaging-based mismatch are required. However, purely subjective assessment of a DWI/PWI mismatch has poor interrater reliability[44] and volumetric assessment is not clinically practical. ASPECTS mismatch on DWI and PWI is a rapid and reliable alternative. A linear correlation between DWI ASPECTS and DWI lesion volume has previously been shown.[45] In a post hoc analysis of the EPITHET data, Butcher and colleagues[46] found 78% (interrater range 72%–84%) sensitivity and 88% (interrater range 83%–90%) specificity for a "DWI-ASPECTS minus PWI-ASPECTS" difference of 2 or more to predict a 20% DWI/PWI mismatch. Applied to CTP, Lin and colleagues[47] have reported 84% (95% CI 65.5%–93.5%) sensitivity and 100% (95% CI 65.9%–100%) specificity of a cerebral blood volume (CBV) ASPECTS minus mean transit time (MTT) ASPECTS difference of 1 or more to identify a volumetric CBV/MTT mismatch of 20% or more. In a study by Parsons and colleagues,[48] ASPECTS applied on CBV parameter maps was more accurate in predicting irreversibly injured tissue and clinical outcome than NCCT or CTA-SI. Moreover, ASPECTS on cerebral blood flow (CBF) parameter maps predicted tissue at risk for infarction without reperfusion (ie, the ischemic penumbra) in this study.

Clinical diffusion mismatch (CDM) has often been used as an alternative to DWI/PWI mismatch in identifying patients with brain tissue at risk of infarction. Volumetric assessment of DWI limits clinical applicability of this paradigm. In a consecutive series of 71 patients with anterior circulation strokes treated with IV tPA, Terasawa and colleagues[45] showed that CDM determined using DWI ASPECTS (NIHSS ≥ 8 and DWI ASPECTS ≥ 7) is associated with neurologic improvement when compared with a group without.

POSTERIOR CIRCULATION NEUROIMAGING SCORES
pc-ASPECTS

A limitation of ASPECTS is its confinement to the MCA territory. To quantify EIC in the posterior circulation, a posterior circulation Acute Stroke Prognosis Early CT Score (pc-ASPECTS) has been developed.[49] pc-ASPECTS allots the posterior circulation 10 points (**Fig. 6**). One point each is subtracted for EIC in left or right thalamus, cerebellum, or posterior cerebral artery territory, respectively, and 2 points each are subtracted for EIC in any part of the midbrain or pons. EIC are defined as focal hypodensity or loss of gray-white differentiation on NCCT. Regions of relatively diminished contrast enhancement are scored as abnormal on CTA-SI.

Similar to the anterior circulation stroke, CTA-SI improved the detection of ischemic tissue in the posterior circulation.[49] pc-ASPECTS on CTA-SI (OR 1.58, 95% CI 1.1–2.2) but not NCCT (OR 1.2, 95% CI 0.8–2.2) predicted functional independence at 3 months. In 46 patients with acute basilar artery occlusion, the extent of hypoattenuation on CTA-SI, quantified with the pc-ASPECTS score dichotomized at >7 versus ≤ 7 predicted favorable functional outcome (RR 12.1; 95% CI 1.7–84.9). This finding was consistent in 21 patients who had angiographic

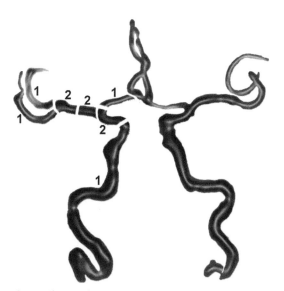

Fig. 6. Clot Burden Score demonstrating extent of clot on CTA in the anterior circulation in patients with acute ischemic stroke. (*From* Puetz V, Dzialowski I, Hill MD, et al. Intracranial thrombus extent predicts clinical outcome, final infarct size and hemorrhagic transformation in ischemic stroke: the clot burden score. Int J Stroke 2008;3(4):230–6; with permission.)

recanalization of the basilar artery within 24 hours from symptom onset (RR 7.7; 95% CI 1.1–52.1).

Pons-Midbrain Index

Schaefer and colleagues[50] developed a CTA-SI score, the pons-midbrain index, that was highly predictive of clinical outcome in patients with acute vertebrobasilar occlusions treated with IA thrombolysis. In an analysis of 16 patients with vertebrobasilar occlusion treated with IA thrombolysis, baseline CTA-SI hypoattenuation in the pons and midbrain, graded as 0 = no hypoattenuation, 1 = <50% hypoattenuation, and 2 = >50% hypoattenuation, were independent predictors of clinical outcome (measured as modified Rankin score at 3 months) (cumulative r = 0.81, $P<.001$). For outcome dichotomized into death versus survival, the CTA-SI pons score (0, 1, 2) (P = .0037) was the only independent predictor.

Application of pc-ASPECTS and the pons-midbrain index could be useful to identify patients with basilar artery occlusion who potentially benefit from thrombolysis, and to stratify patients in trials comparing IV and IA therapy for basilar artery occlusion. However, these scores need validation in other cohorts to allow widespread applicability.

THE CLOT BURDEN SCORE

An oft-ignored but nevertheless significant problem when using ASPECTS is that the site of occlusion may vary. Proximal and distal occlusions in the arterial tree can potentially have similar ASPECTS with significantly different prognosis. Site of occlusion as a prognostic factor could overwhelm treatment effects, especially with IV tPA, which has a variable effect on recanalization depending on occlusion site. In the same IMS-1 post hoc analysis quoted earlier, there was a good correlation between more proximal arterial occlusion and lower ASPECT scores at baseline (Spearman correlation coefficient 0.43, $P<.0001$), thus suggesting that ASPECTS on NCCT could predict occlusion site and therefore effect modification of "time to treatment" on clinical outcome with different treatment modalities.[23]

Proximal occlusions such as the distal internal carotid or proximal MCA infrequently recanalize with IV tPA in the first hours, presumably due to extensive clot burden.[51,52] The authors have developed a CTA-based Clot Burden Score (CBS) for the anterior circulation stroke. The score allots up to 10 points for the presence of contrast opacification on CTA (Fig. 7). A score of 10 indicates absence of visible occlusion on CTA, a score of 0 indicates occlusion of all major intracranial anterior circulation arteries. Patients with higher thrombus burden had higher baseline NIHSS scores and lower baseline ASPECTS scores compared with patients with less thrombus burden. With increasing CBS values (ie, less thrombus burden), patients are significantly more likely to have an independent functional outcome and less likely to die. In addition, final infarct sizes

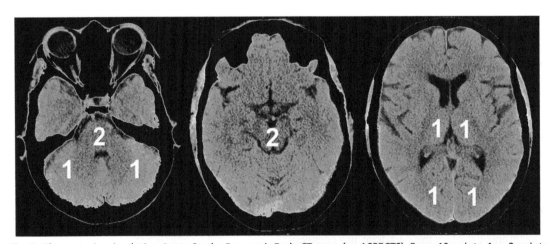

Fig. 7. The posterior circulation Acute Stroke Prognosis Early CT score (pc-ASPECTS). From 10 points, 1 or 2 points each (as indicated) are subtracted for early ischemic changes (NCCT) or hypoattenuation (CTA-SI) in left or right thalamus, cerebellum, or posterior cerebral artery territory, respectively (1 point); any part of midbrain or pons (2 points). pc-ASPECTS=10 indicates a normal scan, pc-ASPECTS=0 indicates early ischemic changes (NCCT) or hypoattenuation (CTA-SI) in all the above territories. (*From* Puetz V, Sylaja PN, Coutts SB, et al. Extent of hypoattenuation on CT angiography source images predicts functional outcome in patients with basilar artery occlusion. Stroke 2008;39(9):2485–90; with permission.)

were smaller and hemorrhagic transformation rates lower.[53] Higher CBS values were associated with higher recanalization rates in a recent study by Tan and colleagues.[54] While useful, the scale is limited because it does not take into account residual flow at the site of arterial occlusion or pial vessel retrograde filling, due to collaterals from anterior cerebral artery-MCA or posterior cerebral artery-MCA.

THE BOSTON ACUTE STROKE IMAGING SCALE

The Boston Acute Stroke Imaging Scale (BASIS) is a combined arterial and parenchymal imaging score. It uses a 2-step algorithm to stratify patients into major and minor stroke. The first step is identification of a proximal artery occlusion, which if identified classifies the stroke as "major." In the second step, if no occlusion is identified on vascular imaging, brain parenchyma is assessed for prespecified lesion extent (>1/3 of MCA territory or ASPECTS 0–7 or bilateral pons or bithalamic involvement), and if present, the stroke is classified as "major." All other strokes are classified "minor." The investigators found highly significant differences in mortality, discharge status, and length of hospital stay in subjects with "major" and "minor" strokes classified as per BASIS using both CT and MR imaging.[55]

LEPTOMENINGEAL COLLATERAL SCORES ON CTA

Viability of brain tissue distal to an arterial occlusion is dependent on the presence of Willisian and leptomeningeal collaterals.[56–58] Leptomeningeal collaterals are direct arteriolo-arteriolar connections between major cerebral arteries that provide a route for retrograde filling of pial arteries distal to an occluded artery. Leptomeningeal collaterals provide a vascular network with the potential to maintain CBF at levels that prolong or indefinitely sustain brain tissue viability beyond an occlusion.[59] Good flow through collateral pathways is associated with a smaller infarct core at baseline,[60,61] and by extending the survival time of penumbra can extend the time window for viable reperfusion. Good collaterals therefore limit infarct core expansion and determine final infarct volumes.

Although the existence of leptomeningeal collaterals has never been doubted and there is growing evidence from animal[62,63] and human microanatomic studies[59,64] for the existence of these small interarteriolar connections in the cortex and subcortical structures, attempts to image them in humans has been difficult. Because leptomeningeal collaterals are responsible for blood flow in pial arteries beyond an occlusion, visualization of pial arteries has been used as surrogate marker for the presence of these collaterals. In MCA occlusions, leptomeningeal collateral scores using digital subtraction cerebral angiography (DSA)[65,66] and CTA[67–69] (**Fig. 8**) emphasize the anatomic extent of opacification of MCA branches, with excellent scores showing flow of contrast right to the distal end of the occluding thrombus.

Does Collateral Status Assessed on Imaging at Baseline Predict Final Infarct Size?

There was an inverse correlation between collateral status on CTA maximum-intensity projection images and infarct volume in a study by Tan and colleagues[67] (correlation coefficient $r = 0.5$). In a retrospective study examining extent of pial collaterals on angiography, Christoforidis and colleagues[66] found that final infarct volumes were significantly lower in patients with better collateral status than those with worse collateral status, regardless of whether they had complete or partial recanalization. In subjects who had complete recanalization, final mean infarct volume was 8.52 cm^3 in the group with good collateral status when compared with 113.93 cm^3 in the

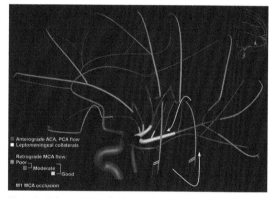

Fig. 8. Schematic of the left cerebral hemisphere arteries, with proximal MCA occlusion (indicated in black) and variable grades of retrograde distal MCA blood flow (*arrows*) via the leptomeningeal collaterals (white). Leptomeningeal collateral scores using digital subtraction cerebral angiography (DSA) and CT angiography (CTA) emphasize the anatomic extent of opacification of MCA branches, with excellent scores showing flow of contrast right to the distal end of the occluding thrombus. (*From* Miteff F, Levi CR, Bateman GA, et al. The independent predictive utility of computed tomography angiographic collateral status in acute ischaemic stroke. Brain 2009;132(Pt 8):2231–8; with permission.)

group with worse collateral status, thus suggesting that collateral status predicts final infarct volumes independent of recanalization status. Kim and colleagues,[70] using a regional collateral score on cerebral angiography based on the ASPECTS template, showed that the presence of collateral flow correlates with lower infarct volume on follow-up CT.

Does Collateral Status Assessed on Imaging at Baseline Predict Final Clinical Outcome?

In a prospective study of patients with MCA ± intracranial internal carotid artery occlusions, Lima and colleagues[71] found that leptomeningeal collateral status on CTA is an independent predictor of good clinical outcome (OR 1.93, 95% CI 1.06–3.34, P = .03). Other studies in the past have also confirmed the role of collateral status at baseline on imaging in predicting final clinical outcomes.[60,61]

Does Collateral Status Assessment have Additional Utility Over and Above Assessment of Baseline Stroke Severity and Assessment of Core and Penumbra in Clinical Decision Making?

Because leptomeningeal collaterals are responsible for blood flow in the ischemic brain region distal to an occlusion, it is intuitive that it should therefore correlate with size of infarct core, size of penumbra and oligemia, and baseline stroke severity. Using multivariable regression techniques to analyze these variables with collateral status is problematic, as they are collinear or highly correlated.[72,73] A multivariable model with correlated predictors may not give valid results about any single variable as a predictor, and therefore does not help us in understanding the relationships between these variables. Many of the studies on collateral status suffer from this drawback, which has resulted in underutilization of imaging-based assessment of collateral status in clinical decision making. Miteff and colleagues[61] highlighted this problem when they commented on the high level of correlation and interaction between predictor variables (NIHSS, collateral status, and reperfusion) and developed a decision tree to illustrate the independent role of collaterals in determining clinical outcome. These investigators found that of 55 subjects with a perfusion CT mismatch ratio of 3 or greater, everyone (17/17) with good collateral status and major reperfusion assessed at 24 hours achieved good clinical outcome. Of 19 patients with mismatch ratio of 3 or greater and reduced collaterals, only 3 with major reperfusion achieved good clinical outcome,

thus suggesting that collateral status has independent predictive utility over and above mismatch status in predicting clinical outcomes.

HOW CAN ASPECTS AND OTHER NEUROIMAGING SCORES BE USED IN CLINICAL DECISION MAKING?

Acute ischemic stroke pathophysiology is a temporally evolving extremely variable process whereby prognosis and treatment effects are dependent not only on intrinsic patient factors like tissue susceptibility to ischemia, Willisian and leptomeningeal collateral status, susceptibility of brain tissue to hemorrhage, age, blood pressure, diabetes, previous strokes/transient ischemic attacks and other comorbidities, but also on variability in treatment approaches and poststroke management. No single variable in isolation can therefore have sufficient predictive ability. Imaging of the brain parenchyma and the vasculature is a composite surrogate for time elapsed from stroke onset, severity of ischemia, collateral status, and extent of thrombus. Imaging is an indication of the effect of these different variables contributing to stroke pathophysiology at a given time point, and is therefore an important prognostic tool available to physicians. Imaging-based classification systems such as ASPECTS and the other neuroimaging scores discussed herein classify different aspects of stroke pathophysiology. It is therefore important from a clinical decision-making perspective to understand the soft interrelationships between these scores and use them appropriately in combination.

Puetz and colleagues[74] used a combined CTA-SI ASPECTS and CBS (best is 20 and worst 0) to identify a large hyperacute stroke population with high mortality and low likelihood for independent functional outcome despite early thrombolysis. Miteff and colleagues[61] used perfusion CT and CTA to identify a group of patients with M1 MCA occlusions and mismatch ratios of less than 3, none of whom achieved good clinical outcome when compared with a group with mismatch ratio of 3 or greater, where collateral scoring helped discriminate clinical outcomes. Accumulated evidence from previous studies suggest that patients with a good scan (ASPECTS >7), high CBS (small clots), and good collateral status may have the best chance of achieving good clinical outcome. The MOSAIC (Multimodal Stroke Assessment using CT) score is an imaging score combining parenchymal assessment on NCCT, vascular imaging on CTA, and tissue perfusion using perfusion CT that showed consistently higher predictive values than the individual CT components in predicting outcome measures.[75] Although these combined scores make intuitive biologic sense, they suffer from either being too detailed or not appropriately weighing individual components, thus sometimes limiting clinical utility. The authors have therefore always used neuroimaging scores in the appropriate clinical context when making clinical decisions in acute ischemic stroke management.

Less than 3 Hours Time Window

Current data do not support exclusion of patients from IV thrombolysis based on ASPECTS. The authors use ASPECTS as a prognostic tool and to guide patient selection for IA recanalizing therapies. Patients with extensive EIC (ASPECTS 0–3) are unlikely to experience a favorable clinical course and are more likely to develop sICH due to thrombolysis. Such patients may further deteriorate because of malignant MCA infarction.[76] Typically, the authors either offer such patients early hemicraniectomy and aggressive rehabilitative or conservative and, most often, palliative stroke care.

Patients with intermediate ASPECTS (4–7) are treated with IV thrombolysis. These patients have a very short time window and there is general equipoise regarding risk versus benefit. The authors advocate an additional IA approach only in exceptional patients (young, disabling clinical deficit, large thrombus burden, and possibly right vs left hemisphere involvement); if based on assessment of the patient's vascular anatomy on CTA including the arch, recanalization can be achieved fast.

About 50% of patients with minor EIC (ASPECTS 8–10) will have a favorable clinical course with IV thrombolysis. Unless a clear hyperdense MCA sign or MCA dot sign are visible,[77,78] the authors perform immediate CTA after NCCT in such patients. In patients with an intracranial arterial occlusion and large clot burden, IV thrombolysis alone is unlikely to achieve recanalization, and early IA thrombolysis or mechanical thrombus removal can be considered.[79,80] Whenever possible, IA treatment approaches should be performed within randomized controlled trials, for example, the IMS-3 trial.[81]

Three to 6 Hours Time Window

Based on the PROACT-II ASPECTS evaluation, the authors hypothesize that patients with a high ASPECTS (ASPECTS >7) in the setting of an MCA occlusion may be ideal candidates for intervention. Specifically, for this highly selected "good-scan-occlusion" population, IV rtPA in the 3- to 4.5-hour time window (based on ECASS-3, the pooled analysis, and the updated Cochrane meta-analysis) is advocated. In patients with large thrombus burden and high ASPECTS, immediate combined IV-IA thrombolysis is considered. Beyond the 4.5-hour time window, based on the good-scan-occlusion paradigm, in a highly select group of patients (young, disabling clinical deficit with very good premorbid functional status, large thrombus burden), IA therapy is advocated. The authors encourage inclusion of patients into clinical trials targeting this group. Assessment of collateral status gives an estimate of potential time window available for recanalization, with patients having intermediate to poor collateral status having short time windows.

Greater than 6 Hours Time Window

ASPECTS might also be useful in the greater than 6-hour time window as well as in patients with so-called wake-up strokes. A subgroup of such patients is likely to have a salvageable penumbra, which can be spared infarction if recanalization can be achieved.[82] The authors hypothesize that those patients with a high admission ASPECTS and proximal occlusion represent a subgroup likely to benefit from delayed thrombolysis, and pilot data in 20 such patients suggest this is the case (Hill, personal communication, 2010). Good outcomes were seen in the Penumbra Pivotal Trial despite recanalization achieved beyond 360 minutes only in the setting of near normal CT scans (ASPECTS 8–10).[20]

Patients with a good NCCT scan (ASPECTS >7) but disabling clinical deficit and intracranial occlusion should be considered for IV-IA or IA treatment approaches with thrombolytic and/or mechanical recanalization strategies. The authors would, however, advocate that patients be treated under a randomized trial protocol for this time window. DIAS (Desmoteplase in Acute Ischemic Stroke) 3 and 4 are extended time window trials designed to demonstrate whether the study drug is effective in the treatment of patients with acute ischemic stroke when given within 3 to 9 hours from onset of stroke symptoms. The study includes only patients with an artery occlusion and excludes patients with extensive EICs on CT or MR imaging, thus relying on a good-scan-occlusion paradigm.

THE GOOD-SCAN-OCCLUSION PARADIGM FOR PATIENT SELECTION IN FUTURE STROKE TRIALS

Imaging-based selection criteria for thrombolytic stroke trials target identification of patients who will likely benefit from thrombolysis, and exclude patients who are unlikely to benefit. The authors propose the use of ASPECTS for definition of a CT-based good-scan-occlusion population as a target for thrombolytic stroke trials. Patients with an NCCT ASPECTS of greater than 7 and the presence of an intracranial arterial occlusion in the M1- or M2-segment could be a target population for IV and/or IA recanalization trials. Comparison studies are needed to assess whether this good-scan-occlusion paradigm provides similar or improved patient selection criteria compared with an MR imaging- and/or CTP-based mismatch paradigm.[83] In phase 2 trials of neuroprotectants, ASPECTS can be used for imaging selection and as a surrogate end point on follow-up scans. Trials on flow augmentation in acute ischemic strokes can use ASPECTS and collateral status estimates for imaging-based selection at baseline. ASPECTS can also be used to adjust for baseline imbalances in post hoc analyses of smaller randomized phase 2 trials.

TRAINING IN THE USE OF ASPECTS AND OTHER NEUROIMAGING SCORES

Training to interpret the often subtle changes on NCCT is crucial in increasing the reliability of ASPECTS.[84–87] Intra- and interrater reliability is an issue not just in the clinical milieu but more still in clinical trial enrollment when using image selection criteria. The authors have designed a Web-based training system (http://www. aspectsinstroke.com) illustrating the ASPECTS methodology, rules of interpretation, desired scan parameters for optimal scan quality, fallacies and potential drawbacks, and a series of examples for training and tests. The authors intend to add other neuroimaging scores to the Web site in the near future.

SUMMARY

Neuroimaging scores such as ASPECTS, CBS, leptomeningeal collateral score, pc-ASPECTS, and BASIS help in conveying pathophysiological information in acute ischemic strokes derived from imaging techniques in a simple, easy to use form that helps clinicians in making appropriate treatment decisions and in determining prognosis with reasonable accuracy. These scores also help in creating an easily understandable numerical scale for use in acute ischemic stroke trials. It is, however, imperative that treating physicians understand the limitations of these scales and use them in the appropriate clinical context when making decisions that affect patient management.

REFERENCES

1. Tissue plasminogen activator for acute ischemic stroke. The National Institute of Neurological Disorders and Stroke rt-PA Stroke Study Group. N Engl J Med 1995;333(24):1581–7.
2. Intracerebral hemorrhage after intravenous t-PA therapy for ischemic stroke. The NINDS t-PA Stroke Study Group. Stroke 1997;28(11):2109–18.
3. Patel SC, Levine SR, Tilley BC, et al. Lack of clinical significance of early ischemic changes on computed tomography in acute stroke. JAMA 2001;286(22): 2830–8.
4. Hacke W, Kaste M, Fieschi C, et al. Intravenous thrombolysis with recombinant tissue plasminogen activator for acute hemispheric stroke. The European Cooperative Acute Stroke Study (ECASS). JAMA 1995;274(13):1017–25.
5. von Kummer R, Allen KL, Holle R, et al. Acute stroke: usefulness of early CT findings before thrombolytic therapy. Radiology 1997;205(2):327–33.
6. Larrue V, von Kummer RR, Muller A, et al. Risk factors for severe hemorrhagic transformation in ischemic stroke patients treated with recombinant tissue plasminogen activator: a secondary analysis of the European-Australasian Acute Stroke Study (ECASS II). Stroke 2001;32(2):438–41.
7. Grotta JC, Chiu D, Lu M, et al. Agreement and variability in the interpretation of early CT changes in stroke patients qualifying for intravenous rtPA therapy. Stroke 1999;30(8):1528–33.
8. Wardlaw JM, Dorman PJ, Lewis SC, et al. Can stroke physicians and neuroradiologists identify signs of early cerebral infarction on CT? J Neurol Neurosurg Psychiatry 1999;67(5):651–3.
9. Butcher KS, Lee SB, Parsons MW, et al. Differential prognosis of isolated cortical swelling and hypoattenuation on CT in acute stroke. Stroke 2007;38(3): 941–7.
10. Demchuk AM, Hill MD, Barber PA, et al. Importance of early ischemic computed tomography changes using ASPECTS in NINDS rtPA Stroke Study. Stroke 2005;36(10):2110–5.
11. Puetz V, Dzialowski I, Hill MD, et al. The Alberta Stroke Program Early CT Score in clinical practice: what have we learned? Int J Stroke 2009;4(5): 354–64.
12. Barber PA, Demchuk AM, Zhang J, et al. Validity and reliability of a quantitative computed tomography score in predicting outcome of hyperacute stroke before thrombolytic therapy. ASPECTS Study Group. Alberta Stroke Programme Early CT Score. Lancet 2000;355(9216):1670–4.
13. Molina CA, Alexandrov AV, Demchuk AM, et al. Improving the predictive accuracy of recanalization on stroke outcome in patients treated with tissue plasminogen activator. Stroke 2004;35(1):151–6.

14. Tsivgoulis G, Saqqur M, Sharma VK, et al. Association of pretreatment ASPECTS scores with tPA-induced arterial recanalization in acute middle cerebral artery occlusion. J Neuroimaging 2008; 18(1):56–61.

15. Dzialowski I, Hill MD, Coutts SB, et al. Extent of early ischemic changes on computed tomography (CT) before thrombolysis, prognostic value of the Alberta Stroke Program Early CT Score in ECASS II. Stroke 2006;37(4):973–8.

16. Barber PA, Hill MD, Eliasziw M, et al. Imaging of the brain in acute ischaemic stroke: comparison of computed tomography and magnetic resonance diffusion-weighted imaging. J Neurol Neurosurg Psychiatry 2005;76(11):1528–33.

17. Hill MD, Buchan AM. Thrombolysis for acute ischemic stroke: results of the Canadian Alteplase for Stroke Effectiveness Study. CMAJ 2005; 172(10):1307–12.

18. Weir NU, Pexman JH, Hill MD, et al. How well does ASPECTS predict the outcome of acute stroke treated with IV tPA? Neurology 2006;67(3):516–8.

19. Penumbra Pivotal Stroke Trial Investigators. The penumbra pivotal stroke trial: safety and effectiveness of a new generation of mechanical devices for clot removal in intracranial large vessel occlusive disease. Stroke 2009;40(8):2761–8.

20. Goyal M, Menon BK, Coutts SB, et al. Effect of baseline CT scan appearance and time to recanalization on clinical outcomes in endovascular thrombectomy of acute ischemic strokes. Stroke 2010;42(1):93–7.

21. Hill MD, Rowley HA, Adler F, et al. Selection of acute ischemic stroke patients for intra-arterial thrombolysis with pro-urokinase by using ASPECTS. Stroke 2003;34(8):1925–31.

22. Furlan A, Higashida R, Wechsler L, et al. Intra-arterial prourokinase for acute ischemic stroke. The PROACT II study: a randomized controlled trial. Prolyse in Acute Cerebral Thromboembolism. JAMA 1999;282(21):2003–11.

23. Hill MD, Demchuk AM, Tomsick TA, et al. Using the baseline CT scan to select acute stroke patients for IV-IA therapy. AJNR Am J Neuroradiol 2006;27(8): 1612–6.

24. IMS Study Investigators. Combined intravenous and intra-arterial recanalization for acute ischemic stroke: the Interventional Management of Stroke Study. Stroke 2004;35(4):904–11.

25. Tanne D, Kasner SE, Demchuk AM, et al. Markers of increased risk of intracerebral hemorrhage after intravenous recombinant tissue plasminogen activator therapy for acute ischemic stroke in clinical practice: the Multicenter rt-PA Stroke Survey. Circulation 2002;105(14):1679–85.

26. Lees KR, Bluhmki E, von Kummer R, et al. Time to treatment with intravenous alteplase and outcome in stroke: an updated pooled analysis of ECASS, ATLANTIS, NINDS, and EPITHET trials. Lancet 2010;375(9727):1695–703.

27. Pexman JH, Barber PA, Hill MD, et al. Use of the Alberta Stroke Program Early CT Score (ASPECTS) for assessing CT scans in patients with acute stroke. AJNR Am J Neuroradiol 2001;22(8):1534–42.

28. Coutts SB, Demchuk AM, Barber PA, et al. Interobserver variation of ASPECTS in real time. Stroke 2004;35(5):e103–5.

29. Mak HK, Yau KK, Khong PL, et al. Hypodensity of >1/3 middle cerebral artery territory versus Alberta Stroke Programme Early CT Score (ASPECTS): comparison of two methods of quantitative evaluation of early CT changes in hyperacute ischemic stroke in the community setting. Stroke 2003;34(5):1194–6.

30. Kalafut MA, Schriger DL, Saver JL, et al. Detection of early CT signs of >1/3 middle cerebral artery infarctions: interrater reliability and sensitivity of CT interpretation by physicians involved in acute stroke care. Stroke 2000;31(7):1667–71.

31. Silver B, Demaerschalk B, Merino JG, et al. Improved outcomes in stroke thrombolysis with pre-specified imaging criteria. Can J Neurol Sci 2001;28(2):113–9.

32. Demaerschalk BM, Silver B, Wong E, et al. ASPECT scoring to estimate >1/3 middle cerebral artery territory infarction. Can J Neurol Sci 2006;33(2):200–4.

33. Dzialowski I, Weber J, Doerfler A, et al. Brain tissue water uptake after middle cerebral artery occlusion assessed with CT. J Neuroimaging 2004;14(1):42–8.

34. Schuier FJ, Hossmann KA. Experimental brain infarcts in cats. II. Ischemic brain edema. Stroke 1980;11(6):593–601.

35. Dzialowski I, Klotz E, Goericke S, et al. Ischemic brain tissue water content: CT monitoring during middle cerebral artery occlusion and reperfusion in rats. Radiology 2007;243(3):720–6.

36. Schramm P, Schellinger PD, Klotz E, et al. Comparison of perfusion computed tomography and computed tomography angiography source images with perfusion-weighted imaging and diffusion-weighted imaging in patients with acute stroke of less than 6 hours' duration. Stroke 2004;35(7): 1652–8.

37. Lev MH, Segal AZ, Farkas J, et al. Utility of perfusion-weighted CT imaging in acute middle cerebral artery stroke treated with intra-arterial thrombolysis: prediction of final infarct volume and clinical outcome. Stroke 2001;32(9):2021–8.

38. Camargo EC, Furie KL, Singhal AB, et al. Acute brain infarct: detection and delineation with CT angiographic source images versus nonenhanced CT scans. Radiology 2007;244(2):541–8.

39. Coutts SB, Lev MH, Eliasziw M, et al. ASPECTS on CTA source images versus unenhanced CT: added value in predicting final infarct extent and clinical outcome. Stroke 2004;35(11):2472–6.

40. Chalela JA, Kidwell CS, Nentwich LM, et al. Magnetic resonance imaging and computed tomography in emergency assessment of patients with suspected acute stroke: a prospective comparison. Lancet 2007;369(9558):293–8.

41. Kimura K, Iguchi Y, Shibazaki K, et al. Large ischemic lesions on diffusion-weighted imaging done before intravenous tissue plasminogen activator thrombolysis predicts a poor outcome in patients with acute stroke. Stroke 2008;39(8): 2388–91.

42. Nezu T, Koga M, Kimura K, et al. Pretreatment ASPECTS on DWI predicts 3-month outcome following rt-PA: SAMURAI rt-PA Registry. Neurology 2010;75(6):555–61.

43. Hill MD, Menon BK. Effect modification and ischaemic stroke treatment. Lancet Neurol 2010;9(7): 649–51.

44. Coutts SB, Simon JE, Tomanek AI, et al. Reliability of assessing percentage of diffusion-perfusion mismatch. Stroke 2003;34(7):1681–3.

45. Terasawa Y, Kimura K, Iguchi Y, et al. Could clinical diffusion-mismatch determined using DWI ASPECTS predict neurological improvement after thrombolysis before 3 h after acute stroke? J Neurol Neurosurg Psychiatry 2010;81(8):864–8.

46. Butcher K, Parsons M, Allport L, et al. Rapid assessment of perfusion-diffusion mismatch. Stroke 2008; 39(1):75–81.

47. Lin K, Rapalino O, Lee B, et al. Correlation of volumetric mismatch and mismatch of Alberta Stroke Program Early CT Scores on CT perfusion maps. Neuroradiology 2009;51(1):17–23.

48. Parsons MW, Pepper EM, Chan V, et al. Perfusion computed tomography: prediction of final infarct extent and stroke outcome. Ann Neurol 2005;58(5): 672–9.

49. Puetz V, Sylaja PN, Coutts SB, et al. Extent of hypoattenuation on CT angiography source images predicts functional outcome in patients with basilar artery occlusion. Stroke 2008;39(9):2485–90.

50. Schaefer PW, Yoo AJ, Bell D, et al. CT angiography-source image hypoattenuation predicts clinical outcome in posterior circulation strokes treated with intra-arterial therapy. Stroke 2008;39(11): 3107–9.

51. del Zoppo GJ, Poeck K, Pessin MS, et al. Recombinant tissue plasminogen activator in acute thrombotic and embolic stroke. Ann Neurol 1992;32(1): 78–86.

52. Saqqur M, Uchino K, Demchuk AM, et al. Site of arterial occlusion identified by transcranial Doppler predicts the response to intravenous thrombolysis for stroke. Stroke 2007;38(3):948–54.

53. Puetz V, Dzialowski I, Hill MD, et al. Intracranial thrombus extent predicts clinical outcome, final infarct size and hemorrhagic transformation in ischemic stroke: the clot burden score. Int J Stroke 2008;3(4):230–6.

54. Tan IY, Demchuk AM, Hopyan J, et al. CT angiography clot burden score and collateral score: correlation with clinical and radiologic outcomes in acute middle cerebral artery infarct. AJNR Am J Neuroradiol 2009;30(3):525–31.

55. Torres-Mozqueda F, He J, Yeh IB, et al. An acute ischemic stroke classification instrument that includes CT or MR angiography: the Boston Acute Stroke Imaging Scale. AJNR Am J Neuroradiol 2008;29(6):1111–7.

56. Brozici M, van der Zwan A, Hillen B. Anatomy and functionality of leptomeningeal anastomoses: a review. Stroke 2003;34(11):2750–62.

57. Liebeskind DS. Collateral circulation. Stroke 2003; 34(9):2279–84.

58. Liebeskind DS. Stroke: the currency of collateral circulation in acute ischemic stroke. Nat Rev Neurol 2009;5(12):645–6.

59. Duvernoy HM, Delon S, Vannson JL. Cortical blood vessels of the human brain. Brain Res Bull 1981; 7(5):519–79.

60. Bang OY, Saver JL, Buck BH, et al. Impact of collateral flow on tissue fate in acute ischaemic stroke. J Neurol Neurosurg Psychiatry 2008;79(6):625–9.

61. Miteff F, Levi CR, Bateman GA, et al. The independent predictive utility of computed tomography angiographic collateral status in acute ischaemic stroke. Brain 2009;132(Pt 8):2231–8.

62. Symon L. Studies of leptomeningeal collateral circulation in Macacus rhesus. J Physiol 1961;159(1): 68–86, 1.

63. Coyle P, Jokelainen PT. Dorsal cerebral arterial collaterals of the rat. Anat Rec 1982;203(3):397–404.

64. Reina-De La Torre F, Rodriguez-Baeza A, Sahuquillo-Barris J. Morphological characteristics and distribution pattern of the arterial vessels in human cerebral cortex: a scanning electron microscope study. Anat Rec 1998;251(1):87–96.

65. Higashida R, Furlan A, Roberts H, et al. Trial design and reporting standards for intraarterial cerebral thrombolysis for acute ischemic stroke. J Vasc Interv Radiol 2003;14(9 Pt 2):S493–4.

66. Christoforidis GA, Mohammad Y, Kehagias D, et al. Angiographic assessment of pial collaterals as a prognostic indicator following intra-arterial thrombolysis for acute ischemic stroke. AJNR Am J Neuroradiol 2005;26(7):1789–97.

67. Tan JC, Dillon WP, Liu S, et al. Systematic comparison of perfusion-CT and CT-angiography in acute stroke patients. Ann Neurol 2007;61(6):533–43.

68. Rosenthal ES, Schwamm LH, Roccatagliata L, et al. Role of recanalization in acute stroke outcome: rationale for a CT angiogram-based "benefit of recanalization" model. AJNR Am J Neuroradiol 2008;29(8): 1471–5.

69. Maas MB, Lev MH, Ay H, et al. Collateral vessels on CT angiography predict outcome in acute ischemic stroke. Stroke 2009;40(9):3001–5.

70. Kim JJ, Fischbein NJ, Lu Y, et al. Regional angiographic grading system for collateral flow: correlation with cerebral infarction in patients with middle cerebral artery occlusion. Stroke 2004;35(6):1340–4.

71. Lima FO, Furie KL, Silva GS, et al. The pattern of leptomeningeal collaterals on CT angiography is a strong predictor of long-term functional outcome in stroke patients with large vessel intracranial occlusion. Stroke 2010;41(10):2316–22.

72. Tu YK, Clerehugh V, Gilthorpe MS. Collinearity in linear regression is a serious problem in oral health research. Eur J Oral Sci 2004;112(5):389–97.

73. Xue X, Kim MY, Shore RE. Cox regression analysis in presence of collinearity: an application to assessment of health risks associated with occupational radiation exposure. Lifetime Data Anal 2007;13(3):333–50.

74. Puetz V, Dzialowski I, Hill MD, et al. Malignant profile detected by CT angiographic information predicts poor prognosis despite thrombolysis within three hours from symptom onset. Cerebrovasc Dis 2010;29(6):584–91.

75. Nabavi DG, Kloska SP, Nam EM, et al. MOSAIC: Multimodal Stroke Assessment Using Computed Tomography: novel diagnostic approach for the prediction of infarction size and clinical outcome. Stroke 2002;33(12):2819–26.

76. Krieger DW, Demchuk AM, Kasner SE, et al. Early clinical and radiological predictors of fatal brain swelling in ischemic stroke. Stroke 1999;30(2):287–92.

77. Barber PA, Demchuk AM, Hudon ME, et al. Hyperdense sylvian fissure MCA "dot" sign: a CT marker of acute ischemia. Stroke 2001;32(1):84–8.

78. Tomsick TA, Brott TG, Olinger CP, et al. Hyperdense middle cerebral artery: incidence and quantitative significance. Neuroradiology 1989;31(4):312–5.

79. Lee KY, Han SW, Kim SH, et al. Early recanalization after intravenous administration of recombinant tissue plasminogen activator as assessed by pre- and post-thrombolytic angiography in acute ischemic stroke patients. Stroke 2007;38(1):192–3.

80. Sims JR, Rordorf G, Smith EE, et al. Arterial occlusion revealed by CT angiography predicts NIH stroke score and acute outcomes after IV tPA treatment. AJNR Am J Neuroradiol 2005;26(2):246–51.

81. Khatri P, Hill MD, Palesch YY, et al. Methodology of the interventional management of stroke III trial. Int J Stroke 2008;3(2):130–7.

82. Baron JC, von Kummer R, del Zoppo GJ. Treatment of acute ischemic stroke. Challenging the concept of a rigid and universal time window. Stroke 1995;26(12):2219–21.

83. Schellinger PD. EPITHET: failed chance or new hope? Lancet Neurol 2008;7(4):286–7.

84. Coutts SB, Hill MD, Demchuk AM, et al. ASPECTS reading requires training and experience. Stroke 2003;34(10):e179 [author reply: e179].

85. Pexman JH, Hill MD, Buchan AM, et al. Hyperacute stroke: experience essential when reading unenhanced CT scans. AJNR Am J Neuroradiol 2004;25(3):516 [author reply: 516–8].

86. von Kummer R. Effect of training in reading CT scans on patient selection for ECASS II. Neurology 1998;51(3 Suppl 3):S50–2.

87. Wardlaw JM, Mielke O. Early signs of brain infarction at CT: observer reliability and outcome after thrombolytic treatment—systematic review. Radiology 2005;235(2):444–53.

Index

Note: Page numbers of article titles are in **boldface** type.

neuroimaging.theclinics.com

Printed and bound by CPI Group (UK) Ltd, Croydon, CR0 4YY

03/10/2024

01040358-0019